Surgical Ophthalmic Oncology

Sonal S. Chaugule
Santosh G. Honavar · Paul T. Finger
Editors

Surgical Ophthalmic Oncology

A Collaborative Open Access Reference

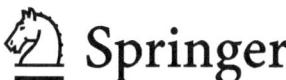 Springer

Editors
Sonal S. Chaugule
Ophthalmic Plastic Surgery,
Orbit and Ocular Oncology
PBMA's H V Desai Eye Hospital
Pune
India

Santosh G. Honavar
Ocular Oncology Service
Centre for Sight Superspeciality
Eye Hospital
Hyderabad
India

Paul T. Finger
The Eye Cancer Foundation, Inc.,
The New York Eye Cancer Center
New York University School of
Medicine
New York, NY
USA

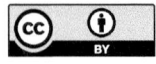

This book is an open access publication.
ISBN 978-3-030-18756-9   ISBN 978-3-030-18757-6   (eBook)
https://doi.org/10.1007/978-3-030-18757-6

This Springer imprint is published by the registered company Springer Nature Switzerland AG
The registered company address is: Gewerbestrasse 11, 6330 Cham, Switzerland

Foreword

The readers are receiving this outstanding book which documents major advancements in the field of ocular oncology. Ocular oncology services are typically provided by highly trained subspecialists. However, general ophthalmologists also need to be sufficiently familiar with early signs, diagnostics, and treatment options to ensure timely management of oncological eye conditions which may progress into vision and life-threatening diseases. Several years of collaborative work have brought together more than 25 authors comprising ophthalmic oncologists, ophthalmic plastic and reconstructive surgeons, vitreo-retinal surgeons, ocular pathologists, and radiation oncologists from many internationally renowned healthcare institutions around the world.

This book was designed to describe symptoms, diagnostic, and treatment approaches for oncologic conditions. It includes indications, pre- and postoperative care, and surgical techniques required to manage various eye cancer ailments with the help of ample illustrations. The text provides a detailed approach to treatment for common and rare diseases and summarizes the key points required for performing the surgeries. The video atlas, comprising of more than 20 well-edited videos, is a valuable opportunity to review the actual surgical steps and enables the readers to understand the procedures in a comprehensive manner. The learning experience of the user is significantly enhanced by these easy-to-follow tutorials.

This book is fully in line with the strategic goals of the International Council of Ophthalmology (ICO) to improve patient's lives and eyesight by improving education and knowledge. General ophthalmologists, ocular oncologists, fellows, and residents as well as students in training will all stand to benefit from this unique collaborative effort. The truly international cooperation, the open-access nature and availability of the book everywhere in the world, and this up-to-date resource as a guiding tool in the field of surgical ophthalmic oncology make it a special delight for the ICO.

Peter Wiedemann, MD
Ivo Kocur, MD
International Council of Ophthalmology
San Francisco, CA, USA

Preface

Ophthalmic oncologists care for the rare and unusual tumors of the eye, lids, and orbit. Around the world, there exist fewer than 300 known eye cancer surgeons. In fact, there are almost 40 countries with no fellowship-trained eye cancer specialist and many more that are underserved.

In 2015, the first Eye Cancer Working Day was held at the Curie Institute in Paris, France. During that meeting, Drs. Honavar and Finger recognized the opportunity to address the needs of the millions of eye cancer patients who do not have access to subspecialty care. It was proposed that a book containing preferred practice guidelines with surgical videos be published in an open-access format to offer ophthalmic surgeons guidance in underserved and unserved countries.

After almost 2.5 years of work, this book is a result of collaborative efforts of more than 25 authors which include ophthalmic oncologists, ophthalmic plastic and reconstructive surgeons, vitreoretinal surgeons, ocular pathologists, and radiation oncologists from various renowned centers spread over in total of five continents. We have enjoyed this unique opportunity to work with all the contributors in collaboration.

> *With the help of 'The Eye Cancer Foundation', this project has materialized into a textbook and video atlas of surgical techniques involved in managing diseases related to ophthalmic oncology. We are hopeful that it would be a valuable resource for general ophthalmologists, surgeons as well as fellows and trainees around the world who encounter these diseases in the care of their patients.* (Paul T. Finger, MD, Chief Executive Officer of the Eye Cancer Foundation (ECF))

The layout of this book has been organized so that it is simple to use as a quick reference. This book covers tumors of the eyelid, cornea, conjunctiva, and orbit as well as intraocular tumors. A chapter dedicated to ophthalmic radiation therapy has been added to describe the eye sparing methods of treatment. It provides vital key points regarding radiation physics to be considered by ophthalmic oncologists during radiation treatment planning. Ophthalmic pathology is an integral part of ophthalmic oncology. A chapter on pathology has been included to guide the operating surgeons with the essential guidelines regarding specimen collection, transport, and interpretation of pathology report.

This book was designed to include indications, pre- and postoperative care, and surgical techniques required to manage the various eye cancer ailments with the help of ample illustrations. The text provides a detailed approach to treatment and summarizes the key points required for performing the surgeries, whereas the video atlas gives an opportunity to review the actual surgical steps as a guiding tool. The atlas comprising of more than 20 well-edited videos would enable the readers to understand the procedures in a more comprehensive manner.

However, we understand that this reference is not a complete compilation of all the existent surgical techniques involved in ophthalmic oncology. The authors aim to provide preferred practice guidelines from their own experience. The surgical techniques may vary between different centers, countries, and areas of the world. We sincerely hope that this book would be able to guide the practitioners from underserved countries with even limited resources to manage the diseases which will allow them to adhere to the oncological principles and achieve optimal outcomes.

Pune, India   Sonal S. Chaugule
Hyderabad, India   Santosh G. Honavar
New York, NY, USA   Paul T. Finger

Acknowledgments

We gratefully acknowledge the important role of Dr. Paul T. Finger and "The Eye Cancer Foundation (ECF)" for supporting the concept of a Collaborative Open Access Surgical Textbook (COAST) at the First Eye Cancer Working Day held at the Curie Institute, Paris, France, in 2015. There, Dr. Santosh G. Honavar and colleagues presented COAST as a method to help eye care professionals in unserved and underserved areas of the world. The project would not have been possible without ECF's generous contributions. In addition, we heartily thank the ECF board, trustees, and donors for underwriting this open-access effort. We also recognize the encouragement from the leadership of the International Council of Ophthalmology (ICO). All have supported the idea behind this book and gave constant encouragement during its execution.

However, it would not have been possible without all our contributors fulfilling their roles as authors in a timely manner. Their willingness as well as enthusiasm to create what has become a relevant and novel ophthalmic oncology resource for ophthalmologists and trainees in developing and underserved areas around the world has been very impressive. We must also acknowledge the reviewers who kindly offered their input for completion of chapters, including Drs. Sonal S. Chaugule, Carol Karp, Daniel Rootman, Steffen Heegaard, and Vikas Khetan. We thank them for donating their time and expertise in reviewing all the chapters.

We are also grateful to the wonderful team of editors at Springer with whom Dr. Sonal S. Chaugule has shepherded this work from inception to production. The final product would not have been possible without her invaluable contribution.

Contents

Contributors

Manab Jyoti Barman, DO, DNB Ocular Oncology Services, Sri Sankaradeva Nethralaya, Guwahati, India

Francesco Bernardini, MD Oculoplastica Bernardini, Genoa, Italy

Kasturi Bhattacharjee, MS, DNB, FRCS Department of Orbit, Ophthalmic Plastic and Reconstructive Surgery, Sri Sankaradeva Nethralaya, Guwahati, India

Sonal S. Chaugule, MBBS, MS Ophthalmic Plastic Surgery, Orbit and Ocular Oncology, PBMA's H V Desai Eye Hospital, Pune, India

Bita Esmaeli, MD, FACS Orbital Oncology and Ophthalmic Plastic Surgery Service, Department of Plastic Surgery, The University of Texas M. D. Anderson Cancer Center, Houston, TX, USA

Ido Didi Fabian, MD Goldschleger Eye Institute, Sheba Medical Center, Tel-Aviv University, Tel-Aviv, Israel

International Centre for Eye Health, London School of Hygiene and Tropical Medicine, London, UK

Paul T. Finger, MD, FACS, LFAAO The Eye Cancer Foundation, Inc., The New York Eye Cancer Center, New York University School of Medicine, New York, NY, USA

Sripurna Ghosh Department of Orbit, Ophthalmic Plastic and Reconstructive Surgery, Sri Sankaradeva Nethralaya, Guwahati, India

Dan S. Gombos, MD, FACS Section of Ophthalmology, Department of Head & Neck Surgery, MD Anderson Cancer Center, Houston, TX, USA

Santosh G. Honavar, MD, FACS Ocular Oncology Service and National Retinoblastoma Foundation, Centre for Sight, Hyderabad, India

Shyamala C. Huilgol, MBBS (Hons), FACD Dermatology Department, Royal Adelaide Hospital, Adelaide, SA, Australia

Zeynel A. Karcioglu, MD Department of Ophthalmology, University of Virginia, Charlottesville, VA, USA

Raghavendra Rao Kolavali, MS Department of Ophthalmology, Post Graduate Institute of Medical Education and Research, Chandigarh, India

Hatem Krema, MD, MSc, FRCS Department of Ophthalmology and Vision Sciences, Princess Margaret Hospital, Toronto, ON, Canada

Fairooz P. Manjandavida, MD Department of Oculoplasty and Ocular Oncology, Horus Specialty Eye Care, Bangalore, India

Hardeep Singh Mudhar, BSc, PhD, MBBChir, FRCpath National Specialist Ophthalmic Pathology Service (NSOPS), Department of Histopathology, Royal Hallamshire Hospital, Sheffield, UK

Raksha Rao, MS, FICO Department of Orbit and Ophthalmic Oncology, Narayana Nethralaya, Bangalore, India

Mark J. Rivard, PhD, FAAPM Department of Radiation Oncology, Brown University School of Medicine, Providence, RI, USA

Svetlana Saakyan, MD Department of Ocular Oncology, Moscow Helmholtz Research Institute of Eye Diseases, Moscow, Russia

Mandeep S. Sagoo, MB, PhD, FRCA (Ed), FRCOphth Ocular Oncology Service, Moorfields Eye Hospital and Retinoblastoma Service, Royal London Hospital, UCL Institute of Ophthalmology, London, UK

Wolfgang A. G. Sauerwein, MD Department of Radiation Oncology, Strahlenklinik, University Hospital Essen, Essen, Germany

Dinesh Selva, MBBS, DHSc, FRACS, PhD, FAICO Ophthalmology Department, Royal Adelaide Hospital, Adelaide, SA, Australia

P. Mahesh Shanmugam, MBBS, DO, FRCSEd, PhD, FAICO Vitreoretinal and Oncology Service, Sankara Eye Hospital, Bangalore, India

Carol L. Shields, MD Ocular Oncology Service, Wills Eye Hospital, Thomas Jefferson University, Philadelphia, PA, USA

Usha Singh, MS Department of Ophthalmology, Advanced Eye Center, Post Graduate Institute of Medical Education and Research, Chandigarh, India

Brent Skippen, MBBS (HONS), B Med Sci, MPH Department of Ophthalmology, Wagga Wagga Rural Referral Hospital, Wagga Wagga, NSW, Australia

Gangadhara Sundar, DO, FRCSEd, FAMS, AB(USA) Orbit and Oculofacial Surgery/Ophthalmic Oncology, Department of Ophthalmology, National University Hospital, National University of Singapore, Singapore, Singapore

Department of Pediatrics, National University Hospital, Singapore, Singapore

Albert Wu, MBBS Dermatology Department, Royal Adelaide Hospital, Adelaide, SA, Australia

Usha Singh and Raghavendra Rao Kolavali

Overview and Epidemiology

Eyelid is a common place for skin cancer to occur and constitute 5–10% of all skin cancers. Eyelid neoplasms comprise a variety of benign and malignant growths (Table 1.1). Significant majority of these growths are benign in nature and constitute 82–98% of all neoplasms (Table 1.2). There is wide, racial, and probable geographical variation reported in the incidence of the various eyelid tumors. Eyelid malignancies vary in distribution and presentation. The most common malignant eyelid tumor in western literature is basal cell carcinoma (BCC) comprising 86–91% incidence among the Caucasians [7, 12]. However, in one of the largest series from China and India this incidence is much lower, consequently sebaceous gland carcinoma (SGC) constitutes 32% of all eyelid tumors [6, 13]. In studies from Asian countries [2, 14, 15] it is the sebaceous gland carcinoma which constitutes the majority (67–77%). The mean age for benign tumor is lower than that of malignant tumors.

Epithelial tumor and dermoid cysts are the most common eyelid tumor in children [16]. Malignant eyelid tumor in children is extremely rare. When it presents, is usually a part of a systemic process, genetic defects or following radiation treatment [17, 18]. Merkel cell carcinomas (MCC) of the eyelid are rare neuroendocrine tumor constituting 5–20% of the head and neck tumor, predominantly in Caucasians [19].

Classification of Eyelid Tumors

Eyelid tumors can arise from various histological layers eyelid is composed of. Eyelid tumors are classified as benign or malignant or according to the tissue or cell of origin (Tables 1.2, 1.3 and 1.4). They can be subdivided into non-melanocytic and melanocytic tumors. Benign epithelial proliferations such as squamous papilloma, pseudoepitheliomatous hyperplasia, seborrheic keratosis, keratoacanthoma cysts and nevi are common. Among the malignant, BCC (Figs. 1.1 and 1.2) is the most common in Caucasians and SGC among the Asians (Fig. 1.3), followed by squamous cell carcinoma (SCC) and malignant melanoma (MM) (Figs. 1.4, 1.5, 1.6, 1.7 and 1.8). The large majority of BCC (93%) was seen in 71% of females [2] SGC has predilection for the upper lid [20]. Merkel cell cancer has higher prevalence in men. Primary malignant melanomas of the eyelid skin are rare and account for 0.2–13% of all reported

U. Singh (✉)
Department of Ophthalmology, Advanced Eye Center, Post Graduate Institute of Medical Education and Research, Chandigarh, India

R. R. Kolavali
Department of Ophthalmology, Post Graduate Institute of Medical Education and Research, Chandigarh, India

© The Author(s) 2019
S. S. Chaugule et al. (eds.), *Surgical Ophthalmic Oncology*,
https://doi.org/10.1007/978-3-030-18757-6_1

Table 1.1 Regional incidence of benign and malignant eyelid neoplasms in the epidemiological studies

	Author, country, year	Study period	Total number of patients	Biopsy proven tumors	Benign (%)	Mean age years (gender preponderance)	Premalignant %	Malignant (%)	Mean age years (gender preponderance)
	Asian studies								
1.	Huang, Taiwan, 2015 [1]	1995–2015	4521	4521	4294 (95.0)	55.4		227 (5)	72.5
2.	Chang CH, Taiwan, 2003 [2]	1994–1998	144	129	126 (87.5)	-(f)	nil	12.5%	61 (f)
3.	Toshida H, Japan, 2012 [3]	1993–2007	118	118	106 (89.8)	47.8 (f)	ns	12 (10.2%)	53.1 (f)
4.	Sihota, India 1996 [4]	1982–1992	313	313	135 (43.1)	ns	ns	178 (56.8)	ns
5.	Rathod A, India, 2015 [5]	2007–2009	100	100	61 (61)	37.02	1	39 (39)	58.59
6.	Ni Z, China, 1996 [6]	1953–1992	3510	3510	2413 (68.7)	na		1097 (31.2)	na
	Western literature								
7.	Deprez, Switzerland, 2009 [7]	1989–2007	4981	4981	4087 (82)	–	18	894 (18)	–
8.	Paul S, USA, 2011 [8]	2004–2007	855	855	649 (75.9)	<60 (nil)		206 (24.1)	>60 (m)
9.	Mclean, AFIP, USA, 1994 [9]	1984–1989	846	456	456 (54)	–	–	390 (46)	
10.	Font, USA, 2006 [10]	1980–1982	1474	NOS	880 (60)		–	594 (40)	–
	Middle East								
11.	Bagheri, Tehran, Iran, 2013 [11]	2000–2010	182	182	82	46.4 (f)		100	63.9 (m)
12.	Gundogan FC, Turkey, 2015 [12]	2008–2012	1502 (1541)	1541	1424 (92.4)	50.08 (f)	6%	22 (1.5%)	68.6 (m)

Table 1.2 Eyelid tumors originating from epidermis

Subtypes	Benign	Premalignant	Malignant
Non-melanocytic	Squamous cell papilloma	Actinic(solar) keratosis	Basal cell carcinoma
	Seborrheic keratosis	Intraepithelial neoplasia	Squamous cell carcinoma
	Inverted follicular keratosis	Sebaceous nevus (of Jadassohn)	Mucoepidermoid carcinoma
	Reactive hyperplasia (pseudoepitheliomatous hyperplasia)	Xeroderma pigmentosa	Keratoacanthoma
		Keratoacanthoma	
Melanocytic	Ephelis or freckles	Congenital dysplastic nevus	
	Lentigo simplex	Lentigo maligna (melanotic freckle of Hutchinson)	Melanoma arising from nevi
	Solar Lentigo		Melanoma arising in lentigo maligna
	Junctional nevus		Melanoma arising de novo
	Intradermal nevus		
	Compound nevus		
	Spitz nevus		
	Balloon cell nevus		
	Blue nevus		
	Cellular blue nevus		
	Oculodermal nevus of Ota		
Eyelid tumors arising from adnexal and cystic lesions			
Sebaceous gland tumors	Sebaceous gland hyperplasia	–	Sebaceous gland carcinoma
	Sebaceous gland adenoma		
Sweat gland and lacrimal gland tumors	Syringoma		Sweat gland (eccrine) adenocarcinoma
	Papillary syringadenoma		Mucinous sweat gland adenocarcinoma
	Eccrine spiradenoma		Apocrine gland adenocarcinoma
	Eccrine acrospiroma		Adenoid cystic carcinoma
			Porocarcinoma
Eyelid tumors arising from hair follicle			
	Trichoepithelioma		Carcinoma of hair follicles
	Trichofolliculoma/trichoadenoma		
	Trichilemmoma		
	Pilomatrixoma (calcifying epithelioma of Malherbe)		
Other cystic lesions			
	Epidermal inclusion cyst		
	Sebaceous cyst		
	Retention cyst		
	Eccrine hidrocystoma		
	Apocrine hidrocystoma		
	Trichilemmal cyst		
	Other benign cystic lesion		

Table 1.3 Fibrous, fibrohistiocystic, and muscular eyelid tumors

	Benign	Intermediate	Malignant
Fibrous	Fibroma		Fibrosarcoma
	Keloid		Congenital fibrosarcoma
	Nodular fasciitis		
	Proliferative fasciitis		
	Fibromatosis		
Fibrous histiocytic	Xanthelasma		Malignant fibrous histiocytoma
	Xanthoma	Atypical fibroxanthoma	Malignant giant cell fibrous histiocytoma
	Dermatofibroma	Dermatofibrosarcoma protuberans	Malignant fibroxanthoma
	Xanthogranuloma	Angiomatoid fibrous histiocytoma	
	Fibrous histiocytoma		
	Juvenile xanthogranuloma		
	Necrotic xanthogranuloma		
	Reticulohistiocytoma		

	Benign	Malignant
Smooth muscle	Leiomyoma	Leiomyosarcoma
	Angiomyoma	
Skeletal muscle	Rhabdomyoma	Rhabdomyosarcoma

Table 1.4 Eyelid tumors arising from vascular, perivascular, neural, lipomatous, cartilage, bone lymphoid tumors, hamartomas, and choristomas

	Benign	Malignant
Vascular	Nevus flammeus (port wine stain)	Angiosarcoma
	Papillary endothelial hyperplasia	Lymphangiosarcoma
	Capillary hemangioma	Kaposi's sarcoma
	Cavernous hemangioma	
	Venous hemangioma	
	Epithelioid hemangioma (angiolymphoid hyperplasia)	
	Arteriovenous malformation	
	Lymphangioma	
Perivascular	Hemangiopericytoma	Malignant hemangiopericytoma
	Glomus tumor	Malignant glomus tumor
Neural	Traumatic neuroma	Malignant peripheral nerve sheath tumor
	Neurofibroma	Merkel cell tumor
	Plexiform neurofibroma	
	Schwannoma (neurilemoma)	
	Neuroglial choristoma	
Lipomatous	Lipoma	Liposarcoma
	Hibernoma	
Cartilage	Chondroma	Chondrosarcoma
	Osteoma	Mesenchymal chondrosarcoma
		Osteosarcoma
Lymphoid	Benign lymphoid hyperplasia	Lymphoma
	Plasmacytoma	Leukemic infiltration
Hamartomas and choristomas	Dermoid cyst	
	Phakomatous choristoma	
	Ectopic lacrimal gland	
Others	Myxoma	

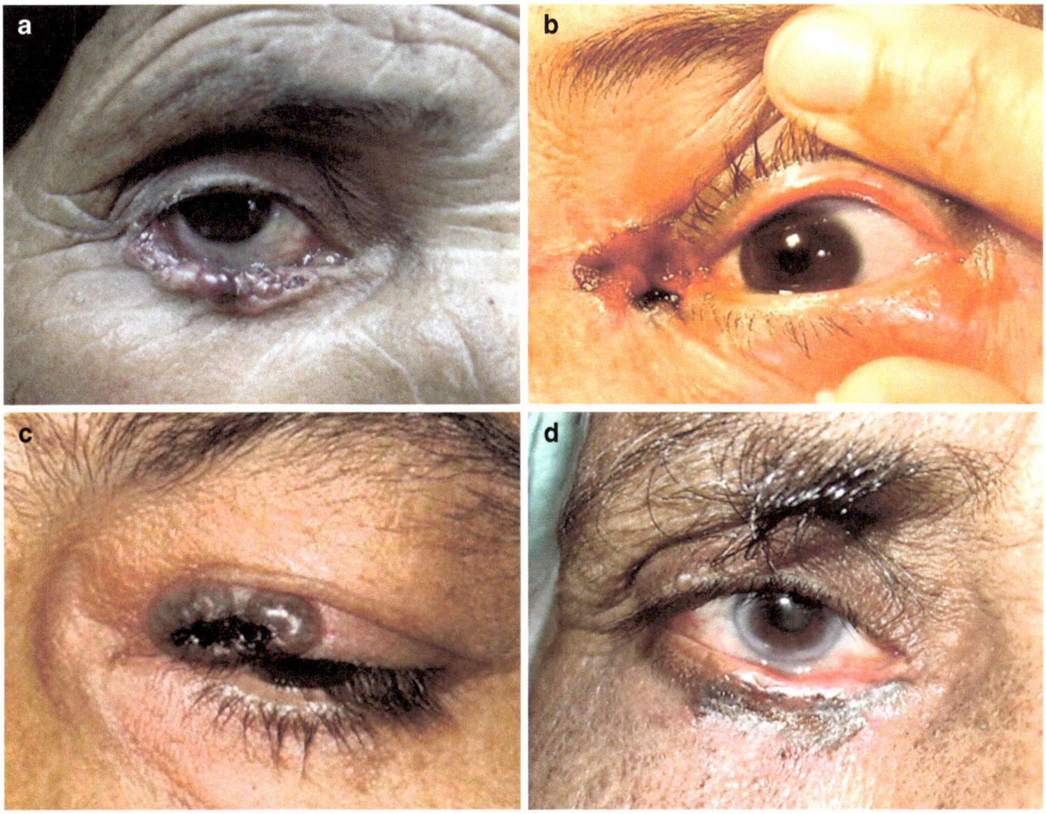

Fig. 1.1 (**a**) Basal cell carcinoma involving the lower lid. (**b**) Ulcerative basal cell carcinoma involving the medial canthus. (**c**) Basal cell carcinoma involving the upper lid with central necrotic area. (**d**) Morpheaform type of basal cell carcinoma involving the lower lid

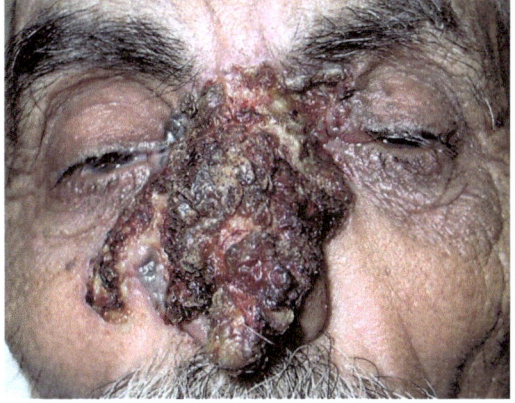

Fig. 1.2 Extensive basal cell carcinoma involving both medial canthi, nose and cheek

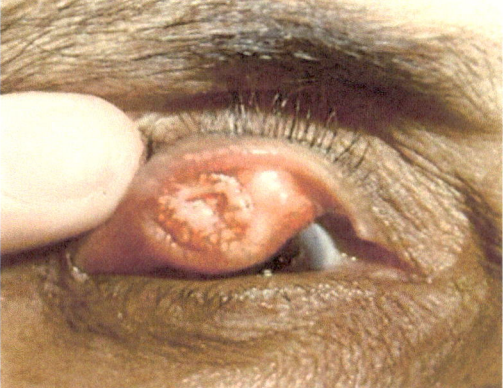

Fig. 1.3 Sebaceous gland carcinoma misdiagnosed as chalazion and surgically intervened

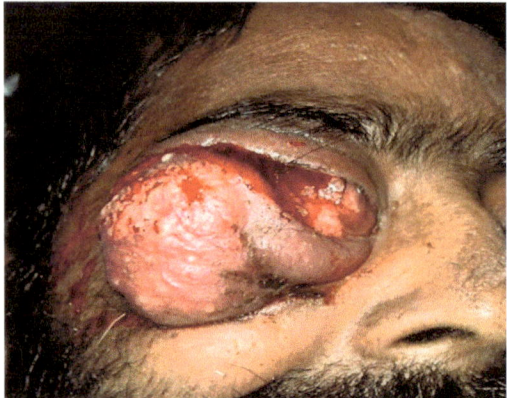

Fig. 1.4 Malignant melanoma involving lower lid and conjunctiva

cases [2, 7]. They occur 20 years later than other non-melanoma tumor and have 2.6 times predilection for the lower lid. Eyelids can also be involved by secondary and metastatic lesions.

All primary carcinomas of the eyelid can be classified based on their clinical and histological presentation using the TNM [tumor, nodes (lymph), metastasis] by AJCC (8th Ed) classification system [21]. TNM staging describes the size of tumor, number and location of regional lymph nodes which have malignant cells in them and whether the malignant cells have spread or metastasized to another part of the body. The TNM classification of eyelid carcinomas reflects both morbidity and mortality risks in order to provide useful guidelines for patient management.

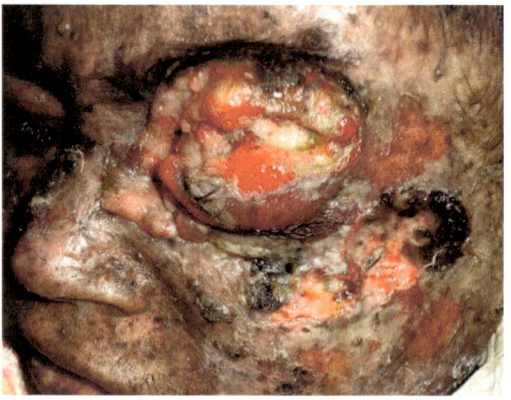

Fig. 1.5 Extensive malignant melanoma involving both the eyelids in a patient with xeroderma pigmentosa

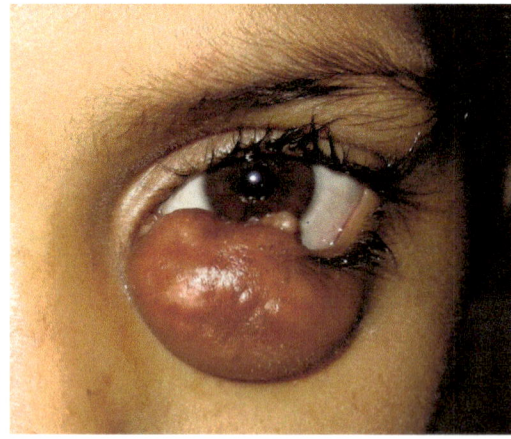

Fig. 1.6 Rapidly growing squamous cell carcinoma of the eyelid and extending to the orbit

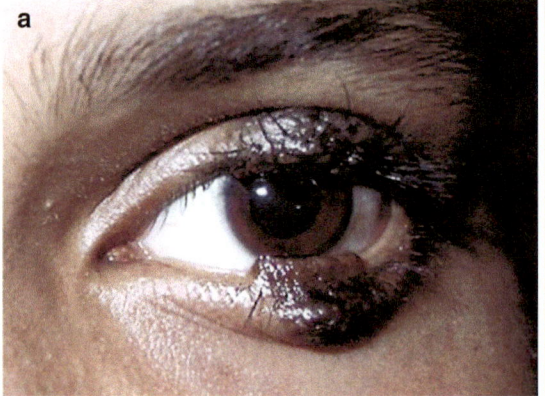

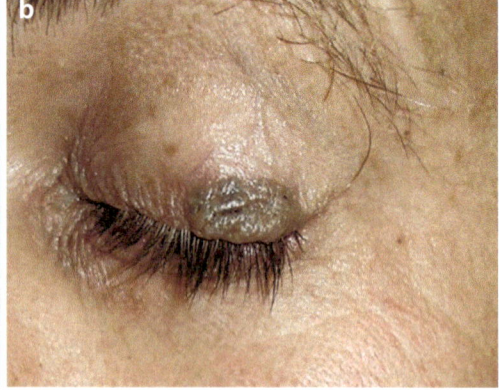

Fig. 1.7 (**a**) Kissing nevus in a young adolescent girl. (**b**) Nevi involving the upper lid in a young adult with a history of recent growth. (**c**) Nevus involving the lid margin in a young adult. (**d**) Keratoacanthoma

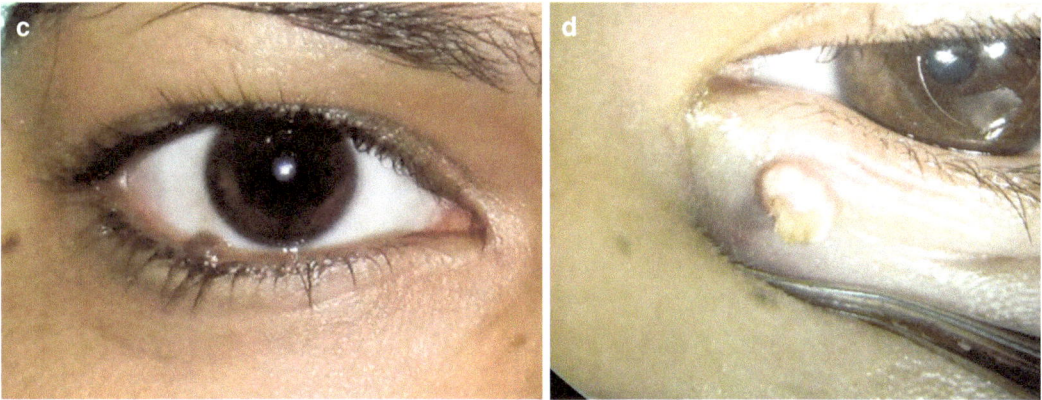

Fig. 1.7 (continued)

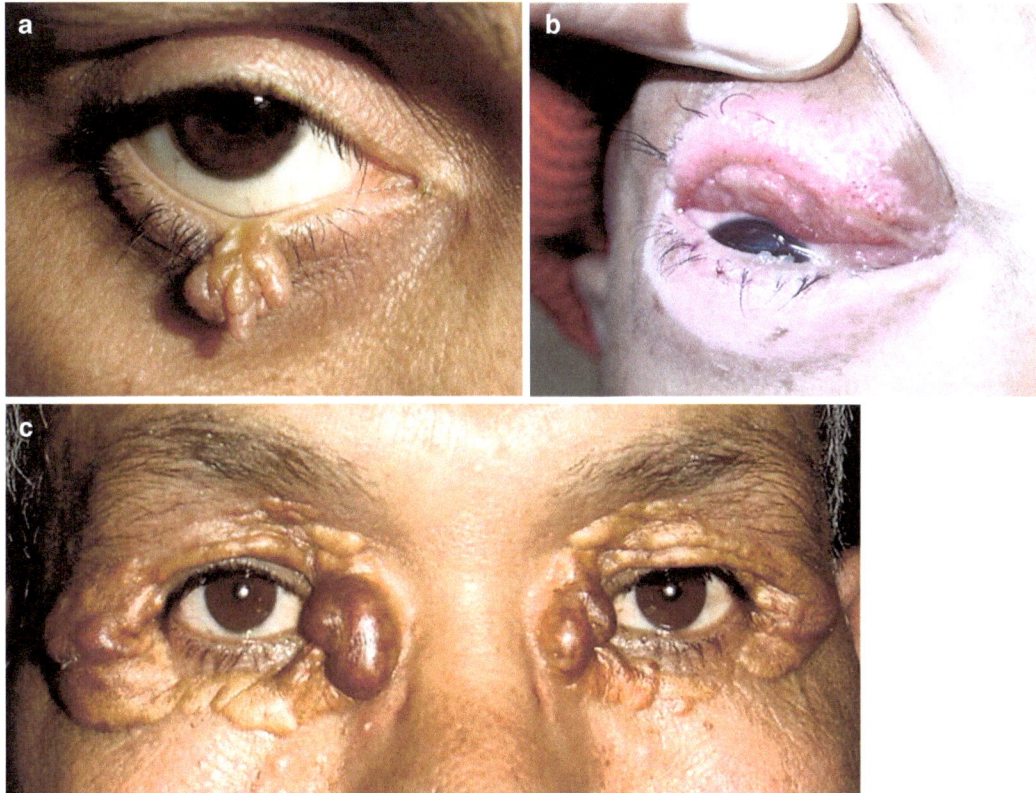

Fig. 1.8 (**a**) Squamous papilloma of the lower eyelid. (**b**) Lymphangioma diffusely involving the lids and orbit. (**c**) Extensive Xanthelesma involving all four lids

References

1. Huang YY, Liang WY, Tsai CC, Kao SC, Yu WK, Kau HC, et al. Comparison of the clinical characteristics and outcome of benign and malignant eyelid tumors: an analysis of 4521 eyelid tumors in a tertiary medical center. BioMed Res Int. 2015;5 pages:453091. https://doi.org/10.1155/2015/453091.
2. Chang CH, Chang SM, Lai YH, Huang J, Su MY, Wang HZ, et al. Eyelid tumors in southern Taiwan: a 5-year survey from a medical university. Kaohsiung J Med Sci. 2003;19:549–54.
3. Toshida H, Mamada N, Fujimaki T, Funaki T, Ebihara N, Murakami A, Okisaka S, et al. Incidence of benign and malignant eyelid tumors in Japan. Int J Ophthalmic Pathol. 2012;1(2):112–4.
4. Sihota R, Tandon K, Betharia SM, Arora R. Malignant eyelid tumors in an Indian population. Arch Ophthalmol. 1996;114(1):108–9.
5. Rathod A, Pandharpurkar M, Toopalli K, Bele S. A clinicopathological study of eyelid tumours and its management at a tertiary eye care center of southern India. MRIMS J Health Sci. 2015;3(1):54–8.
6. Ni Z. Histopathological classification of 3510 cases with eyelid tumor. Zhonghua Yan KeZaZhi. 1996;32:435–7.
7. Deprez M, Uffer S. Clinicopathological features of eyelid skin tumors. A retrospective study of 5504 cases and review of literature. Am J Dermatopathol. 2009;31(3):256–62.
8. Paul S, Vo DT, Silkiss RZ. Malignant and benign eyelid lesions in San Francisco: study of a diverse urban population. Am J Clin Med. 2011;8(1):40–6.
9. McLean IW, Burnier MN, Zimmerman LE, et al. Tumors of the eyelid. In: Tumors of the eye and ocular adnexa. Washington, DC: American Registry of Pathology/AFIP; 1994. p. 7–47.
10. Font RL, Croxatto JO, Rao NA. Tumors of the eyelids. In: Tumors of the eye and ocular adnexa. Washington, DC: American Registry of Pathology/AFIP; 2006. p. 155–22.
11. Bagheri A, Tavakoli M, Kanaani A, Zavareh RB, Esfandiari H, Aletaha M, et al. Eyelid masses: a 10-year survey from a tertiary eye hospital in Tehran. Middle East Afr J Ophthalmol. 2013;20(3):187–92.
12. Gundogan FC, Yolcu U, Tas A, Sahin OF, Uzun S, Cermik H, et al. Eyelid tumors: clinical data from an eye Center in Ankara, Turkey. Asian Pac J Cancer Prev. 2015;16(10):4265–9.
13. Kale SM, Patil SB, Khare N, Math M, Jain A, Jaiswal S. Clinicopathological analysis of eyelid malignancies- a review of 85 cases. Indian J Plast Surg. 2012;45(1):22–8.
14. Prabha DP, Padmavathi P, Ather M. Clinicopathological study of malignant eyelid tumours. Sch J App Med Sci. 2015;3(6A):2165–8.
15. Ho M, Liu DTL, Chong KKL, Ng HK, Lam DSC. Eyelid tumours and pseudotumours in Hong Kong: a ten-year experience. Hong Kong Med J. 2013;19(2):150–5.
16. Hsu HC, Lin HF. Eyelid tumors in children: a clinicopathologic study of a 10-year review in southern Taiwan. Ophthalmologica. 2004;218(4):274–7.
17. Al-Buloushi A, Filho JP, Cassie A, Arthurs B, Burnier MN Jr. Basal cell carcinoma of the eyelid in children: a report of three cases. Eye. 2005;19:1313–4. https://doi.org/10.1038/sj.eye.6701758.
18. Nerad JA, Whitaker DC. Periocular basal cell carcinoma in adults 35 years of age and younger. Ophthalmology. 1988;106:723–9.
19. Lemos BD, Storer BE, Iyer JG, Phillips JL, Bichakjian CK, Fang LC, et al. Pathologic nodal evaluation improves prognostic accuracy in Merkel cell carcinoma: analysis of 5823 cases as the basis of the first consensus staging system. J Am Acad Dermatol. 2010;63(5):751–61.
20. Kaliki S, Ayyar A, Dave TV, Ali MJ, Mishra DK, Naik MN. Sebaceous gland carcinoma of the eyelid: clinicopathological features and outcome in Asian Indians. Eye. 2015;29:958–63.
21. The American Joint Committee on Cancer. In: Amin MB, et al., editors. AJCC cancer staging manual. 8th ed; 2017. p. 779–85. https://doi.org/10.1007/978-3-319-40618-3_64.

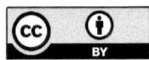

Albert Wu, Shyamala C. Huilgol, and Dinesh Selva

Introduction

Biopsies of eyelid lesions can be performed to establish the diagnosis and may identify high-risk histological tumour subtypes. This may influence management, especially when there is a significant cosmetic impact of excising a large lesion, when non-surgical management can be used or when planning Mohs surgery. Another use is establishing tumour boundaries through mapping biopsies. A biopsy may also assist in determining whether tumour recurrence has occurred following previous treatment [1]. The main types of biopsy are excisional, incisional, punch and shave biopsies. A biopsy may be performed with the intention of excising a lesion, for example, in the case of a very small basal cell carcinoma (BCC) where the clinician feels confident about the diagnosis. It should be borne in mind that biopsies can occasionally provide an inaccurate or incomplete diagnosis due to sampling errors.

Electronic supplementary material The online version of this chapter (https://doi.org/10.1007/978-3-030-18757-6_2) contains supplementary material, which is available to authorized users.

A. Wu (✉) · S. C. Huilgol
Dermatology Department, Royal Adelaide Hospital, Adelaide, SA, Australia

D. Selva
Ophthalmology Department, Royal Adelaide Hospital, Adelaide, SA, Australia

In one study of periocular BCC with aggressive subtypes ($n = 51$), biopsy failed to identify an aggressive component in 52% of cases [2].

Preoperative Considerations

Although biopsies are generally straightforward procedures, the patient's medical history should first be reviewed [1, 3]. General medical history, allergies and medications should be noted. Smoking and medical conditions may impair healing. Antiplatelets, anticoagulants, bleeding disorders and hypertension increase the risk of haemorrhage. Informed consent should be obtained and complications explained such as haemorrhage, infection, scarring, ectropion and pain. The lesion may be outlined with a skin marker pen before the procedure to help identify the lesion following injection of local anaesthesia [1, 3]. A photo with the biopsy site marked and measurements to fixed landmarks such as the canthi or lacrimal puncta are essential for later accurate localisation, especially for smaller lesions which may be very difficult to find after the biopsy.

Biopsy Techniques

The main techniques utilised in the periocular area are excisional, incisional, punch, snip, curette and shave biopsies. Techniques are selected based on lesion characteristics, possible diagnosis, location and surgeon preference. For instance, a snip biopsy may be used for a pedunculated lesion, or a shave biopsy for an elevated lid margin lesion. One study of periocular tumours ($n = 20$) found that incisional biopsy had an accuracy rate of 95% [4]. Similarly, the accuracy rate of punch biopsies in identifying periocular tumours has been reported to be 67–85% [4–6]. Shave biopsy may produce a better cosmetic outcome than a deeper biopsy which may leave a notch in the eyelid if the lesion proves to be benign. However, shave biopsy is not recommended in certain scenarios such as differentiating keratoacanthoma-type squamous cell carcinoma (SCC) from invasive SCC [1, 3] or in suspected melanoma where tumour thickness is an important prognostic factor.

Equipment Required for Biopsy

- Skin preparation materials
- Local anaesthetic with adrenaline 1:100,000
- Forceps
- Scalpel/scissors
- Cautery or other method of haemostasis
- Formalin container(s)

Other equipment can be added as needed, such as disposable punch, blade for shave biopsy and suturing equipment. An eye shield may be used to prevent eye injury.

Incisional Biopsy Technique
(Video 2.1)

1. Aseptic skin preparation.
2. Inject local anaesthetic with adrenaline around the lesion.
3. Using a scalpel blade (No. 11 blade often useful for small lesions), aim to sample a piece of tumour and some adjacent normal tissue. Avoid sampling ulcerated areas which may only provide necrotic tissue and not provide a diagnosis. Also avoid keratinised/crusted areas and remove overlying crust with irrigation/soaking if necessary. An elliptical excision can also be performed.

4. Place specimen in formalin.
5. Cauterise wound or use pressure.
6. Close wound with sutures if necessary but small defects can be left to heal by secondary intention [1, 7, 8].

Punch Biopsy Technique (Video 2.2)

1. Aseptic skin preparation.
2. Inject local anaesthetic with adrenaline around the lesion.
3. Using thumb and index finger, stretch the skin on either side of the lesion away from the lesion. This produces an oval defect which facilitates wound closure. Align the oval defect with skin tension lines.
4. Insert punch into lesion perpendicular to skin with a twisting motion. Aim to sample a non-central part of the lesion away from the margin. Take care not to injure the globe. Consider using an eye shield.
5. Remove the punch perpendicular to skin, leaving behind the whole biopsy specimen.
6. Using forceps, grasp an edge of the specimen gently to avoid crush artefact, and lift the specimen out. The specimen may also be lifted out using a needle, a skin hook or a suture passed through the specimen. This step may be made easier by pushing down on surrounding skin to raise the lesion relative to the surrounding skin.
7. Cut the base of the specimen with scissors or scalpel.
8. Place specimen in formalin.
9. Consider cautery. Haemostasis may also be achieved with sutures and slight pressure. Suture closure produces a better cosmetic outcome but is not always necessary [1, 3, 4, 6, 9].

Shave Biopsy Technique (Video 2.3)

1. Aseptic skin preparation.
2. Inject local anaesthetic with adrenaline intra-dermally, raising the lesion from the surrounding skin.
3. Stretch the skin. When a lesion has limited elevation, the skin may be bunched up to

increase elevation. With raised lesions, forceps may be used to lift the lesion.

4. A scalpel is often used on the eyelid. The blade is used to saw through the lesion horizontally along the skin or the eyelid margin. Razor blades are used elsewhere on the body but are difficult to use on or near the eyelid margin.
5. Place specimen in formalin.
6. Apply light pressure, chemical haemostasis or cautery. Wound re-epithelialisation occurs in around 1 week [1, 3, 7, 8].

Snip Biopsy

Lift the lesion with forceps to snip the base with scissors. The lesion should not be pulled too far, resulting in removal of more skin at the base than necessary. Light pressure may be sufficient for haemostasis [1].

Curette Biopsy

Curette biopsy may be used for soft superficial lesions, including seborrhoeic keratosis, actinic keratosis and some BCC. Stretch the surrounding skin, and scoop down through the lesion with the curette. Avoid this method on lax skin of the eyelid as the curette may tear the skin while attempting to remove the tumour. Light pressure, chemical haemostasis or electrodessication can be used [1].

Communication with Pathologist

The pathology request form and specimen container should be labelled with patient identifying details, date and biopsy site. Ensure the specimen is in the container. The request form should also include details of the requesting clinician, type of biopsy (diagnostic or excisional), and relevant clinical information such as suspected clinical diagnosis and previous treatments to the biopsy site. A diagram or clinical photograph may be included. Specific questions may be included on the request form, and the case may be discussed

with the pathologist if required [1]. The clinician should record all specimens sent to the pathologist, and follow up and act upon pathology results in a timely manner.

Postoperative Care

Vaseline may be applied to the wound site. Topical antibiotics should not be routinely used. The site should be cleaned regularly, and medical advice should be sought if signs of infection develop.

Conclusion

Biopsy of the eyelid is an important skill which assists in diagnosis and management of eyelid tumours. The main techniques are excisional, incisional, punch and shave biopsies, and are selected depending on the clinician's preference and characteristics of the lesion.

References

1. Robinson JK, Hanke CW, Siegel DM, Fratila A, Bhatia A, Rohrer TE. Surgery of the skin: procedural dermatology. 3rd ed. London/New York: Elsevier/Saunders; 2015.
2. Sun MT, Wu A, Huilgol SC, Selva D. Accuracy of biopsy in subtyping periocular basal cell carcinoma. Ophthal Plast Reconstr Surg. 2015;31:449–51.
3. Wheeland RG. Cutaneous surgery. Philadelphia: W.B. Saunders; 1994.
4. Rice JC, Zaragoza P, Waheed K, Schofield J, Jones CA. Efficacy of incisional vs. punch biopsy in the histological diagnosis of periocular skin tumours. Eye (Lond). 2003;17:478–81.
5. Chatterjee S, Moore S, Kumar B. Punch biopsy in the management of periocular basal cell carcinomas. Orbit. 2004;23:87–92.
6. Carneiro RC, de Macedo EM, de Lima PP, Bonatti R, Matayoshi S. Is 2-mm punch biopsy useful in the diagnosis of malignant eyelid tumours? Ophthal Plast Reconstr Surg. 2012;28:282–5.
7. Dutton JJ, Gayre GS, Proia AD. Diagnostic atlas of common eyelid diseases. New York: Informa Healthcare; 2007.
8. Biswas A. Eyelid tumours: clinical evaluation and reconstruction techniques. New Delhi: Springer; 2014.
9. Sassani JW. Punch biopsy technique for the ophthalmologist. Arch Ophthalmol. 1991;109:464–5.

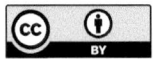

Excision of Eyelid Tumors: Principles and Techniques

Gangadhara Sundar and Fairooz P. Manjandavida

Lesions of the eyelid, benign or malignant, have physical, esthetic and psychological consequences and may on occasion be vision and life threatening. An overview of common and rare conditions affecting the eyelids and a conceptual approach has been described earlier. When the diagnosis is in doubt or when extensive reconstruction or nonsurgical treatment is being considered, an incisional biopsy of the lesion for histopathological confirmation is indicated, which has been described earlier.

Excision of lesions are often performed after an initial diagnosis has been established, thereby being therapeutic [1–3]. Not infrequently, it may be performed as both a diagnostic and therapeutic procedure, especially when preoperative clinical

diagnosis is certain, and reconstruction is straightforward with minimal morbidity. In malignant lesions, wide excisions are performed, which are usually therapeutic followed by reconstruction. Oncological principles for eyelid malignancy are the same as in other malignant neoplasms involving skin and adnexa. The surgical aim should be complete excision with adequate margin clearance to minimize recurrence, metastasis, and mortality. Therefore, clinically confirmed malignant eyelid tumors are often excised with margin control either with frozen section control or by Moh's micrographic surgery followed by formal histopathological confirmation with permanent fixed section [4–6]. Where frozen section facility is unavailable, a wider excision may be performed with margin control with permanent histology and secondary with delayed primary reconstruction after histopathological confirmation of clear margins. Moh's micrographic surgery is a good alternative where available which helps secure clear margins before a delayed primary reconstruction [7]. Conjunctival map biopsy is performed in the presence of suspected intraepithelial invasion of conjunctiva, especially in sebaceous gland carcinoma of eyelid [8].

On occasion, a therapeutic excision of an eyelid tumor, typically infiltrative and aggressive malignant neoplasms, e.g., sebaceous gland adenocarcinoma, melanoma, and Merkel cell carcinoma, may be combined with sentinel lymph node biopsy or a modified radical regional (cervical) lymph node

Electronic supplementary material The online version of this chapter (https://doi.org/10.1007/978-3-030-18757-6_3) contains supplementary material, which is available to authorized users.

G. Sundar (✉)
Orbit and Oculofacial Surgery/Ophthalmic Oncology, Department of Ophthalmology, National University Hospital, National University of Singapore, Singapore, Singapore

Department of Pediatrics, National University Hospital, Singapore, Singapore
e-mail: Gangadhara_sundar@nuhs.edu.sg

F. P. Manjandavida
Department of Oculoplasty and Ocular Oncology, Horus Specialty Eye Care, Bangalore, India

S. S. Chaugule et al. (eds.), *Surgical Ophthalmic Oncology*, https://doi.org/10.1007/978-3-030-18757-6_3

dissection, with adjuvant external beam therapy. The surgeon should thus not only be aware of the indications, but also be familiar with various techniques of excision and reconstruction. They should preferably work in multidisciplinary teams comprising pathologists, head and neck surgeons, Moh's micrographic surgeons, medical and radiation oncologists. Reconstruction, when performed, should not only be functional but should also be esthetically acceptable, with minimal donor site and host site morbidity and minimal downtime.

In general, small benign lesions may be excised with maximal tissue preservation. Unless typical of inflammatory lesions like a chalazion, it is recommended to submit the excised lesions for histopathological examination. Superficial benign epidermal lesions, especially when diagnosis is certain, may also be managed with tissue destructive techniques, e.g., fulguration, electrodessication, etc. [2]

When malignant lesions are excised, a "no touch" technique should be employed to avoid host tissue seeding. Excision should be performed as precisely and delicately as possible with the least tissue destructive technique and maximal hemostasis. It is essential to respect and preserve the anatomical vital structures – medial canthal tendon, lateral canthal tendon, levator aponeurosis, lacrimal sac, etc. The nature of the underlying lesion also determines the margin of resection, e.g., benign lesion, maximal skin and subcutaneous tissue sparing; basal cell carcinoma, minimal 2–4 mm margin depending on the morphological variants; squamous cell carcinoma/sebaceous gland adenocarcinoma, 4–5 mm margin; and melanoma, up to 10 mm margin is recommended as the current standard of care. The commonly used instruments in various excision techniques are shown in Fig. 3.1.

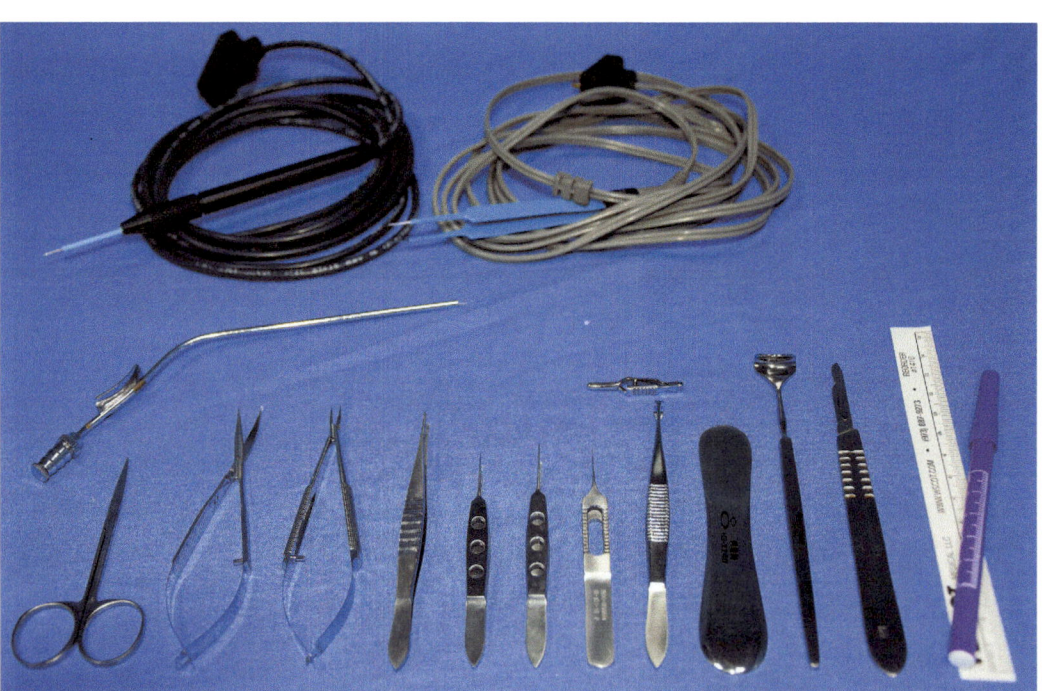

Fig. 3.1 Instrument tray. Instruments, starting lower left: 1, Metzenbaum scissors; 2, Westcott scissors; 3, Castroviejo needle holder; 4, tissue forceps; 5 and 6, Bishop-Harmon forceps; 7, Adson tissue forceps; 8, Graefe forceps; 9, Jaeger lid plate; 10, Desmarres retractor; 11, Bard-Parker knife handle; 12, fine tip marker and ruler; 13, Serrefine-Dienffenbach (bull dog clamps); 14, Frazier suction tip; 15 and 16, radiofrequency cautery monopolar and bipolar tips, 17, single and double skin hooks

Benign Lesions

In general, benign lesions that are asymptomatic and insignificant cosmetically may be observed. When the clinical diagnosis is uncertain, early incisional or excisional biopsy are reasonable options. Most symptomatic benign lesions may be excised safely and easily, with precautions taken to avoid damage to vital ocular and adnexal structures, e.g., canthal tendons, lacrimal puncta and canaliculi, lacrimal sac, ocular surface, etc. Whenever possible a complete excision is recommended (Figs. 3.2, 3.3, 3.4, 3.5, 3.6, 3.7, 3.8 and 3.9, Tables 3.1 and 3.2, Video 3.1).

- Cystic lesions should be excised as to minimize inflammations and recurrences.

- Epidermal lesions are generally excised or fulgurated at the dermo-epidermal junction avoiding scarring, notching and need for wound repair (Video 3.2). Healing occurs by reepithelization of the raw area.
- Dermal lesions and dermal adnexal lesions will require skin excision in addition to complete removal of the lesion (Fig. 3.10a, b). The only exception is a compound or dermal nevus of the eyelid margin, when a shave excision is performed avoiding notching of the eyelid margins.
- Subcutaneous lesions are accessed through skin incisions along the relaxed tension line when possible or through preexisting eyelid creases.

Most eyelid surgeries are clean surgeries, and only topical cleansing of the eyelid with postoperative topical antibiotics is indicated.

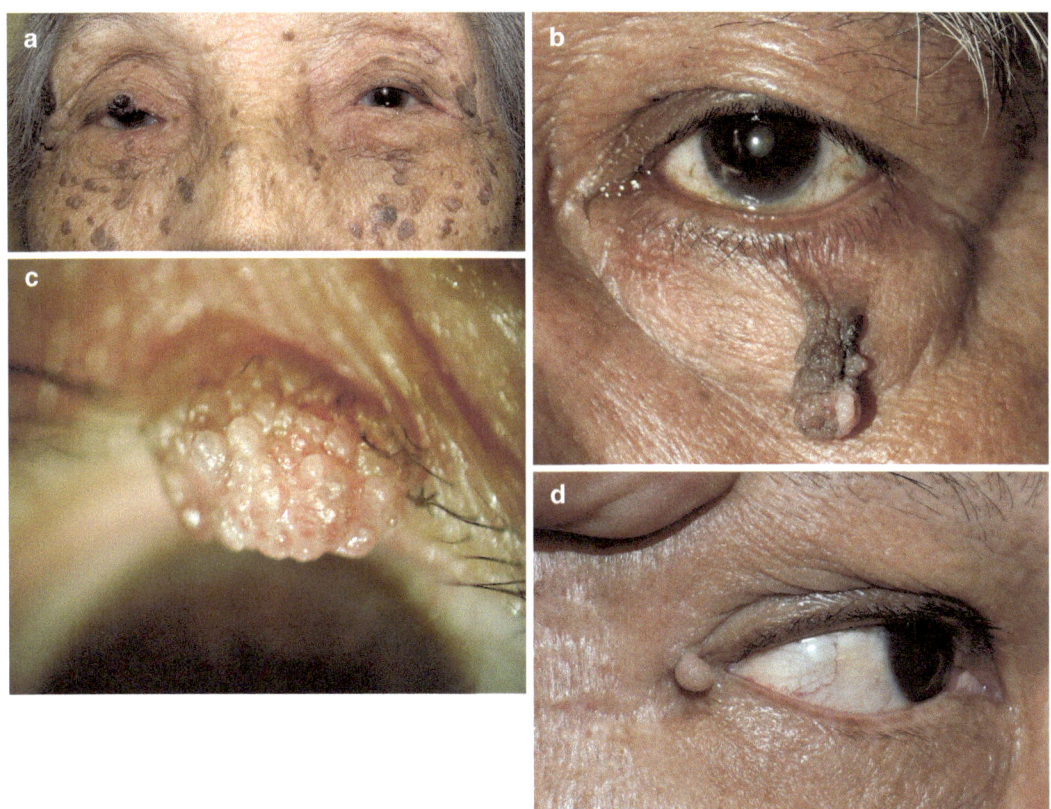

Fig. 3.2 (**a**) Seborrheic keratosis. (**b**) Fibroepithelial polyp. (**c**) Verruca vulgaris. (**d**) Acrochordon (skin tag)

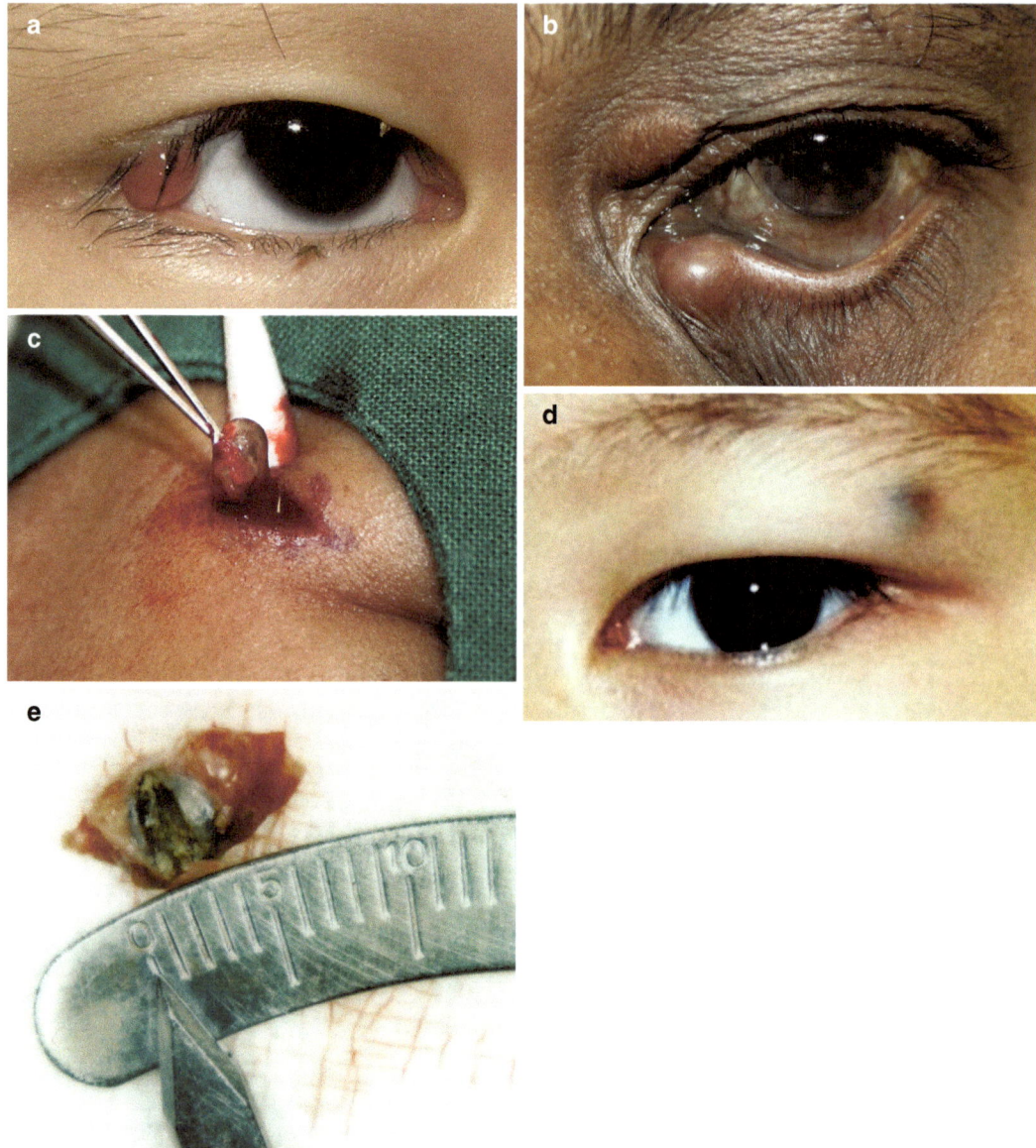

Fig. 3.3 (**a**) Chalazion with pyogenic granuloma. (**b**) Hidrocystoma Trichoepithelioma. (**c**) Complete excision. (**d**) Pilomatrixoma. (**e**) Excised specimen of pilomatrixoma

Premalignant Lesions

It is essential for the clinician to recognize potential premalignant lesions. Although these are more common in the Caucasian population, they may present in all ethnic groups and various skin types and pigmentation. In general, there should be a low threshold for performing a biopsy of suspicious lesions. At risk patients (e.g., actinic keratosis – squamous cell carcinoma, lentigo maligna – melanoma, xeroderma pigmentosa (Fig. 3.11) – basal cell carcinoma, squamous cell carcinoma, melanoma) should also be advised against ultraviolet light/sun exposure. Clinically evident change in size, thickness, color and vascularity may indicates malignant transfor-

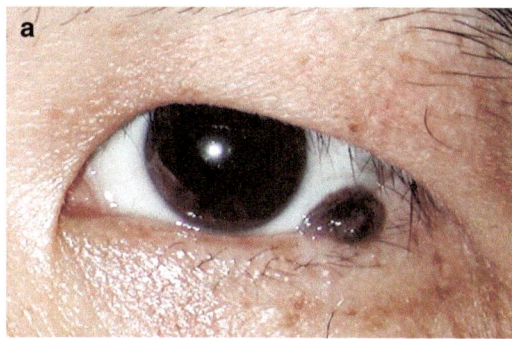

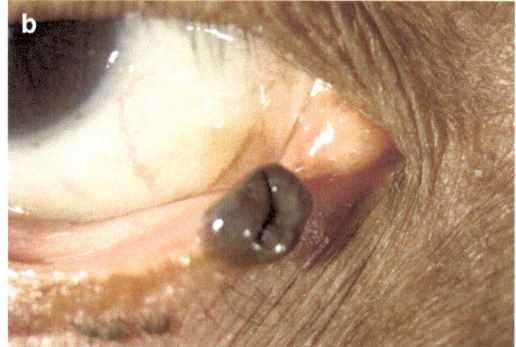

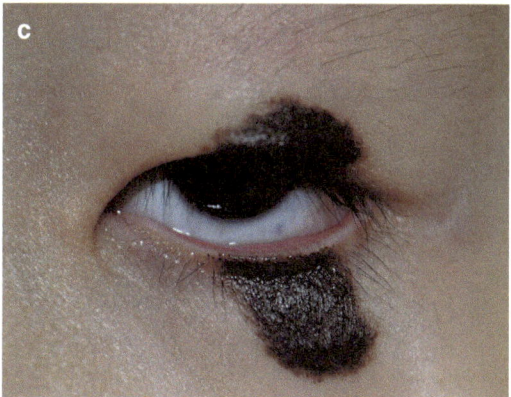

Fig. 3.4 (**a**) Eyelid margin pigmented nevus. (**b**) Peripunctal nevus. (**c**) Kissing nevus

mation, which may need surgical intervention (Figs. 3.11 and 3.12, Table 3.3).

Malignant Eyelid Tumors

In general, malignant lesions of the eyelids and periocular region are far less common than benign lesions [9]. While basal cell carcinomas are the most common in all ethnic groups, occurring primarily in sun-exposed areas, the prevalence of squamous cell carcinomas [10] and sebaceous gland adenocarcinomas are different between the Caucasian and the Asian populations. In eyelid malignancies other than basal cell carcinoma, regional lymph nodes, and systemic screening is mandated clinically and preferably by imaging as well. The decision to perform wide excision biopsy with clear margins, regional lymph node/sentinel node biopsy (sebaceous gland adenocarcinoma, melanoma, Merkel cell carcinoma, etc.), cryotherapy of the edges, and ocular surface map biopsy (Sebaceous gland adenocarcinoma) depends on the nature of the primary malignancy. Some salient differences and some examples are shown in Table 3.4 (Figs. 3.13, 3.14, 3.15, 3.16, 3.17, 3.18, 3.19, 3.20, 3.21, 3.22 and 3.23).

Basal Cell Carcinoma (BCC)

Basal cell carcinomas are the most common malignant neoplasms of the eyelids and the face, globally. While most are sporadic and related to sun exposure especially in Caucasians of the lower Fitzpatrick skin types, they are seen in all ethnic and geographical regions with minor variations. Early lesions, typically nodular, are either ignored or misdiagnosed unless lesions are routinely sent for histopathological examination. In pigmented races, a pigmented form of BCC is often mistaken for a melanoma (Fig. 3.24). While the common type is a nodular or nodulo-ulcerative type, rare forms include the morphea-form, infiltrative BCC (Fig. 3.25) or even the multicentric or superficial basal cell carcinoma. The latter are often diagnosed late and managed poorly as obtaining clear margins are difficult with local excision.

When localized, small and early, a simple excision with margin of 2–3 mm with frozen section control will suffice with primary reconstruction. Lid margin lesions will require a full thickness block resection (and not wedge resection) ideally under frozen section control with primary reconstruction [11]. Principles of wound healing and reconstruction include the laissez-faire technique, use of adjacent (eyelid, cheek, forehead) or regional flaps/grafts.

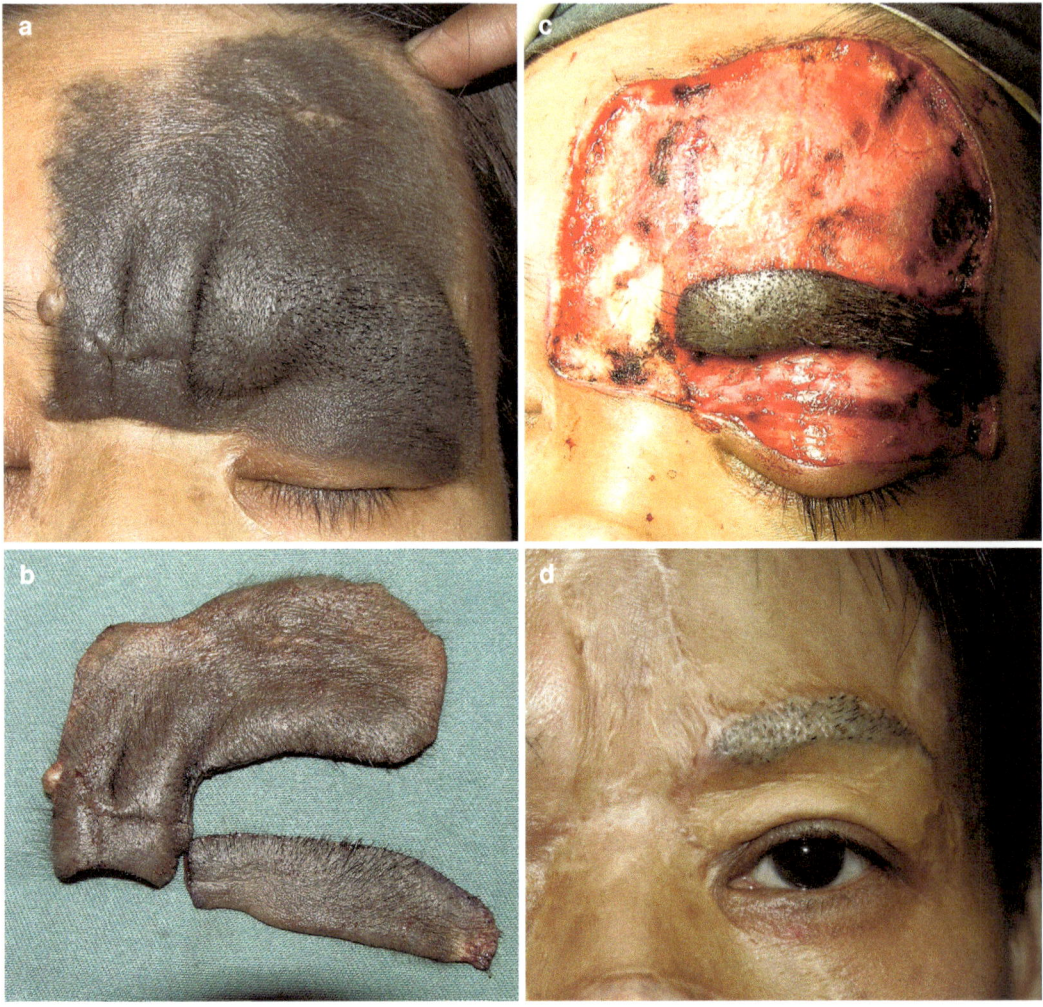

Fig. 3.5 (**a**) Giant hairy nevus. (**b**) Excised lesion of giant hairy nevus. (**c**) Post-excision with eyebrow preservation. (**d**) Post-reconstruction with suprapubic skin graft and laser treatment for eyebrow

Large lid margin defects may require complex reconstruction using either composite graft-flap techniques or lid sharing procedures and are discussed in detail in the following chapter. Large extensive and inoperable lesions away from the globes may be amenable to external beam radiation [12]. While it may obtain tumor control, tissue destruction is not often addressed by this modality of treatment. In the recent years, extensive and invasive basal cell carcinomas have been shown to be responsive to targeted therapy with hedgehog pathway inhibitors and,

may be considered for extensive, recurrent and the rare metastatic lesions [13].

Squamous Cell Carcinoma (SCC)

Less frequent, but more challenging to diagnose and manage are SCC of the eyelid and adnexa. They are typically more common among the light pigmented races and those with predisposing conditions like actinic keratosis and xeroderma pigmentosa. While typi-

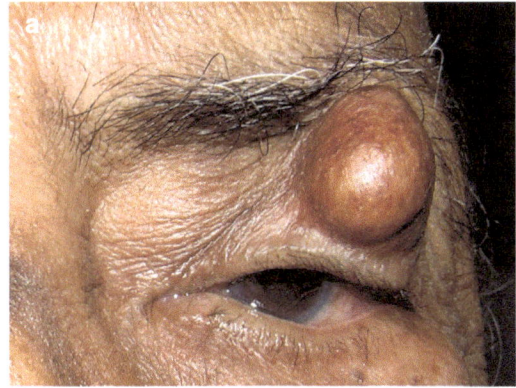

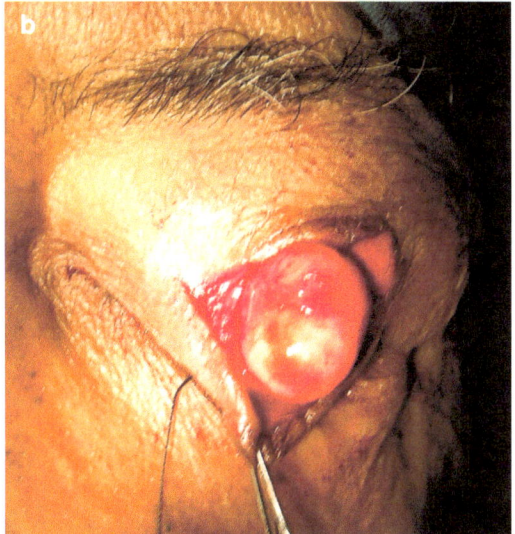

Fig. 3.6 (**a**) Epidermal cyst. (**b**) Dissected epidermal cyst

cal presentations are easily suspected, atypical presentations often result in late diagnosis and thus delay in management with a poorer prognosis [10]. Principles of management include wide excision with 3–4 mm margins under frozen section control, followed by reconstruction or Moh's micrographic surgery if available. Extensive lesions, deeper invasion, positive margins and inoperable lesions may

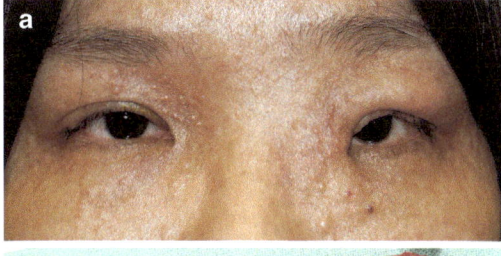

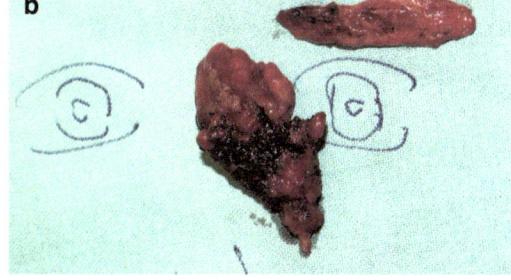

Fig. 3.8 (**a**) Neurofibroma. (**b**) Excised neurofibroma (templet method)

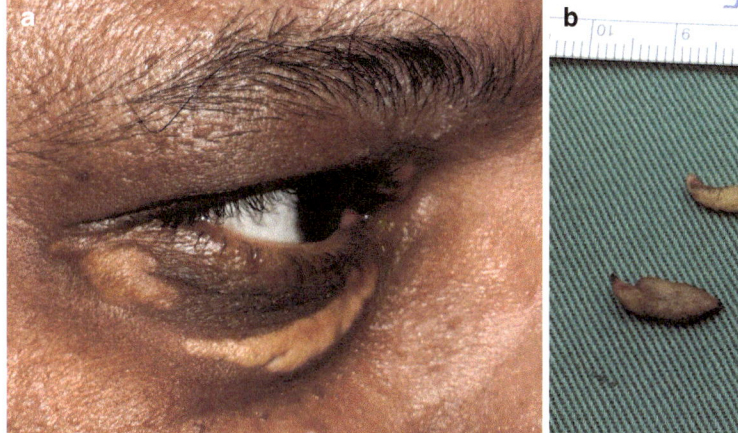

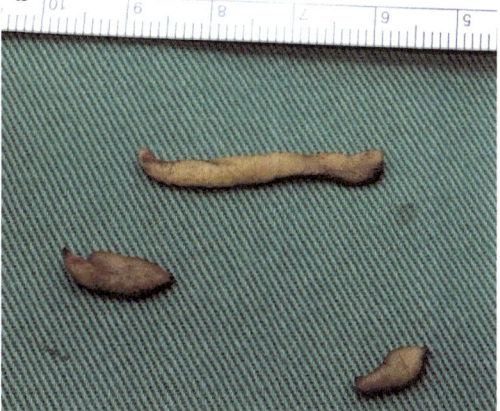

Fig. 3.7 (**a**) Eyelid xanthelasma. (**b**) Xanthelasma post-excision

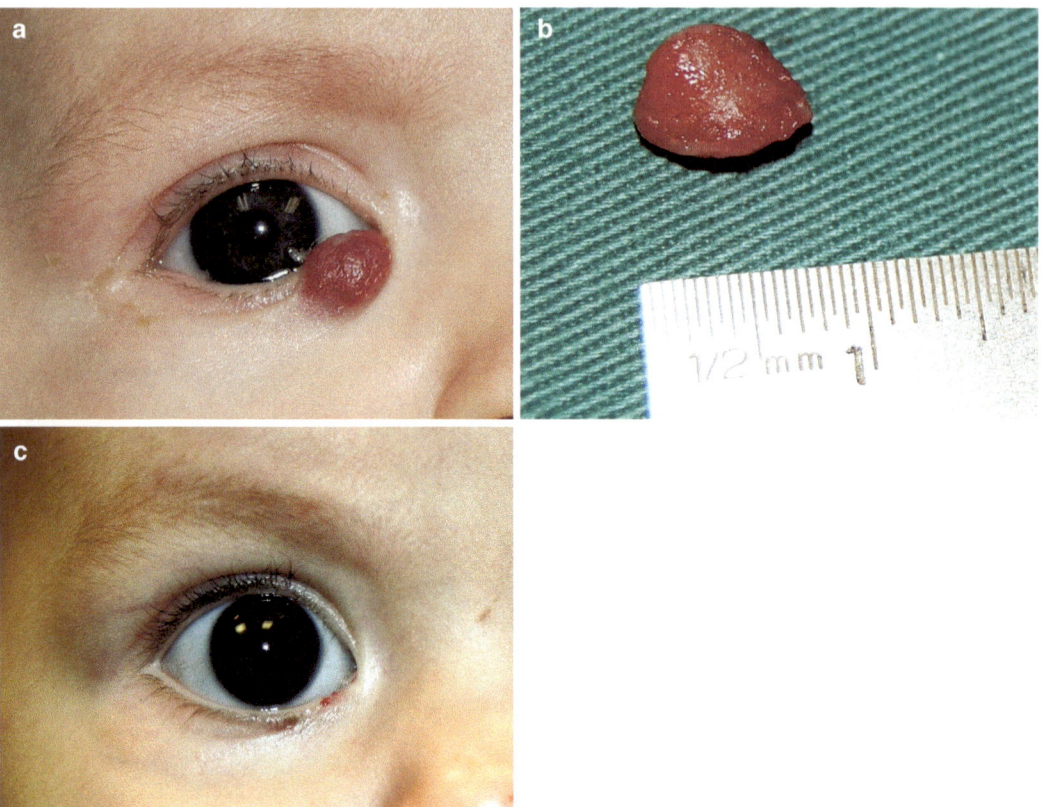

Fig. 3.9 (**a**) Partially involuted infantile hemangioma. (**b**) Excised partially involuted infantile hemangioma. (**c**) Postoperative image

Table 3.1 Spectrum of anesthetic techniques for various lesions of the eyelid and ocular adnexa

Type of anesthesia	Principle	Typical indication	Technique
None	Brief, momentary, simple procedure	Acrochordons (skin tags), pedunculated verruca	–
Topical	Superficial epidermal, sessile, multiple lesions	Syringomas, seborrheic keratosis, etc.	Topical lidocaine – prilocaine application with occlusive dressing for 15–20 min
Local/infiltrative (lidocaine with epinephrine, with or without bupivacaine)	Nerve blocks	Larger eyelid lesions, planned reconstruction	Frontal nerve block, infraorbital nerve block, infraorbital fan block etc.
	Regional blocks		
	Fan blocks		
General anesthesia	Extensive resections/ reconstruction, regional lymph node dissection, distal donor site harvesting, uncooperative patients	Exenteration, extensive reconstruction, cervical lymph node dissection, etc.	

Table 3.2 Principles of management: benign eyelid lesions

Type of lesion	Principles of management
Epidermal lesions	
Seborrheic keratosis (Fig. 3.2a)	Observation, electrodessication, cautery with curettage
Pseudoepitheliomatous hyperplasia	
Fibroepithelial polyp (Fig. 3.2b)	Simple excision
Verruca vulgaris (Fig. 3.2c)	Excision with no touch technique
Acrochordons or skin tags (Fig. 3.2d)	Snip excision (Video 3.1)
Benign adnexal tumors	
Hordeolum internum	Systemic antibiotics, warm compresses
Hordeolum externum	Lash epilation, pus expression
Chalazion: without or with pyogenic granuloma, chalazion externum (Fig. 3.3a)	Incision, curettage, subconjunctival steroid injection, pyogenic granuloma excision
Sebaceous adenoma	Excision
Eccrine sweat gland origin	
Eccrine hidrocystoma	Marsupialization, complete excision
Syringoma	Chemical peel, surface treatment
Pleomorphic adenoma	Excision
Apocrine sweat gland origin	
Apocrine hidrocystoma	Marsupialization, complete excision
Hair follicle origin	
Trichoepithelioma (Fig. 3.3b)	Complete excision (Fig. 3.3c)
Trichofolliculoma	Excision
Tricholemmoma	Excision
Pilomatrixoma (Fig. 3.3d)	Excision (Fig. 3.3e)
Benign melanocytic lesions	
Lid margin involving-	
Single margin involving (Fig. 3.4a)	Shave excision
Peripunctal nevi (Fig. 3.4b)	Limited excision with punctal preservation
Kissing nevi (Fig. 3.4c)	Observation, excision with preservation of lid margin
Non-lid margin involving nevi	
Simple nevi	Observation, excision with skin grafting, pigment laser treatments
Hairy nevi	
Giant nevi (Fig. 3.5a–d)	
Freckle	Observation, pigment laser applications
Lentigo simplex	
Solar lentigo	
Blue nevus	
Dermal melanocytosis	
Others	
Cysts (Fig. 3.6a): Epidermal cyst, implantation cysts, inclusion cysts, dermal adnexal cysts	Excision with intact cyst (Fig. 3.6b)
Xanthogranuloma	Excision
Xanthelasmata (Fig. 3.7a)	Excision (Fig. 3.7b) with primary wound closure
Neurofibromas (Fig. 3.8a)	Excision (template technique) (Fig. 3.8b)
Capillary hemangioma (Fig. 3.9a–c)	Observation, systemic beta blockers, systemic/intralesional steroids, excision

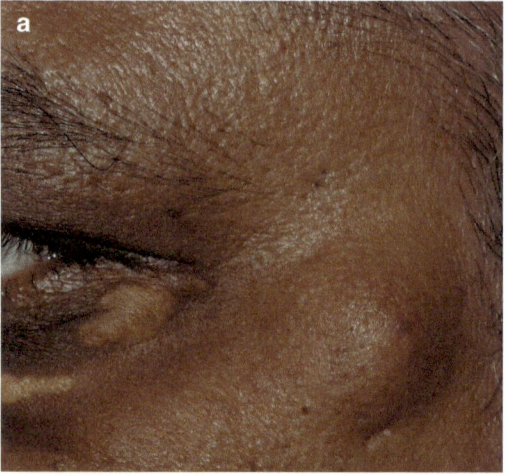

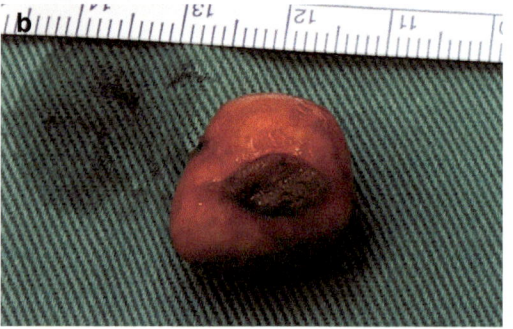

Fig. 3.10 (**a**) Dermal adnexal cyst. (**b**) Excised dermal adnexal cyst

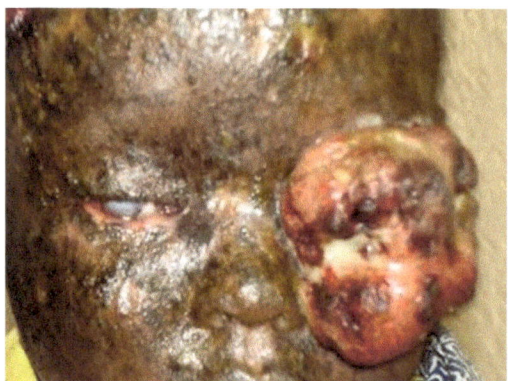

Fig. 3.11 Xeroderma pigmentosa

be candidates for radiation therapy. Epidermal growth factor receptor (EGFR) inhibitors have shown promising results recently [13].

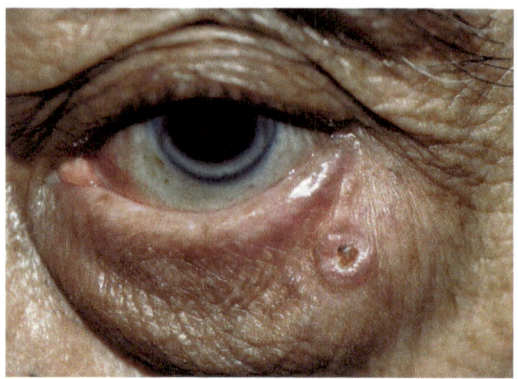

Fig. 3.12 Keratoacanthoma

Table 3.3 Principles of management: premalignant/in situ malignant eyelid lesions

Type of lesion	Principles of management
Actinic keratosis	Observation with serial follow-up, biopsy of suspicious lesions
Lentigo maligna	Observation with serial follow-up, biopsy of suspicious lesions
Keratoacanthoma (Fig. 3.12)	Excision biopsy
Xeroderma pigmentosa (Fig. 3.11)	Close observation and biopsy of suspicious lesions

Sebaceous Gland Carcinoma (SGC)

These are far more common among Asians, being increasingly recognized compared to the past when they were either misdiagnosed as squamous cell carcinomas or even chronic blepharoconjunctivitis [14, 15]. Most commonly arising from the meibomian glands situated in the posterior lamellae, they may even arise from the Zeis glands and caruncle. Seen most commonly in the upper eyelid, involving the tarsal meibomian glands, they are notorious for pagetoid spread with skip lesions rendering frozen sections less reliable and frequently involve the ocular surface. Late presentations may also present with anterior orbital extension, regional (preauricular and cervical lymph nodes) spread, or even systemic metastasis [16].

Table 3.4 Principles of management: malignant eyelid lesions

Type of lesion	Principles of management
Basal cell carcinoma (Figs. 3.13a–c, 3.14a, b and 3.15a–d)	Wide excision with 2–4 mm margin, frozen section control, primary reconstruction
	Moh's micrographic excision with delayed primary reconstruction.
	External beam radiation (inoperable lesions)
	Hedgehog pathway inhibitors (for inoperable, non-radiatable BCCs)
Squamous cell carcinoma (Fig. 3.16)	Wide excision 3–4 mm margins, frozen section control, primary reconstruction
	Moh's micrographic excision with delayed primary reconstruction
	Radiotherapy
	Exenteration (extensive eyelid lesion with orbital invasion)
	Imiquimod therapy (superficial, extensive, recurrent SCC)
	Epidermal growth factor receptor inhibitors
Sebaceous gland adenocarcinoma (Figs. 3.17a–c and 3.18a–e)	Wide excision with wide margins (4 mm), under frozen section control (less reliable), cryotherapy of edges, conjunctival map biopsy, primary reconstruction. Sentinel lymph node biopsy in lesions >10 mm in size, regional lymph node dissection (spread, PET-CT positive)
	Chemoreduction with local excision
	Orbital exenteration
Mucinous carcinoma (Fig. 3.19a–d)	Excision with wide margins, frozen section control, primary reconstruction
Merkel cell carcinoma (Fig. 3.20a, b)	Wide excision with 4 mm margins under frozen section
	Moh's micrographic excision
	Sentinel lymph node biopsy
	Regional lymph node dissection, adjuvant chemotherapy, radiotherapy
Melanoma (Fig. 3.21a, b)	Wide excision (10 mm if possible), primary reconstruction, sentinel lymph node biopsy, orbital exenteration, palliative therapy
Lymphoma (Fig. 3.22)	Radiation and chemotherapy
Metastasis (Fig. 3.23)	External beam radiotherapy, targeted therapy where applicable

Principles of management include preoperative systemic evaluation to rule out regional and systemic spread followed by wide excision with margin clearance of at least 4 mm [17] (Video 3.3). Frozen section control is challenging in the presence of conjunctival intraepithelial (pagetoid) spread. A few examples of eyelid sebaceous gland carcinoma excision and reconstruction are shown in Videos 3.4, 3.5, 3.6 and 3.7.

In the presence of clinically suspicious intraepithelial spread with conjunctival hyperemia (tarsal and/or bulbar) and lid margin thickening, a conjunctival map biopsy is indicated to ensure ocular surface is free of the tumor and guide further management if indicated [18]. The location of the map biopsy varies according to the clinical presentation. These include forniceal conjunctival (upper and lower), bulbar conjunctival (upper and lower), perilimbal conjunctival (four quadrants) and the caruncle. Invasion of the orbit is often considered an indication for orbital exenteration.

Recent evidence suggests a possible benefit of systemic "chemoreduction" minimizing the need for mutilating exenteration with early orbital invasion [19]. With obvious cervical node involvement, a modified radical lymph node dissection is often indicated. A recent trend toward sentinel lymph node biopsy (SNLB) is practiced in some centers around the world. SNLB is indicated in tumors that are clinically measured >10 mm in size. Despite a better understanding, greater awareness and improved techniques, locoregional recurrences and distant metastases are not uncommon resulting in higher mortality compared to the above neoplasms.

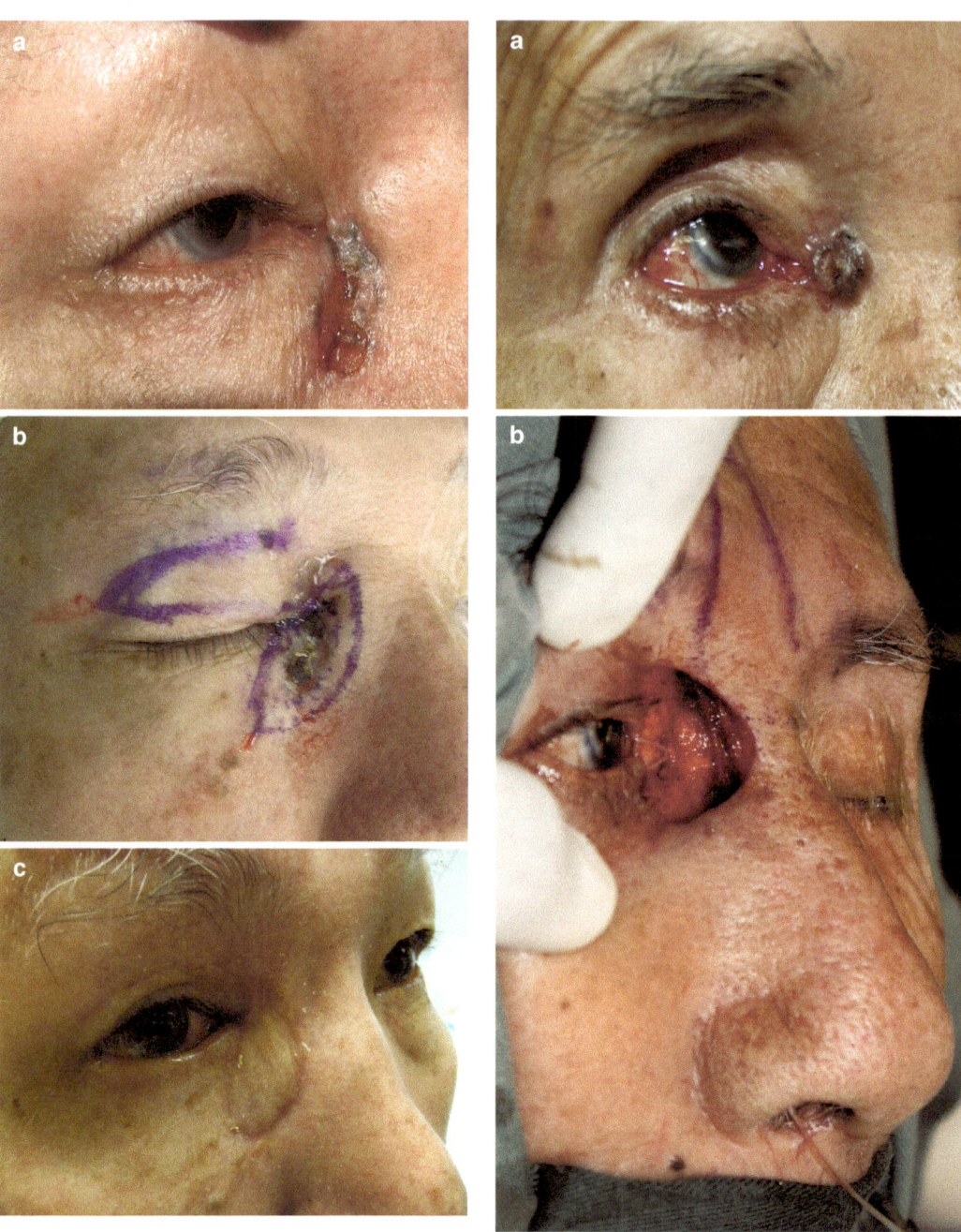

Fig. 3.13 (**a**) BCC at medial canthus. (**b**) BCC at medial canthus repaired with regional flap. (**c**) Postoperative image

Fig. 3.14 (**a**) BCC at medial canthus. (**b**) Basal cell carcinoma medial canthus repaired with paramedian forehead flap. Note the reconstruction of lacrimal system

Eyelid Melanoma

Melanomas of the eyelid are rare and may be either a nodular melanoma or superficial spreading melanoma (arising from a lentigo maligna), and can be primary or secondary. They are commonly associated with a poorer prognosis as recurrence rates are high, and the presence of regional or systemic spread even at or soon after presentation.

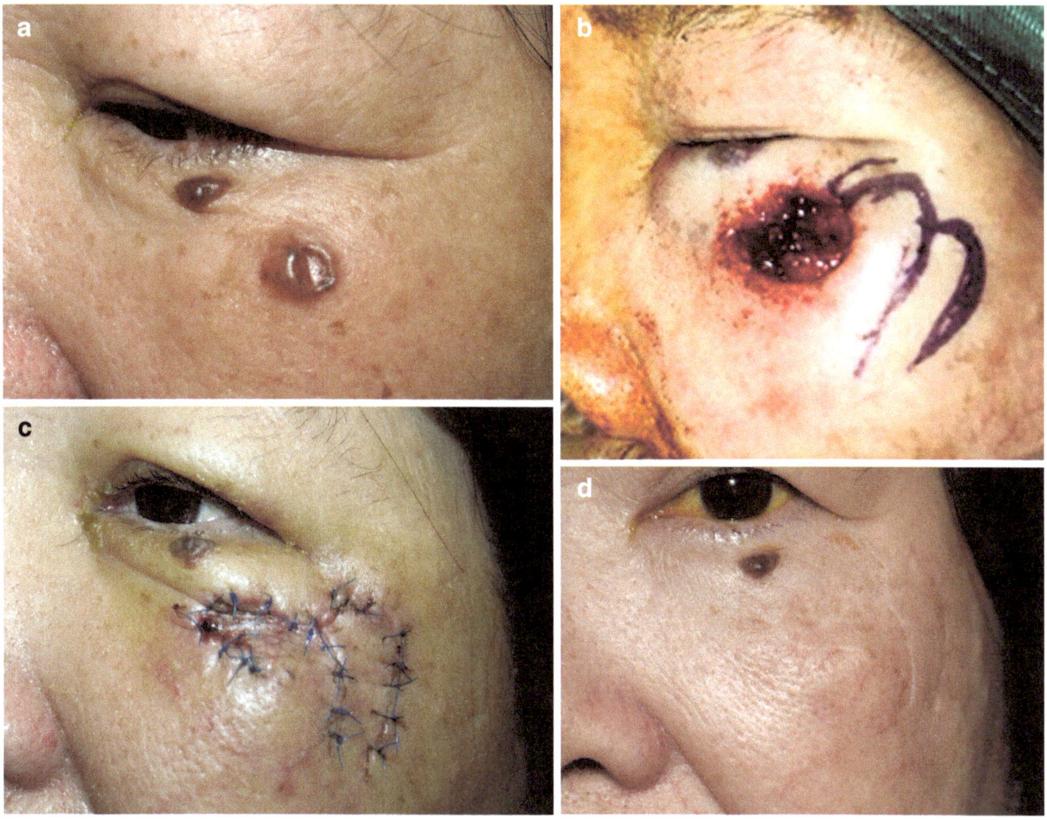

Fig. 3.15 (**a**) Basal cell carcinoma left cheek. (**b**) Basal cell carcinoma left cheek with markings for reconstruction. (**c**) Basal cell carcinoma left cheek post-reconstruction. (**d**) Postoperative image

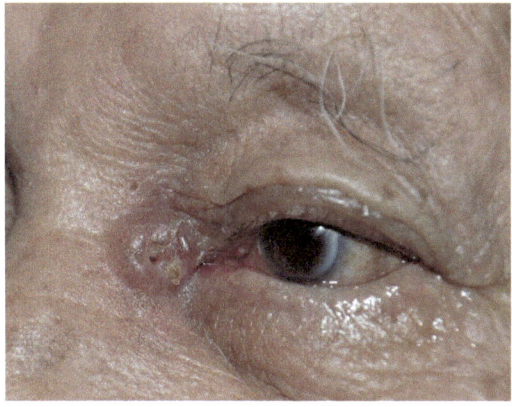

Fig. 3.16 Squamous cell carcinoma at medial canthus

In keeping with melanoma elsewhere, whenever possible a wide excision with at least 5–10 mm margin may be indicated, making reconstruction challenging [20]. Video 3.7 demonstrates management of lower eyelid melanoma. Histopathological features of lymphatic or vascular invasion, lesions ≥1 mm thick, >1 mitotic figure/high power field and/or ulceration and Breslow grading of more than 1000 microns are common indications for sentinel node biopsy and regional lymph node dissection. There is no role for cryotherapy with melanomas of the eyelid. When the systemic spread is present, the prognosis for life is usually guarded. The recent introduction of targeted therapy with BRAF inhibitors and MEK inhibitors in conjunctival melanoma is yet to be validated in eyelid melanomas.

Merkel Cell Carcinoma

These rare but aggressive neoplasms also commonly involve the upper eyelids and are often diagnosed as recurrent chalazia. Because of their late recognition and aggressive nature, they fre-

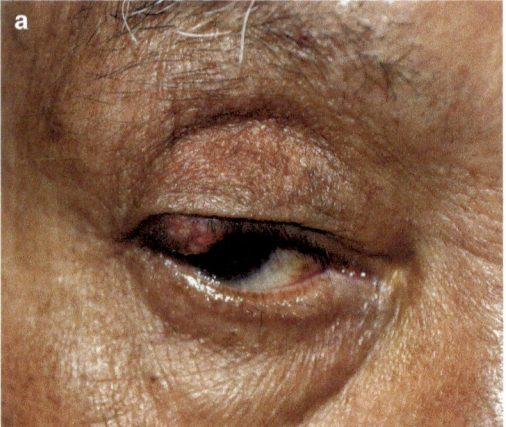

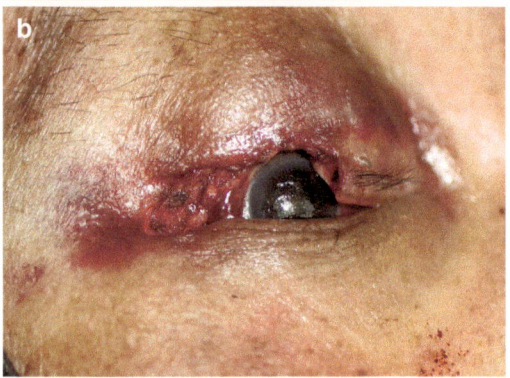

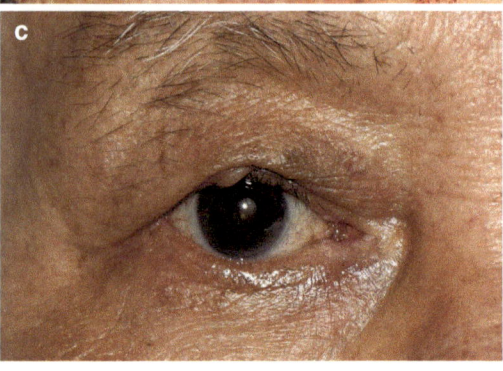

Fig. 3.17 (**a**) Sebaceous gland carcinoma Right upper eyelid. (**b**) Post-resection Sebaceous glands carcinoma. (**c**) 3-month postoperative follow-up image

quently spread regionally and even systemically, even at initial presentation resulting in early mortality. Localized lesions, after initial incisional biopsy, should undergo wide excision and reconstruction with sentinel node biopsy where possible. Radiotherapy and immuno-chemotherapy play an important role with regional and systemic spread, despite their guarded prognosis [21–23].

Postoperative Care

As in most surgeries, postoperative care is important to avoid complications such as infection, bleeding, and to maintain wound integrity especially with extensive reconstructions. Therefore, immediate postoperative wound care plays a major role.

- Local cleaning with 5–10% povidone-iodine solution and topical antibiotic ointment is recommended 2–3 times per day starting the day after the surgery to prevent infection until 3 weeks.
- To avoid bleeding, the patient is advised to refrain from strenuous physical activities and avoid drugs that may prolong bleeding. Traditional medicines including gingko, garlic, ginseng, and even high doses of Vitamin E can alleviate bleeding tendencies.
- Postoperative swelling can be minimized with immediate use of ice packs that mostly subsides within 3 days postoperative.

Follow-Up

Despite meticulous surgical approach, recurrence may occur in eyelid tumors, be it benign or malignant. Unlike the benign variants, malignant eyelid tumors warrant strict follow up to detect early recurrence and metastasis. It includes postoperative follow-up at 1 week, 3 weeks, and 6 weeks. For the first year 3 monthly follow-up is recommended for lethal eyelid malignancies, followed by 6-monthly up to next 2 years and yearly thereafter lifelong.

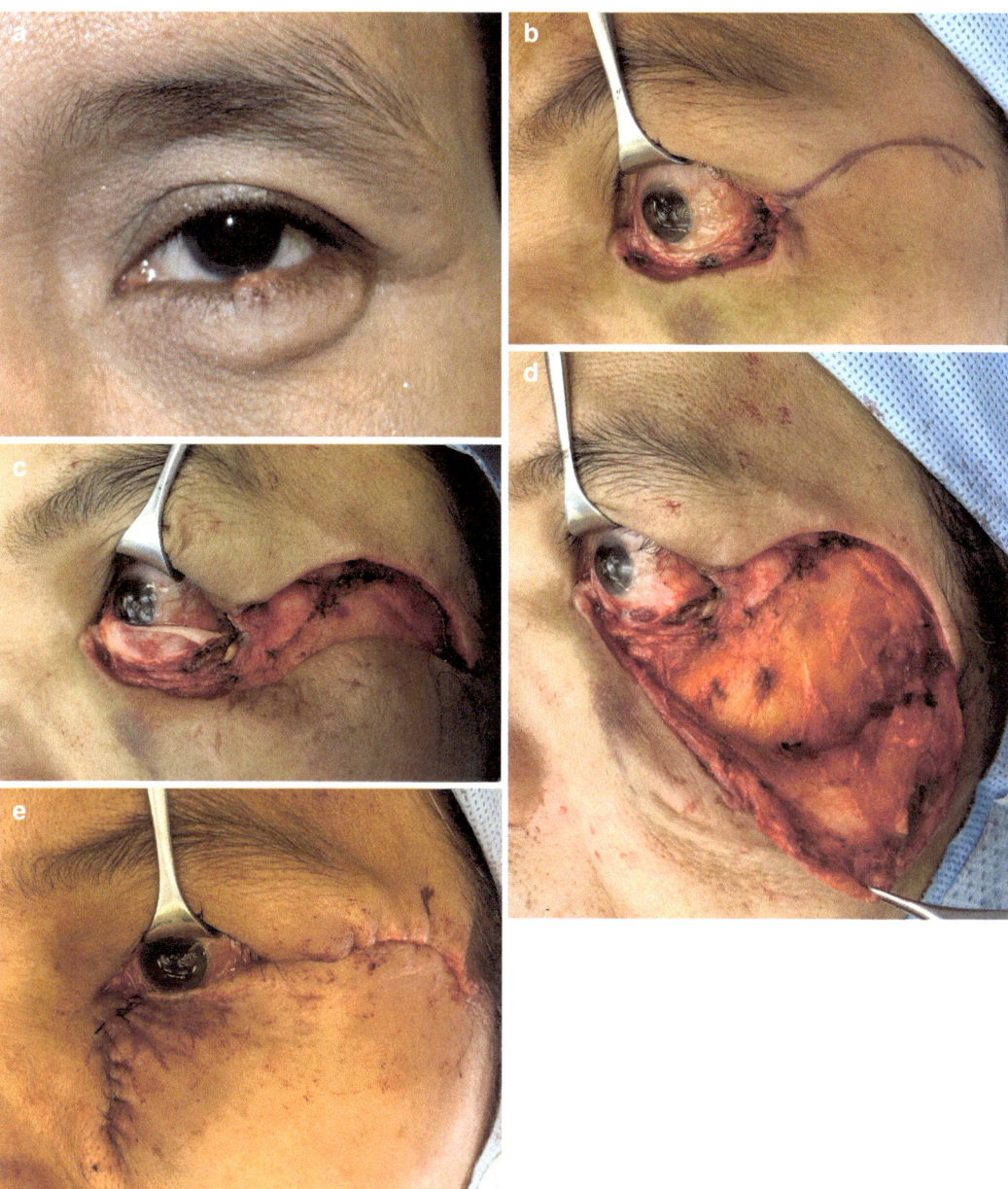

Fig. 3.18 (**a**) Sebaceous gland carcinoma lower eyelid. (**b**) Post-resection. (**c**) Posterior lamellar reconstruction with hard palate mucosal graft. (**d**) Cheek rotation flap. (**e**) Post-reconstruction

In summary, lesions of the eyelid may be benign (inflammatory, developmental or true neoplasms) or malignant. A high degree of clinical suspicion, incisional or excisional biopsy when suspected, regional and systemic assessment when indicated followed by tailored approaches to reconstruction and management are essential to deliver the most optimal outcome. Long-term follow-up is warranted in detecting early recurrence and metastasis in eyelid malignancies.

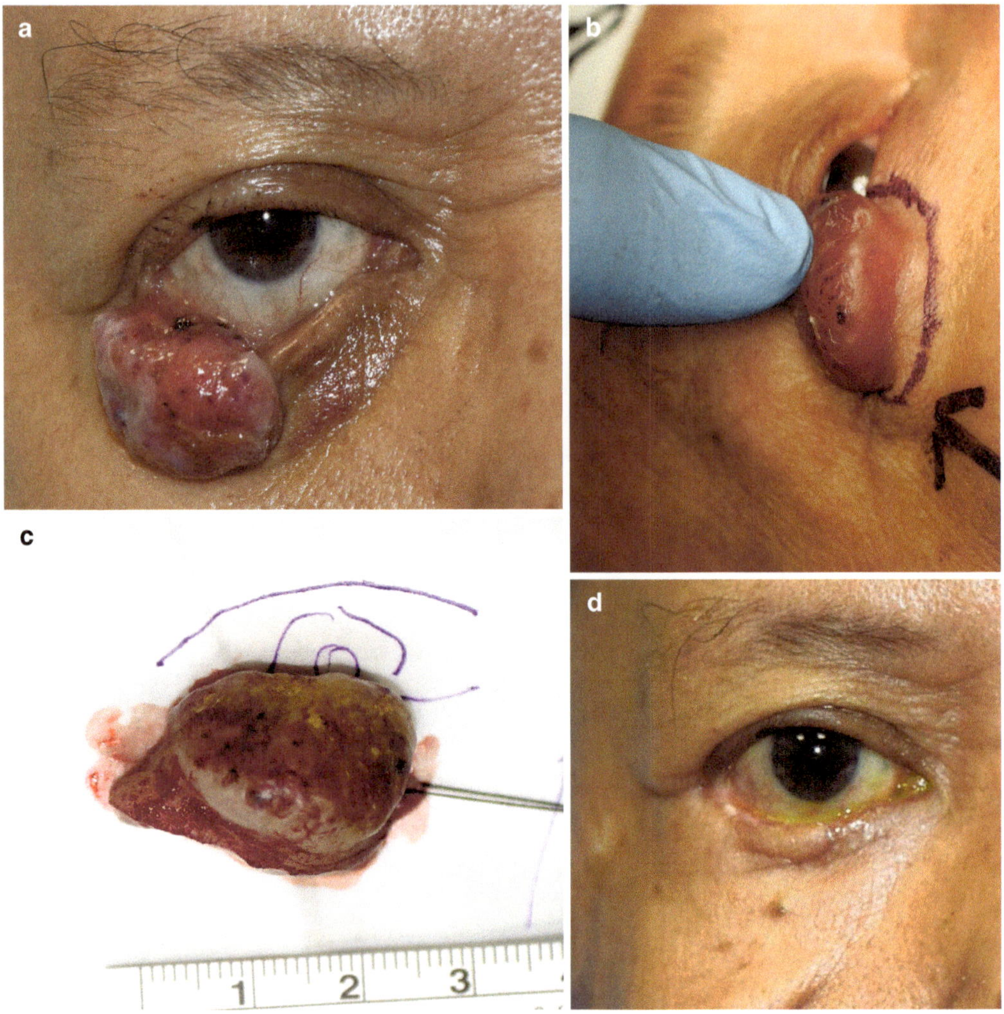

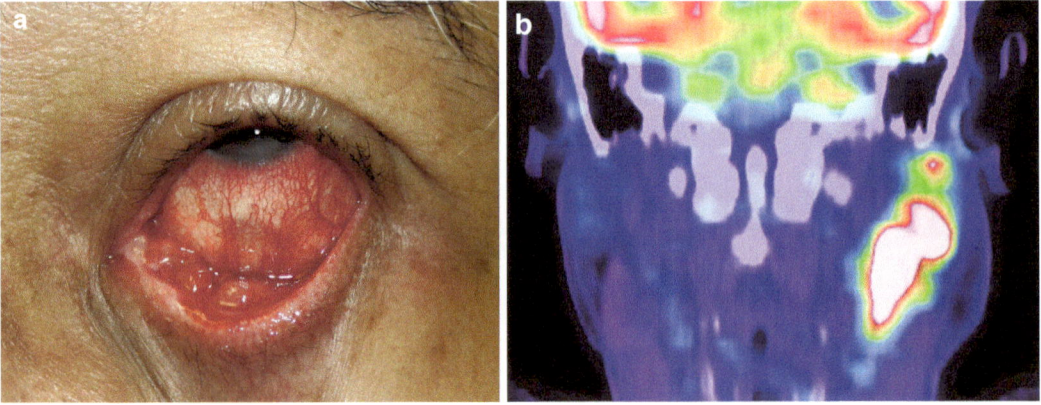

Fig. 3.19 (**a**) Mucinous carcinoma right lower eyelid. (**b**) Intraoperative marking with 4 mm margin. (**c**) Intraoperative specimen. (**d**) Late postoperative view

Fig. 3.20 (**a**) Merkel cell carcinoma. (**b**) PET-CT Merkel cell carcinoma with regional lymph node involvement

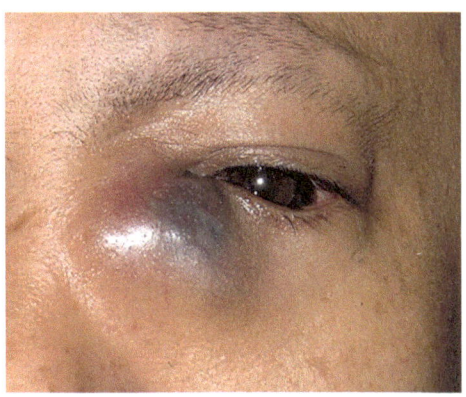

Fig. 3.21 Melanoma eyelid and medial canthus

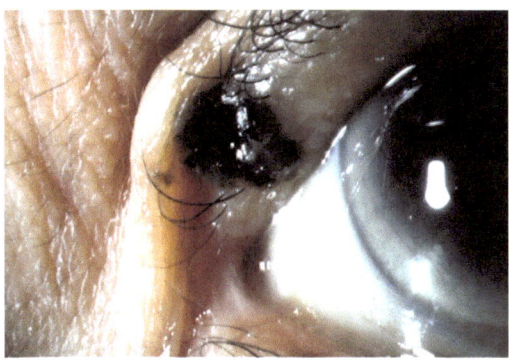

Fig. 3.24 Pigmented basal cell carcinoma referred as melanoma

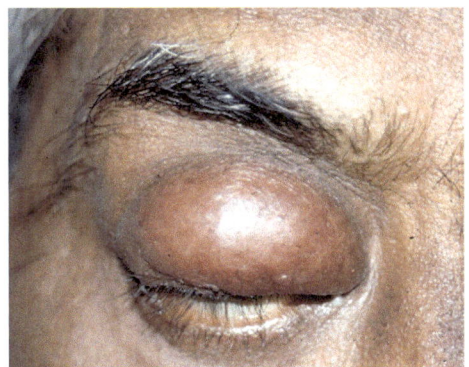

Fig. 3.22 Lymphoma involving eyelid

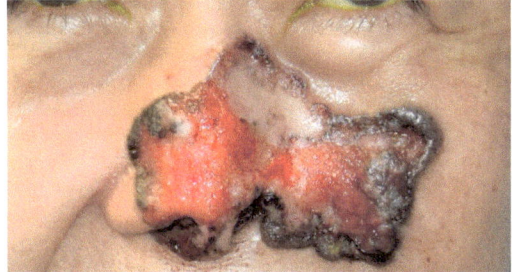

Fig. 3.25 Infiltrative basal cell carcinoma

Acknowledgment Videos 3. 4–3.7 have been included with contribution from Santosh G Honavar, MD, FACS, and Ankit Singh Tomar, MD, Ocular Oncology Service, Centre for Sight, Banjara Hills, Hyderabad, India.

References

1. Cook BE Jr, Bartley GB. Treatment options and future prospects for the management of eyelid malignancies: an evidence-based update. Ophthalmology. 2001;108(11):2088–98.
2. Bernardini FP. Management of malignant and benign eyelid lesions. Curr Opin Ophthalmol. 2006 Oct;17(5):480–4.
3. Rene C. Oculoplastic aspects of ocular oncology. Eye (Lond). 2013 Feb;27(2):199–207. https://doi.org/10.1038/eye.2012.243.
4. Gayre GS, Hybarger CP, Mannor G, Meecham W, Delfanti JB, Mizono GS, Guerry TL, Chien JS, Sooy CD, Anooshian R, Simonds R, Pietila KA, Smith DW, Dayhoff DA, Engman E, Lacy J. Outcomes of excision of 1750 eyelid and periocular skin basal cell and squamous cell carcinomas by modified en face frozen section margin-controlled technique. Int Ophthalmol Clin. 2009. Fall;49(4):97–110.

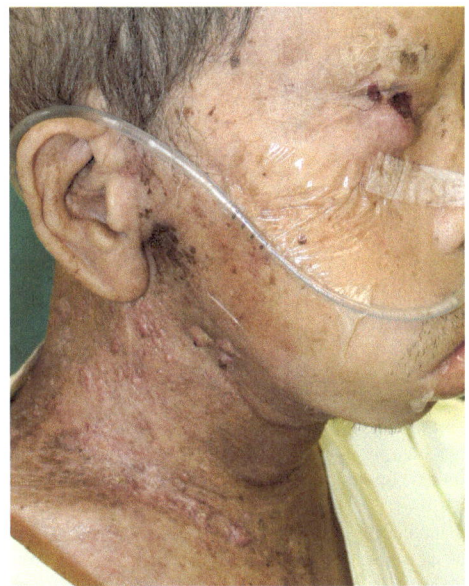

Fig. 3.23 Recurrent sebaceous gland carcinoma with loco-regional & systemic spread

5. Giordano Resti A, Sacconi R, Baccelli N, Bandello F. Outcome of 110 basal cell carcinomas of the eyelid treated with frozen section-controlled excision: mean follow-up over 5 years. Eur J Ophthalmol. 2014;24(4):476–82.

6. Mohs FE. Micrographic surgery for the microscopically controlled excision of eyelid cancers. Arch Ophthalmol. 1986;104(6):901–9.

7. While B, Salvi S, Currie Z, Mudhar HS, Tan JH. Excision and delayed reconstruction with paraffin section histopathological analysis for periocular sebaceous carcinoma. Ophthalmic Plast Reconstr Surg. 2014;30(2):105–9.

8. McConnell LK, Syed NA, Zimmerman MB, Carter KD, Nerad JA, Allen RC. Shriver EM. An analysis of conjunctival map biopsies in sebaceous carcinoma. Ophthalmic Plast Reconstr Surg. 2017;33(1):17–21.

9. Cook BE Jr, Bartley GB. Epidemiologic characteristics and clinical course of patients with malignant eyelid tumors in an incidence cohort in Olmsted County, Minnesota. Ophthalmology. 1999;106(4):746–50.

10. Nemet AY, Deckel Y, Martin PA, Kourt G, Chilov M, Sharma V, Benger R. Management of periocular basal and squamous cell carcinoma: a series of 485 cases. Am J Ophthalmol. 2006;142(2):293–7.

11. Frank HJ. Frozen section control of excision of eyelid basal cell carcinomas: 8 1/2 years' experience. Br J Ophthalmol. 1989;73(5):328–32.

12. Rodriguez-Sains RS, Robins P, Smith B, Bosniak SL. Radiotherapy of periocular basal cell carcinomas: recurrence rates and treatment with special attention to the medical canthus. Br J Ophthalmol. 1988;72(2):134–8.

13. Yin VT, Pfeiffer ML, Esmaeli B. Targeted therapy for orbital and periocular basal cell carcinoma and squamous cell carcinoma. Ophthalmic Plast Reconstr Surg. 2013;29(2):87–92.

14. Watanabe A, Sun MT, Pirbhai A, Ueda K, Katori N, Selva D. Sebaceous carcinoma in Japanese patients: clinical presentation, staging and outcomes. Br J Ophthalmol. 2013;97(11):1459–63.

15. Kaliki S, Ayyar A, Dave TV, Ali MJ, Mishra DK, Naik MN. Sebaceous gland carcinoma of the eyelid: clinicopathological features and outcome in Asian Indians. Eye (Lond). 2015;29(7):958–63.

16. Shields JA, Saktanasate J, Lally SE, Carrasco JR, Shields CL. Sebaceous carcinoma of the ocular region: the 2014 Professor Winifred Mao lecture. Asia Pac J Ophthalmol (Phila). 2015;4(4):221–7.

17. Brady KL, Hurst EA. Sebaceous carcinoma treated with Mohs micrographic surgery. Dermatol Surg. 2017;43(2):281–6.

18. Honavar SG, Shields CL, Maus M, Shields JA, Demirci H, Eagle RC Jr. Primary intraepithelial sebaceous gland carcinoma of the palpebral conjunctiva. Arch Ophthalmol. 2001;119(5):764–7.

19. Honavar SG. Sebaceous gland carcinoma: can we do better? Indian J Ophthalmol. 2018;66(9):1235–7.

20. Chan FM, O'Donnell BA, Whitehead K, Ryman W, Sullivan TJ. Treatment and outcomes of malignant melanoma of the eyelid: a review of 29 cases in Australia. Ophthalmology. 2007;114(1):187–92.

21. Herbert HM, Sun MT, Selva D, Fernando B, Saleh GM, Beaconsfield M, Collin R, Uddin J, Meligonis G, Leatherbarrow B, Ataullah S, Irion L, McLean CJ, Huilgol SC, Davis G, Sullivan TJ. Merkel cell carcinoma of the eyelid: management and prognosis. JAMA Ophthalmol. 2014;132(2):197–204.

22. Colombo F, Holbach LM, Jünemann AG, Schlötzer-Schrehardt U, Naumann GO. Merkel cell carcinoma: clinicopathologic correlation, management, and follow-up in five patients. Ophthalmic Plast Reconstr Surg. 2000;16(6):453–8.

23. Stagner AM, Jakobiec FA. Updates on the molecular pathology of selected ocular and ocular adnexal tumors: potential targets for future therapy. Semin Ophthalmol. 2016;31(1–2):188–96.

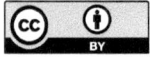

Francesco Bernardini and Brent Skippen

Principles of Periocular Reconstruction

The end goal of eyelid reconstruction is both functional and aesthetic restoration of the eyelid and periocular area while minimizing surgical morbidity. Attention to reconstruction of the bilamellar eyelid structure is essential [1]. Reconstructive surgical planning is determined by several factors including the nature of the defect, the health and age of the patient, the availability and integrity of surrounding tissues, and the surgeon's experience and preferences.

A preoperative consultation is mandatory to determine possible sites from which flaps and grafts may be obtained to minimize surgical morbidity [1].

In general, the following principles help achieve successful eyelid and periorbital reconstruction [2]:

1. If both anterior and posterior eyelid lamellae are to be reconstructed, only one can consist of a graft, the other must be composed of a vascularized flap. Graft on graft reconstruction has a high failure probability because of lack of vascular supply.
2. Aim to provide adequate canthal fixation to support the reconstructed eyelid/globe apposition.
3. Provide sufficient horizontal and vertical eyelid dimensions for maximal function, i.e., avoid vertical tension on the lower eyelid.
4. Perform any appropriate direct closure of the defect prior to sizing a graft.
5. Match tissue characteristics as best as possible for grafts and flaps.
6. Balance complexity of technique(s) with improvement(s) in outcome.
7. Eyelid closure adequate to avoid exposure sequelae.
8. Optimal eyelid symmetry and cosmesis (tissue of appropriate color, texture, and thickness).

Box 4.1 General Principles
- Recognize full-thickness vs. anterior lamella defects
- Anterior lamella defects:
  - Always prefer primary closure with or without undermining
  - Flaps over grafts
  - Grafts possibly from eyelid skin when available
  - Full-thickness skin grafts (FTSGs) to the eyelids and canthus require

---

Electronic supplementary material The online version of this chapter (https://doi.org/10.1007/978-3-030-18757-6_4) contains supplementary material, which is available to authorized users.

F. Bernardini (✉)
Oculoplastica Bernardini, Genoa, Italy
e-mail: francesco@oculoplasticabernardini.it

B. Skippen
Department of Ophthalmology, Wagga Wagga Rural Referral Hospital, Wagga Wagga, NSW, Australia

ideally a thinner than those used on other areas of the face. Thankfully, the periocular region is well-vascularized, with typically excellent wound healing.

- Small to medium size full-thickness defects of the lower lid can usually be repaired by direct closure, adding canthotomy and cantholysis or semicircular Tenzel flap if necessary.
- Larger defects (>50%) are usually repaired in at least two layers (posterior and anterior lamella) using flaps or grafts.
- Medial canthal defects are more challenging to repair to preserve the lacrimal system function.
- Lateral canthal defects can also have particular challenges.

Note: Some general principles are useful to guide the progression in eyelid reconstruction, from basic to more advance.

Reconstruction of Eyelid Defects

The type of surgery depends upon extent of tissue removed.

Preferred Anesthesia

For most surgeries the anesthesia used is the same:

- Local anesthesia with propofol sedation
- 27G–30G needle, 1% ropivacaine or 0.5% bupivacaine with 1:100,000 adrenaline

Basic instruments and necessary equipment are shown in Fig. 4.1.

Anterior Lamella Defects

Partial thickness anterior lamellar defects can be left to heal by secondary intention if small [3]. Larger defects may warrant direct closure or a simple sliding flap or graft to avoid rota-

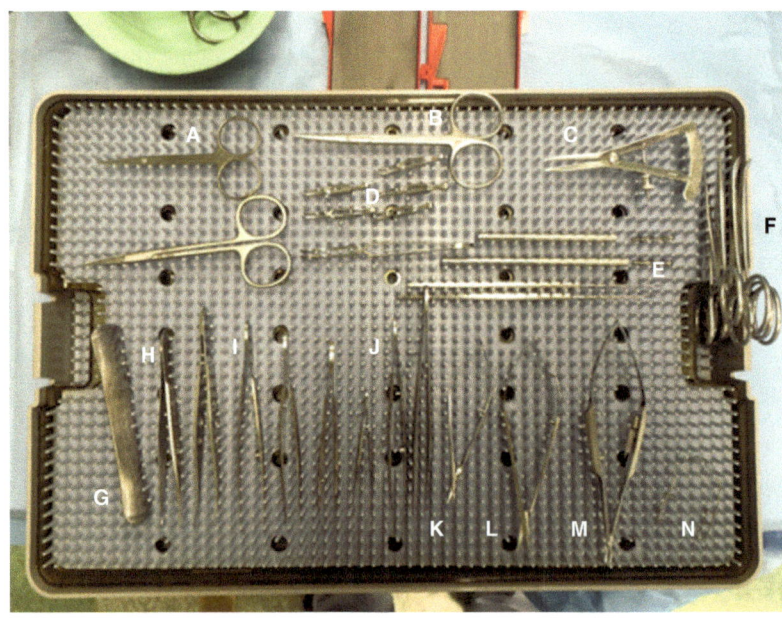

Fig. 4.1 Basic instruments and necessary equipment. A, iris (straight, sharp-tipped) scissors; B, Stevens (curved, blunt-tipped) scissors; C, surgical calipers; D, bulldog clamps; E, skin retractors, single and double pronged; F, artery forceps, curved; G, Jaeger lid plate; H, small fine-tooth tissue forceps; I, small, non-tooth forceps; J, large tooth forceps (Adson); K, Vannas spring scissors, curved; L, Westcott tenotomy scissors, curved; M, Castroviejo needle holder, with catch; N, eyelid speculum

tion of the eyelashes. Options for reconstruction of partial thickness periocular defects include:

1. Laissez-faire (small): Healing by secondary intention or granulation
2. Topical imiquimod 5% for 1 month
3. Direct closure
4. Flap or graft
   - Flaps: e.g., transposition, advancement, rotation, bilobed, rhomboid, z-plasty, V-Y plasty, Y-V plasty
   - Grafts: Full-thickness skin graft, split-thickness skin graft

Laissez-Faire

Laissez-faire is also known as healing by secondary intention or granulation. Fox and Beard described their good results following healing by secondary intention in six medial canthal defects [4]. Mehta reported 11 cases of satisfactory healing by secondary intention with defects involving the lower lid and medial canthus [5]. Da Costa and Jones described one patient having an excellent outcome following excision of a lateral canthal lesion [6]. Da Costa and Jones also showed that the technique of laissez-faire can be extended to larger defects with a good outcome [6]. One patient in their series had an excellent functional and aesthetic outcome following healing of a large upper eyelid defect.

Shankar et al. reported a series of 25 periocular defects with healing by secondary intention [7]. A "good" or "very good" result was obtained in 92% of their cases. Only one patient required secondary surgery for cicatricial ectropion [7]. A patient satisfaction survey in their study showed high patient satisfaction with the aesthetic outcome and postoperative follow-up required for healing by laissez-faire.

Indications for a laissez-faire approach to periocular skin tumors also include [8]:

1. Medial canthal lesions, especially after radiotherapy, where the skin may be unsuitable for flaps or free skin grafts.

2. Patients with primary skin precancerous conditions like xeroderma pigmentosa.
3. Patients with poor general health, who may not be fit for general anesthesia or prolonged surgical procedures involving complex skin flaps or skin grafting under local anesthesia.
4. For tumor surveillance where detection of tumor recurrences beneath or adjacent to the reconstructed area may be delayed.
5. Simplicity of wound management for patient care associated with this technique [7].
6. Also, in cases of large defects that are closed partially with flaps and grafts but not entirely, a small part of the defect can be left to heal by secondary intention.
7. Not indicated in patients with poor compliance for follow-up.

Disadvantages of Laissez-Faire Include

1. Prolonged healing time
2. Small risk of a secondary surgical intervention
3. Causing lower lid cicatricial ectropion and subsequent watery eye
4. Poor suitability for large upper lid defects where there may the risk of exposure keratitis during wound healing

Direct Closure

Direct closure may be useful for both partial and full-thickness eyelid defects following tumor excision. The immediate postoperative distortion is temporary thanks to spontaneous tissue expansion brought about by the steady pressure of the displaced globe against the reconstructed eyelid [9]. The surgery is often simple and the functional and cosmetic results can be excellent. In the event of histologically incomplete tumor resection, subsequent re-excision for additional clearance would not present the problems that other reconstructive techniques might. Should postoperative wound dehiscence occur, the defect may be allowed to granulate as in the "laissez-faire" method. Subsequent excision of any notch or delayed reconstruction would still be viable options and made easier by the decrease in defect size [9].

The factors that make direct closure possible are [9]:

1. Preexisting eyelid and canthal tendon laxity.
2. Inherent eyelid elasticity.
3. Straightening of the normal lid curvature (arc to chord conversion) by globe displacement.
4. The "mechanical tissue creep" phenomenon talked of in relation to tissue expander use under the skin [10].
5. Mechanical creep is one of the factors that makes direct closure under tension possible (Fig. 4.2).

Although the operated eyelid may be under considerable tension at the end of surgery, as long as the tension is horizontal, it usually relaxes within a matter of days without running the risk of eyelid malposition [9]. Generally, by 2 months postoperatively, the eyelid has expanded to normal proportions.

Full-Thickness Skin Graft

Indication for Surgery Skin grafting is a relatively easy procedure that any reconstructive surgeon should master before undertaking tumor excision. Even though the best functional and aesthetic results are achievable with local flaps, there are occasions where a skin graft is the best option as in cases of elongated oval-shaped central eyelid defects (Fig. 4.3). In the eyelid region, skin grafting means full-thickness skin graft (FTSG). FTSGs are best when harvested from the upper eyelid skin when available; other potential donor areas include the preauricular or postauricular areas, inner brachial, and supraclavicular areas. When harvesting FTSGs from areas other than the upper eyelid, there are some disadvantages include the potential for color/thickness mismatch; risk of potential complications such as graft contracture, scar hypertrophy, and more rarely graft failure. Figure 4.3c demonstrates the use of a bolster associated with Frost sutures to improve graft survival and overall better graft uptake. It is always a good idea to use a firm pressure dressing for 48–72 h.

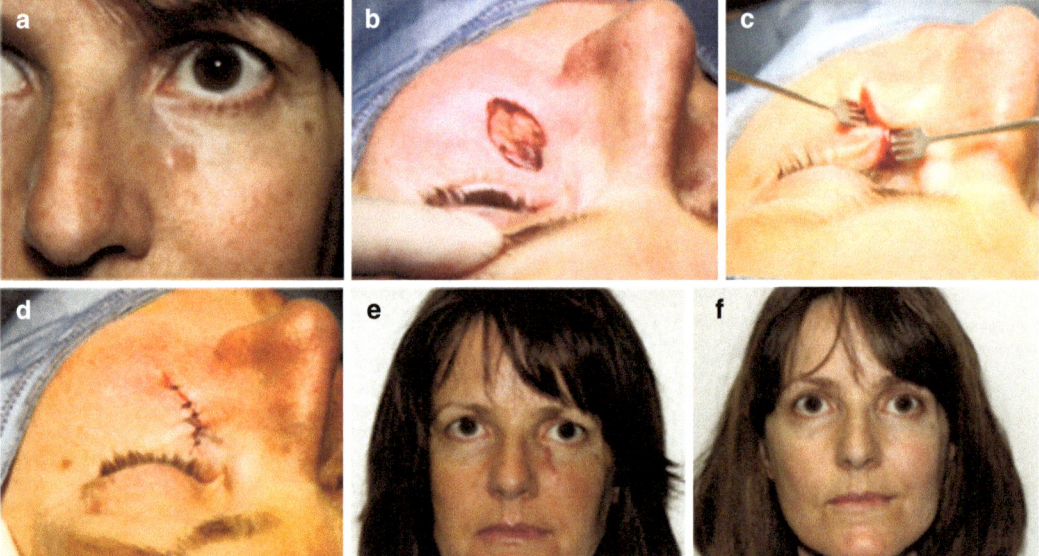

Fig. 4.2 (a–f) Direct closure of a lower lid-cheek junction defect

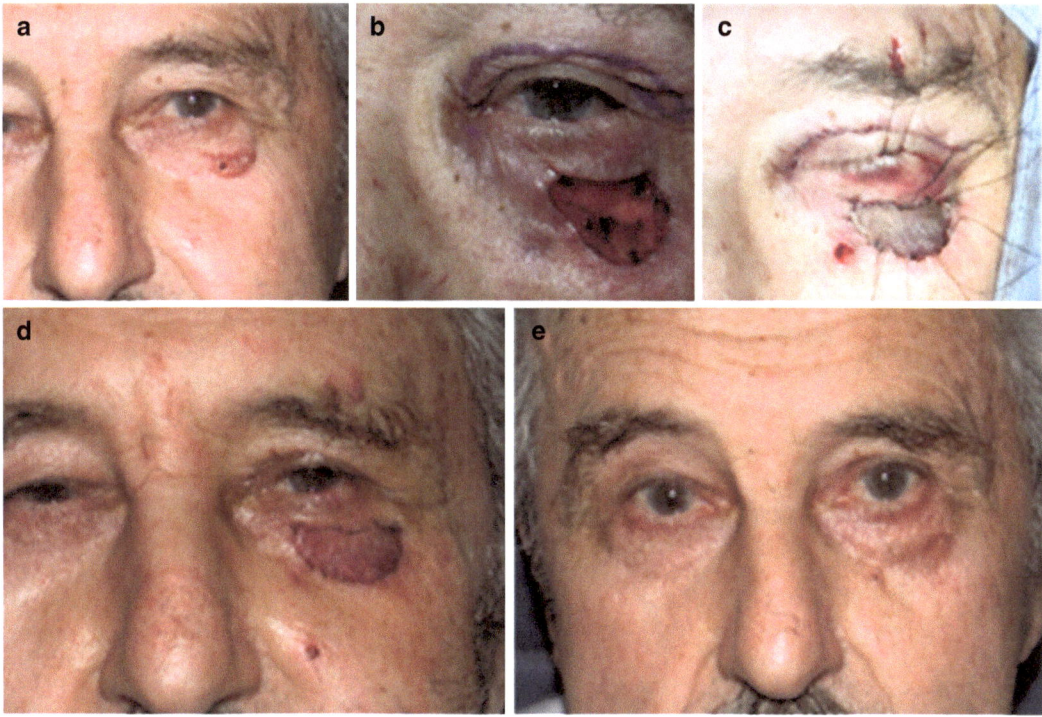

Fig. 4.3 (a–e) Upper lid full-thickness skin graft for closure of lower lid-cheek junction defect

Standard Surgical Technique

- A template is used to measure the size of the defect and match to the area being harvested.
- The FTSG is harvested, taking care not to button-hole the tissue.
- The FTSG is then thinned posteriorly, using Westcott scissors to remove subcutaneous tissue.
- The thinned graft is then secured to the defect, first using 3–4 cardinal sutures of 6-0 Vicryl.
- The rest of the graft is sutured into place using 7-0 Vicryl which can be used in an interrupted or continuous fashion.
- A bolster associated with longer Frost sutures to keep it in place may assist graft survival (Fig 4.3c).
- A firm pressure dressing should be used for 48–72 h whether or not the bolster was used (Fig. 4.3).

Full-Thickness Defects (Anterior Lamella and Posterior Lamella)

Full-thickness eyelid defects require reconstruction of both the anterior and posterior lamellae. Both lamellae can't be grafts since at least one of them must have a blood supply. The correct options include:

1. Anterior graft + posterior flap OR
2. Anterior flap + posterior graft OR
3. Anterior + posterior flap

Upper Lid Full-Thickness Defect

The surgeon's choice depends upon extent of tissue removed and especially upon the horizontal extent of the defect (Table 4.1).

Two major factors determining the repair are the horizontal extent of the defect and how much

Table 4.1 Treatment of full-thickness upper eyelid defect

Horizontal defect (% of total lid length)	Surgical options
<33%	Direct closure
33–66%	Lateral cantholysis Tenzel semicircular flap

>66%	Full thickness lower to upper eyelid flap repair, e.g., Cutler–Beard procedure
	    2 stages, divide at 2–6 weeks
	    Posterior lamella defect: graft—opposite tarso-conjunctiva, ear, palate
	    Cannot use if other eye has poor vision
	Periosteal strip
	Anterior lamella advancement from upper lid + posterior lamella graft (2 stage)
	"Bucket handle" flap
	Sliding upper eyelid tarsoconjunctival flap
	Mustarde total lid switch

tarsal plate remains [3]. Repair of the upper eyelids is more important than the lower as it is the upper eyelid that is the main protector of the cornea during blinking and eye closure [3]. Once an upper eyelid defect can no longer be closed by direct suture, tissue must be added back to the eyelid, and there have been numerous techniques described including full-thickness flaps and grafts from the surrounding tissues (including the lower eyelid); anterior lamella advancement, sliding, and rotational flaps; and combined upper and lower lid advancement flaps. Numerous grafts have been described including skin, mucous membrane, hard palate, nasal mucosa, and auricular cartilage [3].

Depending on the laxity of the eyelid tissues, full-thickness defects of the eyelid margin involving up to one-third of the horizontal length may be closed with direct closure. Residual tension can be released with a lateral canthotomy or cantholysis [11]. Direct closure of a wound affecting one-third to two-thirds of the eyelid may be done if there is enough horizontal laxity of the eyelid. If the wound is too tight, then a canthotomy and cantholysis should be consid-

ered [3]. If the temporal skin can be mobilized, then a semicircular advancement (Tenzel) flap technique can be utilized [12]. If the lateral canthus has been lost, then a local tarsoconjunctival flap may be used along with a periosteal strip [13, 14]. The anterior lamella can be replaced with a full-thickness skin graft or myocutaneous flap. If there is enough anterior lamella to support a graft, then alternatives may be used to recreate the posterior lamella, such as a free tarsal graft from the contralateral upper eyelid or hard palate.

When there is insufficient local upper eyelid tissue to reconstruct the full-thickness defect, distal flaps must be constructed to provide a blood supply for any reconstruction. The classic upper eyelid reconstruction when more than two-thirds of the eyelid is missing is a Cutler-Beard procedure, which is a two-stage bridging procedure [11].

Direct Closure

Indication for Surgery. For smaller defects of the upper eyelids, the same principles of repair for a lower eyelid apply to the upper. The amount of upper eyelid tissue that can be excised with direct closure to follow is generally 8–10 mm (up to 50%), but this depends on the age of the patient and the degree of eyelid laxity. Assessment includes pulling the edges of the defect together to confirm the wound is not under too much tension [3].

In selected cases, direct eyelid closure may be achieved after considerably larger eyelid margin resections than conventionally taught. The immediate postoperative distortion and reduction in palpebral aperture (ptosis) is temporary thanks to spontaneous tissue expansion brought about by the steady pressure of the displaced globe against the reconstructed eyelid. The surgery is simple and the functional and cosmetic results are excellent [15].

Standard Surgical Technique

– 7-0 polygalactin (Vicryl) sutures placed in the tarsus, gray line to gray line with a vertical mattress suture; a slight eversion of the wound edges is desirable to avoid the risk of notching of the eyelid margin (Fig 4.4b).

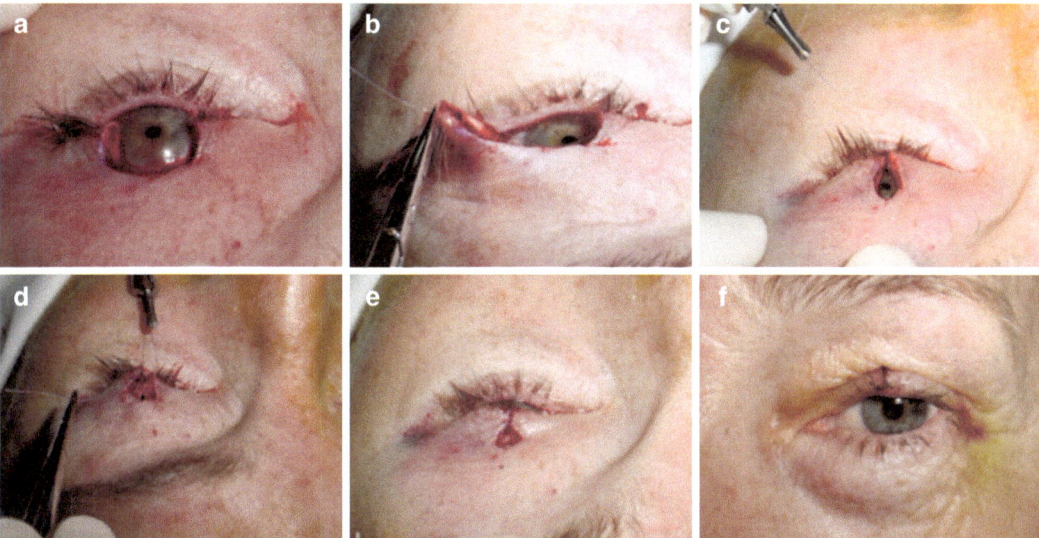

Fig. 4.4 (**a–f**) Direct closure of a full-thickness upper eyelid wound 33–50% horizontal length

- A second 7-0 Vicryl suture is used to approximate the anterior lash line.
- Two to three deep tarsal sutures are passed partial thickness through the tarsal plate to take the horizontal tension off the eyelid margin—one close to the eyelid margin and a second parallel and 1–2 mm from the first (Fig. 4.4c).
- Skin sutures are then placed in an interrupted or continuous fashion, using 7-0 Vicryl (Fig 4.4f).

Lateral Semicircular Skin Flap or Tenzel Flap

Indication for Surgery. The amount of skin flap that is rotated into the upper eyelid may be small as the main benefit of this procedure is the undermining of tissue lateral to the canthus, reducing the horizontal tension from direct eyelid advancement. The goal of the rotation flap is to use the skin lateral to the canthus to form the lateral eyelid and to mobilize the residual eyelid tissues centrally in contact with the eye. In elderly patients with more extensive upper eyelid tumors, rather than submitting the patient to a more complicated procedure, the superior limb of the medial canthal tendon can also be released [3].

Standard surgical technique (applicable for upper and lower eyelids) (see also surgical details for Tenzel flap reconstruction of the lower lid):

- First assess the eyelid tension to exclude the ability to close the defect via direct closure.
- A semicircular incision is marked out with a surgical marking pen starting at the lateral canthus, curving inferiorly for approximately 3 cm and laterally for approximately 2 cm, or as much as possible taking care to remain within the lateral orbital rim with the semicircular flap dissection or less than 2 cm passed the rim to avoid injuring the frontal branch of the temporalis nerve (Fig 4.5b).
- The skin incision is made using a number 15 Bard Parker blade (Fig 4.5c).
- The flap is then undermined using blunt-tipped Stevens scissors to the depth of the mid-dermis (Fig 4.5d).
- A canthotomy and cantholysis are usually also required [16].
- The lateral canthus is suspended to the lateral orbital rim periosteum with a buried 5-0 Vicryl.
- The primary defect is closed first by way of simple primary closure followed by the repair of the semicircular defect. 6-0 Vicryl can be used, tarsal plate first and then lash line and anterior lamella.
- The lateral angle is then reformed fixating the rotated skin to the upper eyelid right at the corner.

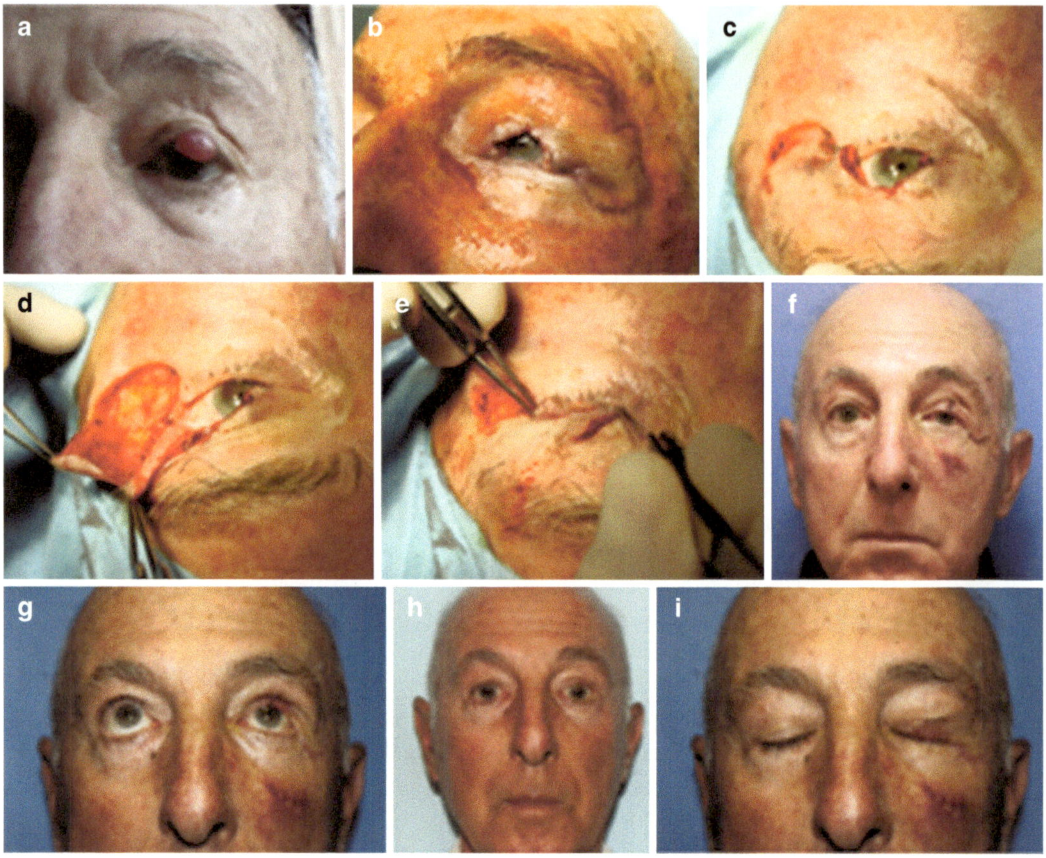

Fig. 4.5 (a–i) Tenzel semicircular flap repair of an upper eyelid defect

Full-Thickness Lower to Upper Eyelid Flap Repair

Indication for Surgery. The Cutler-Beard procedure uses a full-thickness advancement flap from the lower eyelid [13]. The method is only useful for vertical defects of the upper eyelid. Unfortunately, there is minimal to no tarsus added to the new upper lid margin, which is where the structural support is required and consequently upper lid entropion may result. Despite some postoperative problems, the Cutler-Beard procedure continues to be used by many surgeons and can be used for defects of 100% of the horizontal eyelid length [7] (Fig. 4.6).

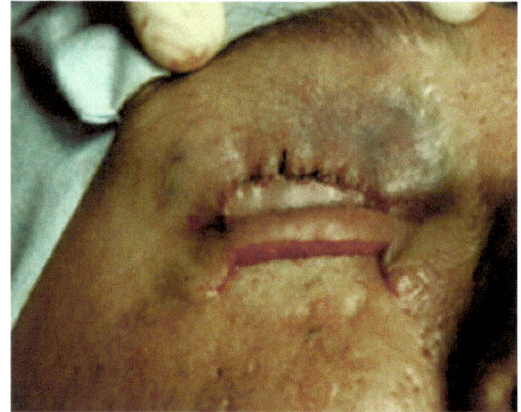

Fig. 4.6 End of stage 1 of Cutler-Beard procedure

Standard Surgical Technique

– The lower eyelid margin is left intact with inferior full-thickness incision made to advance a skin–muscle conjunctiva into the upper eyelid underneath this bridge of tissue.

– A three-sided inverted U-shaped incision is marked on the lower eyelid using a surgical marking pen, beginning 4–5 mm below the eyelid margin [16].

- A silk traction suture is passed through the gray line of the lower eyelid, which is then everted over a Desmarres retractor.
- A conjunctival incision is made below the tarsus.
- A conjunctival flap is created and dissected inferiorly into the lower fornix and onto the globe.
- A free tarsal graft is harvested from the contralateral upper eyelid and sutured to the tarsal remnants and to the upper fornix conjunctiva and the lower edge of the levator muscle.
- The flap is advanced into the upper eyelid defect and sutured to the free tarsal graft using 6-0 Vicryl sutures, taking care to bury the knots to avoid corneal irritation.
- The edges of the graft are sutured edge to edge to either tarsal remnants or to local periosteal flaps using 5-0 Vicryl sutures [16].
- An incision is then made horizontally through the lower eyelid skin and orbicularis muscle just inferior to the tarsus and extended inferiorly to create a skin–muscle advancement flap [16].
- The lower eyelid skin–muscle flap is advanced posterior to the bridge of lower lid tarsal and eyelid margin tissue to cover the graft and sutured to the residual upper eyelid skin using 6-0 Vicryl sutures [16].

Postoperative Medications and Wound Care: Pattern of Follow-Up Visits and Evaluation

- Antibiotic ointment applied to wound and in the eye (check for allergies), firm double pad.
- Remove pad at home after 48 h and apply antibiotic ointment three times a day to wound.
- Follow-up in 1–2 weeks.
- The flap is divided 2–8 weeks after reconstruction with repair of the lower eyelid donor site and repair of the new eyelid margin to prevent entropion [11].
    - Earlier division of the flap at 2 weeks has been reported without problem except in large defects or when the lower lid skin is tight such as in younger patients [17].
    - For patients with a poor vascular supply (e.g., post-radiotherapy treatment or

trauma), a longer interval between primary surgery and flap division is more suitable.

Periosteal Strip: Adjunct Procedure

Indication for Surgery. A strip of periosteum can be reflected from the zygoma nasally to function as a lateral canthal tendon and posterior lamella of the temporal eyelid. This is a useful adjunct procedure for larger upper eyelid defects >66% of horizontal eyelid length.

Note: This is an adjunctive procedure to help with some eyelid reconstruction but not a standalone posterior lamella substitute.

Standard Surgical Technique

- After the lateral orbital rim is exposed with blunt dissection, a rectangular periosteal strip with an intact base is fashioned with a scalpel blade and separated from bone with a Freer elevator.
- The periosteal incisions are slanted 45° downward for upper eyelid reconstructions so that the strip follows the contour of the upper eyelid after it is reflected superonasally.
- The strip should be at least 1 cm wide and long enough to reach the residual tarsal stump with adequate tension.
- The strip is reflected nasally to position the outer periosteum against the globe and sutured to the anterior surface of the residual tarsal stump with 5-0 polygalactin 910 (Vicryl) sutures.
- The anterior lamella needs to then be reconstructed by advancing a myocutaneous flap or FTSG over the strip.
- Residual conjunctiva in the fornix is sutured to the inferior edge of the strip with 7-0 polygalactin 910 sutures, and the side of the strip facing the eye is allowed to re-epithelialize.

Bucket-Handle Flap

Indication for Surgery. This has been described as a solution for reconstruction of total or semi-total full-thickness upper eyelid defects which is both relatively simple and utilizes well the potential vascularity of the transferred tissue [18]. This flap is also useful in patients with compromised healing abilities [18].

Standard Surgical Technique [18]

- A free tarsal graft is harvested from the contralateral upper eyelid and sutured to the remnants of the tarsal plate medially and laterally (Fig 4.7d). In case of a shortage of residual tarsal plate, a periosteal flap can be formed and used to anchor the free tarsal graft.
- The conjunctiva from the upper fornix is advanced and sutured to the upper tarsal border, as is the levator muscle (Fig 4.7e).
- A bucket handle bipedicle flap of orbicularis muscle and eyelid skin from just below the brow hair is transferred onto the lower edge of the upper eyelid defect to cover a free tarsal graft harvested from the contralateral upper eyelid (Fig 4.7f).
- The superior limb of the incision is made along the margin of the inferior brow with a number 15 Bard Parker blade with a horizontal extension as to adapt to fill the defect.
- The inferior limb of the incision corresponds to the upper edge of the eyelid defect.
- The medial and lateral ends of the flap are flared slightly to maximize the blood supply at each end of the flap.
- The flap is raised in the sub-orbicularis plane of dissection until it is mobile enough to allow for tension-free insertion into the upper eyelid defect.
- A FTSG is then harvested, possibly from the contralateral upper eyelid skin, and sutured to cover the sub-brow anterior lamella defect (Fig. 4.7g, h). Video 4.1- Reconstruction with free tarsal graft and flap.

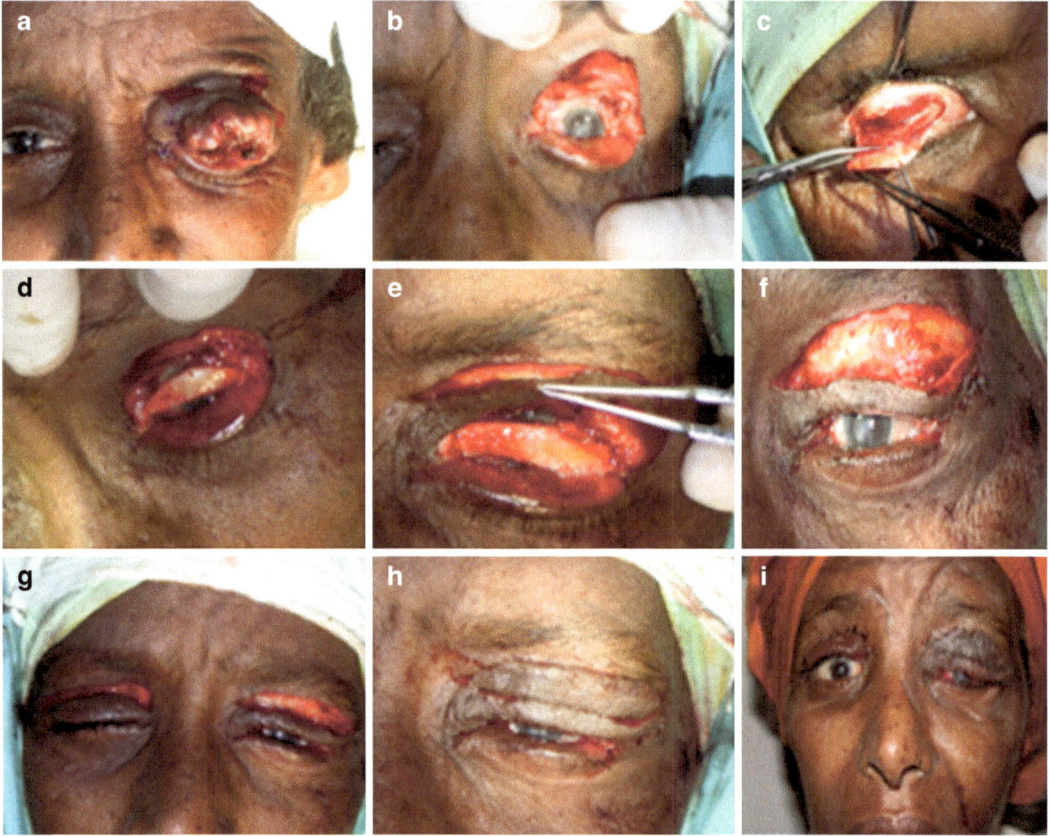

Fig. 4.7 (**a–i**) Bucket handle flap for left upper eyelid reconstruction

Postoperative Medications and Wound Care: Pattern of Follow-Up Visits and Evaluation

- Double pad, antibiotic ointment to wound and in the eye (check first for allergies).
- Remove pad at home after 48 h and apply antibiotic ointment three times a day to wound.
- Follow-up in 1 week.
- Usually 2–3 weeks later the pedicles are divided and the flap insetting completed [18].

Sliding Upper Eyelid Tarsoconjunctival Flap

Indication for Surgery. In our opinion a bucket handle flap or an upper eyelid tarsoconjunctival flap (Hughes to the upper eyelid) is always preferable to a Cutler-Beard procedure as it is a single-stage procedure with a much better aesthetic result and avoids complications of the Cutler-Beard such as entropion, lower eyelid retraction, and scarring [19, 20]. The upper eyelid sliding tarsoconjunctival flap is possible when some tarsus is preserved after Mohs excision. The residual tarsal plate slides, still attached to the upper conjunctival flap, is displaced inferiorly to repair the posterior lamella and is subsequently covered with a skin graft.

Potential complications of an upper eyelid sliding tarsoconjunctival flap include eyelid retraction, eyelid margin abnormality, lack of cilia, and abnormal eyelid contour. In comparison, direct (primary) closure avoids disrupting the eyelid margin contour and eyelash loss, but it often leads to residual upper eyelid ptosis.

Standard Surgical Technique

- A tarsoconjunctival flap is formed similarly to what happens for the lower eyelid from the upper half of the tarsal plate adjacent to the defect; vertical cuts are made continued superiorly into the conjunctiva toward the fornix to completely release the tarsoconjunctival flap.
- The extent of the incisions into the conjunctiva depends on the extent of flap mobilization required to close the defect under minimal/modest tension.
- The conjunctiva is then released from the levator aponeurosis and Muller's muscle [20].
- The flap is then moved to fill the posterior lamellar defect and stored medially and laterally to the tarsal remnants.
- The tarsoconjunctival flap should be overcorrected inferiorly by about 1 mm beyond the anticipated new eyelid margin to allow for shrinkage.
- A FTSG or an upper eyelid skin–muscle advancement flap is used to repair the anterior lamella.
- The new anterior lamella is sutured to tarsus along the eyelid margin using 7-0 Vicryl sutures, taking care to avoid corneal irritation with the suture knots.

Lower Lid Full Thickness

Knowledge of different reconstructive options allows for planning of the surgical repair. Lower eyelid defects can be categorized by:

1. Amount of full-thickness eyelid defect (as percent of eyelid margin)
2. Degree of nonmarginal eyelid involvement
3. Total size of defect
4. Canthal involvement
5. Lacrimal involvement

Depending on the laxity of the eyelid tissues, full-thickness defects of the eyelid margin involving up to one-third of the horizontal length may be closed with direct closure (Table 4.2). Minimal tension can be released with a lateral canthotomy or cantholysis [1]. Larger defects may require use of the Tenzel or Hughes flaps.

Options for anterior lamellar reconstruction include skin grafts and local skin flaps. Skin graft sites include upper eyelids, postauricular, preauricular, supraclavicular, neck, or inner

Table 4.2 Treatment of full-thickness lower eyelid defect

Full-thickness defect size	Primary techniques	Adjunct techniques
Small (20–30%)	Direct closure Canthotomy with closure Lateral advancement flap	– – –
Medium (30–40%)	Lateral advancement flap	Canthal fixation Canalicular reconstruction Periosteal flap
Large (>40–50%)	Lateral advancement flap Hughes tarsoconjunctival flap Mustarde cheek flap	– FTSG Autogenous tarsal graft or hard palate mucosal graft Medial canthotomy/cantholysis

arm. One should consider the type and distribution of hair in the donor graft [21]. Skin flaps include advancement, rotation, and transposition flaps. Flaps may have a base, direct pedicle, tubed or pedicle or be an island flap. Specific local eyelid flaps include O-to-T, V-to-Y, and rhombic flaps.

Periorbital flaps include transposition and rotation cheek flaps (Tenzel, Mustarde, etc.), glabellar flaps, paramedian forehead flaps, and temporal forehead flaps (Fricke). Flaps may need to be divided or inset as a second stage procedure several weeks after the initial repair, e.g., Hughes procedure [21].

Options for posterior lamellar reconstruction also include grafts or flaps [22, 23]. Flaps include tarsoconjunctival flap and can be central such as in a Hughes flap or lateral-based; in either case there is a pedicle of conjunctiva that provides vascular supply to the flap. Grafts may include tarsoconjunctival grafts, tarsomarginal grafts, hard palate grafts, and auricular cartilage grafts.

Direct Closure: Wedge Excision

Indication for Surgery. An eyelid defect of 25% or less may be closed directly, and some authors have reported excellent results for defects much larger than this, closing the defect under considerable tension [4–6]. In patients with marked eyelid laxity or through the use of lateral canthotomy with or without cantholysis, a defect even larger than 50% of the eyelid may sometimes be able to be closed directly.

Standard Surgical Technique

– Initial wedge excision of the lesion with margin control
– Primary closure entails first repair of the tarsus with 2× buried 6-0 or 5-0 Vicryl sutures
– Then a 6-0 Vicryl lash line suture
– Sometimes a gray line suture (7-0 Vicryl, cut knot short to avoid corneal irritation)
– Finally repair of the anterior lamella with interrupted or continuous 6-0 Vicryl sutures [16, 23]

Cantholysis: Adjunct Procedure

Indication for Surgery. The size of the defect that can be repaired in the lower eyelid can be increased if necessary by the addition of a lateral cantholysis. In elderly patients, eyelid defects of up to half the horizontal length of the eyelid or 14 mm can be directly repaired. This is sometimes a useful adjunct to direct closure.

Standard Surgical Technique

– Canthotomy is made with a size 15 blade or Westcott scissors.
– The lower limb of the lateral canthal tendon is released.
– The eyelid is slit at the gray line for at least 6 mm.
– The lower canthal tendon fibers are released, but the upper lid tendon fibers must remain intact to avoid distortion of the canthus postoperatively.
– A traction (Frost) suture to elevate the lower lid for 48–72 h is sometimes useful (Fig. 4.8).

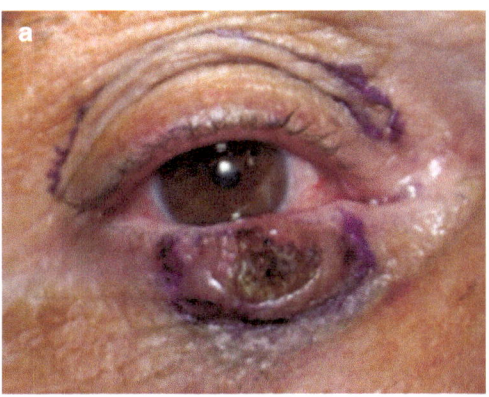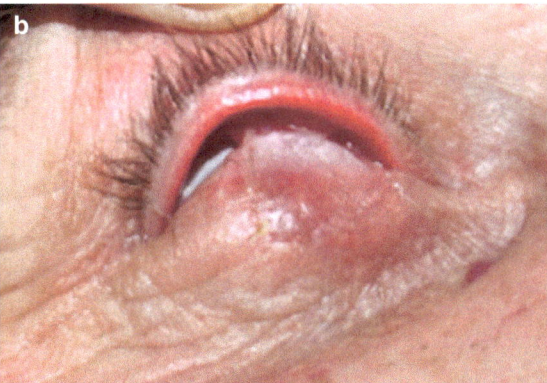

Fig. 4.8 (**a**, **b**) Inferior cantholysis adjunct to direct closure

Tenzel Semicircular Flap

See upper eyelid description.

Indication for Surgery. The main indication for a Tenzel flap is a larger full-thickness lower eyelid defect with up to half of the eyelid length involved; however, it may be used for defects up to 70% if the lower eyelid retractors and inferior orbital septum are identified and severed from their attachments [12].

Hughes Tarsoconjunctival Flap

Indication for Surgery. The original Hughes procedure was reported in 1937[25] since which time some modifications have been made [25–29]. A modified Hughes tarsoconjunctival flap can be used for full-thickness defects of more than half the lower eyelid length [16, 25]. This procedure can be used for defects involving the entire horizontal length of the lower eyelid. The integrity of the upper eyelid margin is retained by leaving the lower 4 mm of the upper tarsal plate intact [23].

One-eyed (monocular) patients and children in the amblyogenic age, whose vision may be affected by the temporary eyelid closure, are better served with single stage advancement flaps.

Standard Surgical Technique

– The defect should be assessed under gentle tension.
– A silk traction suture is passed through the gray line of the upper eyelid, which is everted over a Desmarres retractor [16].
– The tarsal conjunctiva incision line is marked with a surgical marking pen 4 mm above the eyelid margin.
– A superficial horizontal incision is made along the conjunctiva and tarsus 4 mm above the eyelid margin using a number 15 Bard Parker blade [16].
– The incision is deepened through the full thickness of the tarsus using the number 15 blade, and the horizontal incision is completed with Westcott scissors. Vertical relieving cuts are then made at both ends of the tarsal incision [16].
– Tarsus and conjunctiva are dissected free from Müller's muscle and the levator aponeurosis up to the superior fornix. The tarsoconjunctival flap is advanced into the lower eyelid defect to reconstruct the posterior lamella of the lower eyelid.
– The flap tarsus is sutured to the remaining lower eyelid tarsus edge with interrupted 6-0 Vicryl sutures. The lower eyelid conjunctival edge is sutured to the inferior border of the mobilized tarsus with a continuous or interrupted 6-0 Vicryl suture.
– A FTSG (preferred by us because it reduces the risks of cicatricial ectropion) or advancing a myocutaneous flap from the cheek can be used to reconstruct the anterior lamella. The graft or flap is sutured into place with 6-0 Vicryl sutures.

- The skin edge is sewn to the superior aspect of the tarsus using interrupted 7-0 Vicryl sutures.
- The occasional use of oblique medial and lateral periosteal flaps in conjunction with the Hughes flap enables the repair of maximal defects of the lower eyelid [28]. Video 4.2-Reconstruction with Hughes flap.

Postoperative Medications and Wound Care: Pattern of Follow-Up Visits and Evaluation

- Remove pad at home after 48 h, and apply antibiotic ointment three times a day to wound.
- At a second operation, the conjunctival pedicle is cut and the lower eyelid margin reconstructed.
- Although the second operation has typically been performed 3–4 weeks after the first operation [25], the tarsoconjunctival pedicle may be safely divided at 2 weeks [29] and even as early as 7 days [29].

Second Stage

- Local anesthesia with propofol sedation.
- 27G–30G needle, 1% ropivacaine with 1:100,000 adrenaline, injected into the upper and lower eyelids.
- Next, one blade of a pair of Westcott scissors is inserted just above the desired level of the new eyelid border, and the flap is cut open[16] (Fig. 4.9).
- The upper eyelid is then everted, and the residual flap is excised using Westcott scissors.
- The anterior and posterior lamellar margin are sutured together with 7-0 Vicryl sutures.

Single-Stage Advancement Flaps +/− Free Grafts

Indications for Surgery. Disadvantages of the Hughes flap are not insignificant and include [30]:

1. The eye is closed postoperatively for 1–2 weeks or longer.
2. A second stage is required.
3. There is a loss of eyelashes in the area of the flap.
4. The edge of the flap can be persistently erythematous.

These disadvantages have prompted the search for alternative single-stage procedures. Reconstruction of the anterior lamella in full-thickness eyelid defects can be accomplished by a number of different techniques, each with some variations. FTSGs may be utilized if the tarsal flap has a vascular supply (Hughes flap) or when an orbicularis muscle flap is advanced. A myocutaneous pedicle flap will typically result in a better color and thickness match [31]. Free tarsoconjunctival (TC) flaps associated with myocutaneous advancement flaps are less likely to lead to complications of eyelid margin erythema and subsequent revision surgery than Hughes TC flaps with FTSGs [32]. They are also single stage procedures and thus useful for monocular patients.

Other single-stage alternative procedures to the Hughes flap for reconstruction of large lower eyelid defects have recently gained favor and include lateral-based full-thickness advancement flaps [33] and

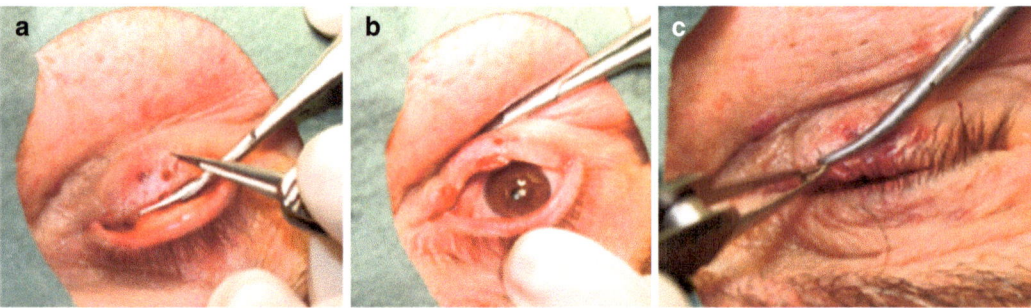

Fig. 4.9 (**a–c**) Stage 2 of the Hughes procedure

free tarsoconjunctival graft and myocutaneous transposition flap [34]. Perry and Allen described successful single-stage reconstruction of large full-thickness defects of the lower eyelid which involve 50–75% of the horizontal length of the eyelid [30]. The procedure employs lateral stabilization of the posterior lamella with a periosteal strip, medial transposition of the lateral posterior lamella for central and medial defects, and a myocutaneous advancement flap to stabilize the anterior lamella. For defects ≥66% of the lower eyelid, a free tarsal graft is often necessary in addition to the periosteal strip to complete posterior lamellar reconstruction [30].

Standard Surgical Technique: Lateral-Based Full-Thickness Advancement Flap

Indication
Full-thickness lower eyelid defect greater than 50% eyelid width with no tarsus remaining;

minimum 25% full-thickness lateral lower eyelid intact for medial advancement [33] (Fig 4.10a).

Technique
– The horizontal dimension of the lower eyelid defect is measured along with the residual lateral full-thickness lower eyelid. Lateral incisional markings are then drawn [33] (Fig 4.10b).
– A full-thickness advancement flap, based laterally, is created. The skin height in the flap is made 1–2 mm greater than the skin height in the defect [33] (Fig 4.10c).
– The conjunctiva and retractor–orbital septum fused complex are incised along the inferior border of the tarsal plate and then incised vertically, 1 mm or so anterior to the lateral fornix recess, cutting down onto the periosteum of the lateral orbital rim [33].
– The lateral palpebral raphe tissue at that point is lysed, until the posterior lamella is

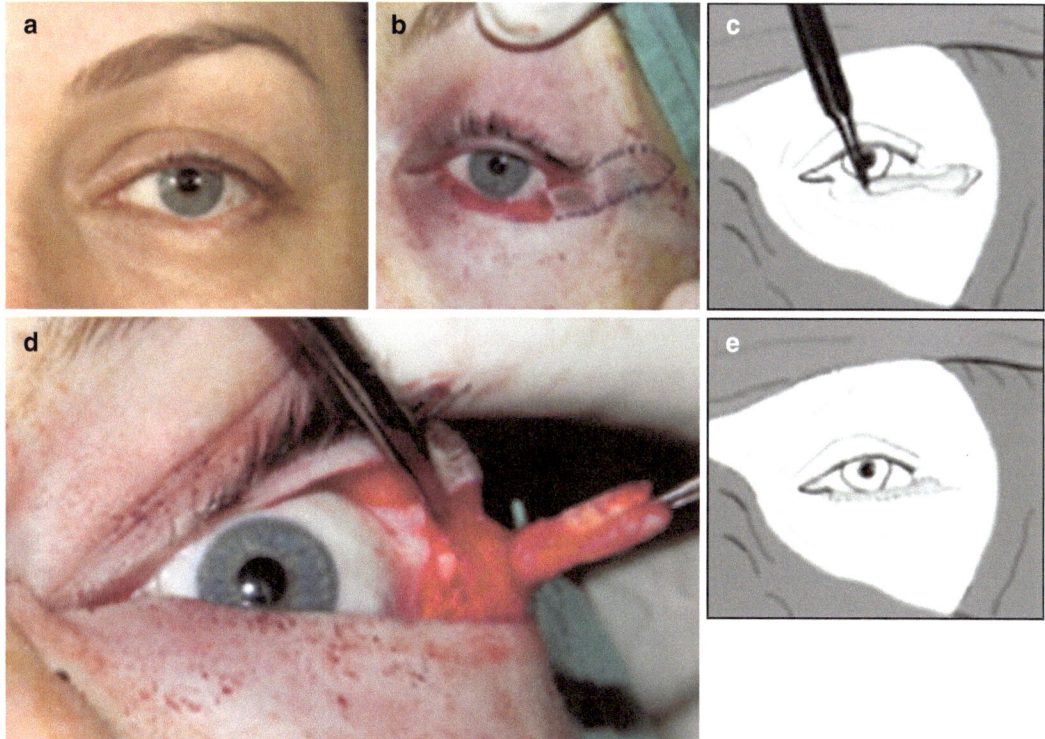

Fig. 4.10 (a–g) Single staged flap. (From Skippen et al. [33], with permission)

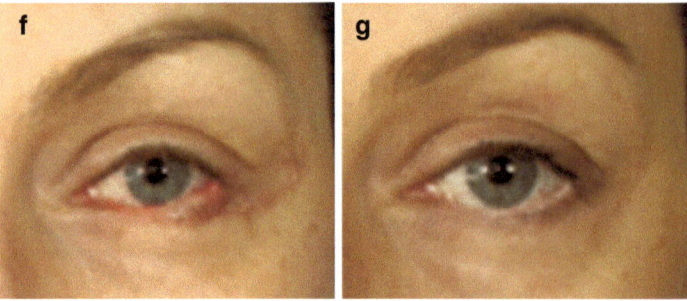

Fig. 4.10 (continued)

completely mobilized from the orbital rim (Fig 4.10d).

– From the lateral eyelid wound edge, the skin is incised laterally, superiorly, and inferiorly in parallel with the curve of the eyelid margin. The full-thickness eyelid flap is then advanced medially to ascertain whether there needs to be further mobilization of the lateral skin base in a V-Y manner [33].

– The medial tarsal edge of the full-thickness flap is sutured to the medial edge of the defect with two 6-0 Vicryl interrupted sutures. A continuous 6-0 Vicryl suture is run along the inferior conjunctival margin of the flap with the knots buried away from the ocular surface [33].

– The anterior lamella of the flap is sutured to the skin edge of the defect with 6-0 Vicryl sutures (Fig 4.10e).

Another means of laterally located large, full-thickness repair of large lower eyelid defects consists of the creation of a lateral-based tarso-conjunctival flap with vascular supply coming from the lateral conjunctiva; the tarso-conjunctival flap is severed from the donor eyelid as if it was a free tarsal graft, except for the lateral most part attached to the conjunctiva; the flap can be fully mobilized to reach the recipient bed in the lower eyelid and anchored into the new position; subsequently a FTSG or better a skin/muscle flap from the same upper eyelid (Fig. 4.11), providing the best functional and cosmetic result.

Mustarde's Cheek Rotation Flap. A large lower eyelid defect, also involving the cheek, can classically be reconstructed with Mustarde's cheek rotation flap, which utilize the lateral cheek and zygomatic skin to cover a posterior lamellar graft [16, 23]. Excision of a significant amount of normal tissue is required in the cheek area to avoid a dog ear deformity and this flap is reserved for large lower eyelid defects extending to the cheek, rather than isolated lower eyelid defects. The flap size needs to be 3–4 times the area of the primary defect. It is important to remember that this is a rotation flap rather than a simple advancement and thus requires a very significant degree of undermining.

Medial Canthus Reconstruction

Reconstruction of the medial canthus after the excision of cutaneous malignancy is challenging not only from an aesthetic aspect, but also due to the complexity of the medial canthal anatomy and its importance for vision and eyelid function. Furthermore, there is minimal laxity of skin in this region, often precluding primary closure of defects. In addition to consideration of eyelid and medial canthal skin reconstruction, the naso-lacrimal apparatus requires attention to avoid or treat potentially disabling epiphora [35]. Primary closure is sometimes possible, depending on the excision technique used, i.e., Moh's, frozen section, and delayed paraffin.

For larger anterior defects, or those lacking a vascular bed for FTSG survival, various transposition or advancement flaps can be employed, such as a glabellar forehead flap or paramedian

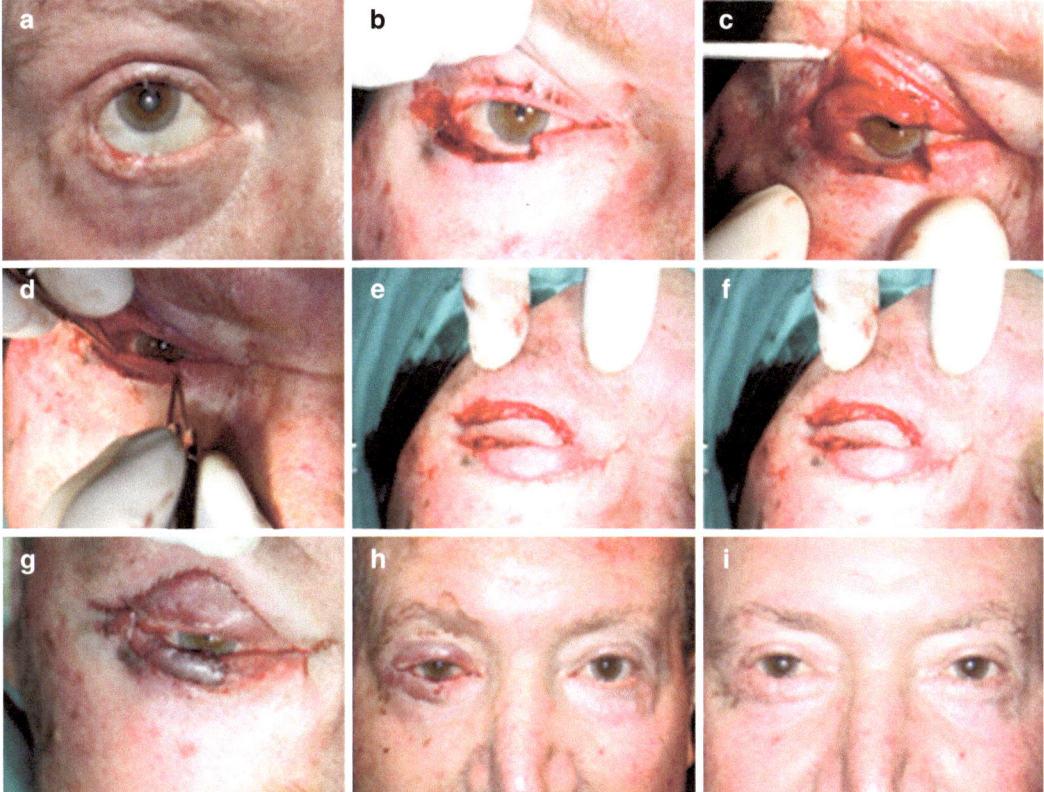

Fig. 4.11 (a–i) Large lower eyelid defect repair using lateral-based tarso-conjunctival flap

forehead flap [2, 36]. When the defect involves full-thickness medial eyelid(s) or sacrifice of the medial canthal tendon, the remaining eyelid must be reapproximated and fixated to periosteum or bone [38]. When the medial canthal tendon is interrupted or completely lost, the remaining eyelid portion of the tendon must be fixated to the area of the tendinous origin to ensure proper alignment and support of the eyelid(s). If only the anterior limb of the tendon is disrupted, it may not cause malposition of the medial canthus if the posterior limb remains intact [24]. If any tendon remains on the anterior or posterior lacrimal crest, direct reattachment with polygalactin (Vicryl) or polypropylene (Prolene) suture is possible.

Reconstruction Options

1. Laissez-faire (small, shallow defects)
2. Direct closure
3. Glabellar or bilobed flaps (if poor vascular support; need to be thinned)
4. Paramedian forehead flap [37]
5. Combination flaps for deeper defects [36]
6. FTSG (if good vascular support; larger defects)

Some of the problems encountered in reconstruction in this area include [35]:

1. A difference in skin color between host tissue and skin grafts used for reconstruction
2. Differing skin textures, for example, thick skin from the glabellar region is often a poor match for medial canthal skin
3. Poor eyelid motility and function, which requires adequate canthal tendon fixation in the appropriate position and at the correct tension
4. Loss of volume in the concavity of the medial canthus, which tends to be cosmetically obvious

5. Limited globe motility, typically reduced abduction, which may result from a conjunctival cicatrix
6. Chronic epiphora, which may result from secondary corneal exposure, an abnormal lid position or damage to the nasolacrimal system

Laissez-Faire (Spontaneous Granulation)

After its initial description by Fox and Beard in 1964, the laissez-faire method has become well-established as a method of medial canthal reconstruction, with excellent cosmetic results [42]. Excess scar formation may occasionally occur, which may lead to difficulties in subsequent tumor surveillance, but this may be dealt with surgically using standard techniques. Scarring may be reduced in defects that symmetrically bisect the medial canthal tendon with appropriate contouring and alignment along the relaxed skin tension lines (RSTL) [35].

Direct Closure of the Defect

Where possible, direct closure of the edges of a defect typically provides excellent cosmetic results, however, the use of this technique has traditionally only been used for small defects due to concern about closing defects under tension and subsequent unacceptable distortion of the palpebral apertures. However, it has recently been shown that even when eyelid defects are closed under extreme tension, intraoperative, and postoperative tissue expansion allows the dimensions of the palpebral apertures to return to normal after a period of a few months [15].

Mobilization of Nasal Skin into a Medial Canthal Defect

Indication for Surgery. A variety of techniques involving flaps have been described, permitting mobilization of infraglabellar nasal skin into a medial canthal defect, all of which allow defect closure within a single aesthetic facial unit [35].

The Rhomboid Transposition Flap

This provides a simple and versatile method for medial canthal reconstruction [38]. Custer also described a transnasal flap, similar in construction to a rhomboid flap but triangular in shape, which has been reported to provide excellent cosmetic results in 22 patients [39].

Advantages of using a rhomboid flap include:

– Scar length minimized
– Tissue excision minimized
– Easier to work with straight defect sides

Standard Surgical Technique

– The defect, which may be an irregular shape, is conceptualized as a rhomboid shape, with its long-axis perpendicular to the relaxed skin tension lines (RSTL).
– Short diagonal of excised rhomboid on the same line with RSTL.
– A flap adjacent to typically the upper half of the defect (greater skin motility superiorly) is mobilized, which is then transposed into the defect.
– Base of triangle of donor flap perpendicular to RSTL.
– After flap advancement, the greatest tension lies in closing the triangular donor site.
– Undermining of tissues allows closure of the secondary defect.
– Tissue closure with interrupted 6-0 Vicryl sutures.

The Bilobed Flap

This is an alternative versatile option to the rhomboid flap and uses two lobes of skin on a shared pedicle and is thus a double transposition flap [40]. This technique permits movement of more skin over longer distance than possible with single transposition flap.

Standard Surgical Technique

– Each lobe of the defect is tethered to a cutaneous pedicle.
– The proximal lobe is transposed into the defect, whereas the second lobe is rotated into the defect created by the first.
– The first lobe is designed to be equal to the width of the original defect.

- The defect arising from the second pedicle can usually be closed directly, in a linear fashion.
- This defect bears the greatest closure tension and is best placed in a natural skin crease where possible.
- Tissue closure with interrupted 6-0 Vicryl sutures.

Mobilization of Forehead or Glabellar Tissue

Mobilization of tissue as a flap from the forehead or glabellar area can be achieved through a bilobed flap [40] as described above, or a glabellar flap as described by McCord and Wesley [41]. The underlying rich vascular supply of this region allows for a very robust flap. Such forehead flaps can preserve their vascular pedicle along an axial pattern, such as a paramedian forehead flap.

Mobilization of Upper Eyelid Anterior Lamella

Skin and/or orbicularis may be mobilized from the upper eyelid using a variety of flap techniques [42]. Dermatochalasis may provide a large amount of redundant skin that can be mobilized with little local morbidity in a cosmetically acceptable manner. Tissue flaps can be advanced through a rotation flap, hinged laterally, or more commonly through a medially based pedicle, which allows the movement of larger quantities of skin and or muscle; this latter technique, when used bilaterally, can also be used in the reconstruction of the entire superficial upper half of the nose. Thin eyelid skin, however, does not always allow adequate volume replacement of the medial canthal hollow [35].

Mobilization of Cheek, Forehead, and Midface Tissue

Upward movement of nasolabial, cheek, and midfacial tissue into a medial canthal defect can be achieved through rotation and/or transposition flaps, but is perhaps more simply achieved

with a subcutaneous island pedicle advancement flap [43]. The design of the flap is "V-Y," with the lower part of the defect being closed to form the limb of the "Y." Such flaps provide well-vascularized tissue and are easily combined with other techniques, such as a forehead or glabellar flap, for larger defects. Disadvantages include a downward vector of the flap, which may predispose to subsequent medial ectropion [35].

Paramedian Forehead Flap

Indication for Surgery. For large medial canthal defects, a paramedian forehead flap can be useful [37]. The paramedian forehead flap method elevates the flap with the supratrochlear vessels and nerves, ensuring an abundant blood supply. The common paramedian forehead flap utilizes the contralateral supratrochlear artery as the pedicle and has the merit of not bending the artery severely due to its large rotation arc. A paramedian forehead flap method utilizing the ipsilateral supratrochlear artery has also been described, with good results [37].

Disadvantages of the paramedian forehead flap include the procedure needing two stages and the relatively poor aesthetic outcome compared to other techniques. The pedicle crossing the skin of the nose like a tube requires second stage flap division, usually after 2–3 weeks [37].

Combination Flaps

Indication for Surgery. For larger, deeper medial canthal defects [36].

Standard Surgical Technique

- Lacrimal system intubated with Crawford tubes during tumor excision
- Medial canthal angle recreated first with 4-0 Vicryl onto periosteum of posterior lacrimal crest then medial part of the eyelid defect
- Glabellar rotational flap used for superomedial part of the defect
- Lateral-based upper eyelid advancement flap used for lateral part of defect
- Posterior parts of both flaps fixated to periosteum in medial canthus with 5-0 Vicryl sutures
- Skin incisions closed with 6-0 Prolene and 5-0 fast absorbing gut sutures (Fig. 4.12)

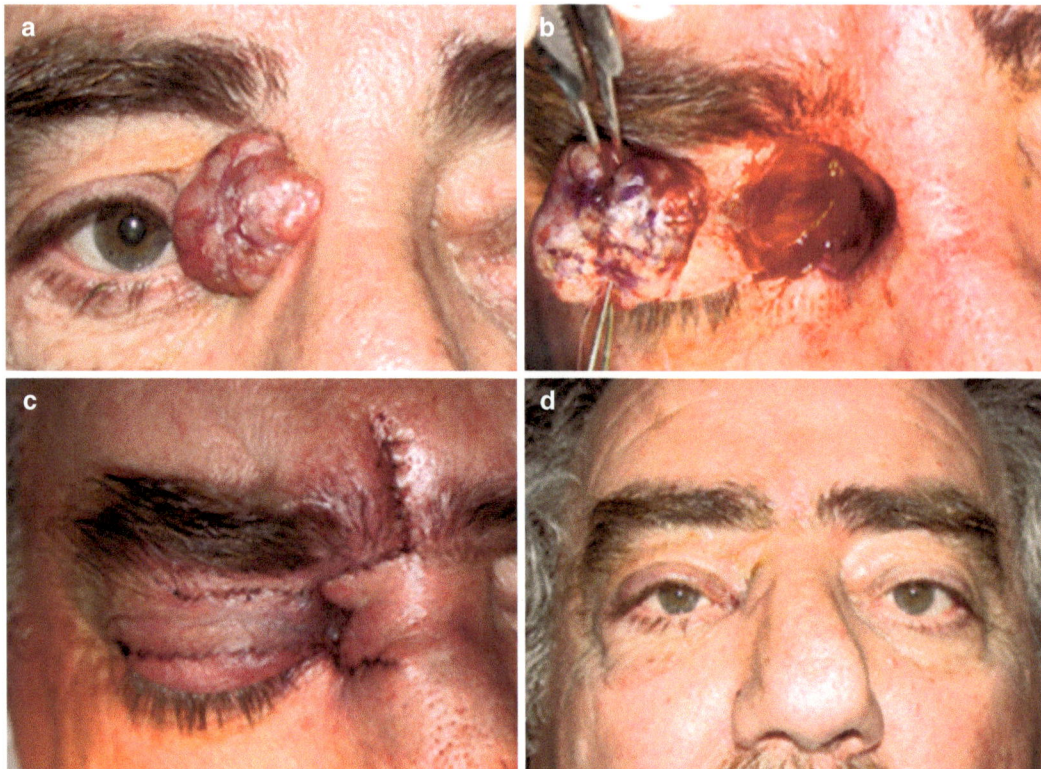

Fig. 4.12 (**a–d**) Combination flaps for large, deep right medial canthal defect

Skin Grafting

Indication for Surgery. Medial canthal defects can also be effectively covered by means of skin grafting, which can be either a split-thickness graft (SSG) or more typically a FTSG [44]. Contracture of skin grafts seems to occur more frequently as the thickness of the graft decreases, which often precludes the use of SSG in this region. FTSGs for the medial canthal region are typically harvested from the upper eyelid skin, preauricular or postauricular areas, inner brachial, and supraclavicular areas [44].

Lateral Canthus Reconstruction

Reconstruction of the lateral canthus, or canthoplasty, is not as well described as that of the medial canthus. Reconstruction of the lateral canthus is dependent upon the extent of injury to the surrounding tissues. The key to adequate reconstruction is correct recognition of the extent of injury and the correct fabrication of the damaged or missing structures [45]. Options for skin-only defects differ from options for full-thickness defects. The lateral canthal angle needs to be reformed. If eyelid laxity is present, then options include lateral canthopexy and a lateral tarsal strip. Other considerations in this region include skin rotation flaps for anterior lamella and periosteal flaps for posterior lamella.

Commonly used surgical procedures in this region include (done after complete clearance of the tumor, with adequate margins):

– Primary closure
– Advancement flap, rhomboid flap, rotation flap, transposition flap
– Combination flaps
– Lateral periosteal flaps can be helpful if lateral upper lid or lower lid tarsal loss
– FTSG

Skin-Only Defects

Primary Closure

For small lesions, primary closure is the best method of reconstruction. Closing the defect in the direction of relaxed skin tension lines is typically the best orientation to perform primary closure. However, in the area of the lateral canthus, facial rhytids are described to occur in a crow's feet distribution. These rhytids do not always follow the relaxed skin tension lines and care should be taken to orient the scars with regards to the crow's feet orientation [45].

Rhomboid Flap

Indication for Surgery. Initially described by Limberg, the rhomboid flap is useful for skin reconstruction at the lateral canthus [46]. Advantages of the flap are its ability to minimally distort important adjacent anatomic structures while providing a similar skin for the defect reconstruction.

Standard Surgical Technique

- Excise the defect as a rhomboid so that its 120° angle is located at the area of greatest skin excess.
- A line is then drawn out into this skin excess from the apex of the 120° angle equal to the length of one side of the rhomboid.
- A 60° cut is then drawn at the end of this line.
- This line will be parallel and equal in length to the side of the rhomboid defect.
- The flap is then cut and transposed so that the apex of the 60° cut is inserted in the 60° angle of the rhomboid defect.
- Undermining of tissues allows closure of the secondary defect.
- Tissue closure with interrupted 6-0 Vicryl sutures.

Fricke Flap

The Fricke flap is an inferiorly based transposition flap designed in the forehead or temporal skin area and rotated medially to cover skin defects at the lateral canthus [47]. It can also be used for large lower eyelid full-thickness defects.

When the flap is narrow the donor site can be closed primarily but care should be taken not to move the eyebrow laterally or the hairline anteriorly. Larger flaps may require FTSG closure of the donor site, which may leave an aesthetically unsatisfactory result.

An alternative for primary donor site closure is the use of a bipedicle flap instead of the Fricke flap transposition. Other forehead flaps with/without preservation of the vascular pedicle (i.e., paramedian forehead, axial pattern flaps, etc.) may be useful [45].

Lateral Canthal Tendon Repair

Reestablishment of the attachment of the lateral canthal tendon to the internal aspect of the lateral orbit at Whitnall's tubercle is a surgical goal if the continuity of these two structures has been disrupted. The vector that has been described for representing the lateral canthus is one of a superior and lateral direction with periosteal fixation [48]. If both upper and lower eyelid structures are involved laterally, periosteum from both the upper and lower lateral orbital rim may be required to reconstitute the lateral canthal structure [49].

Full-Thickness Defects

Full-thickness loss at the lateral canthus almost always involves loss of adjacent structures such as the eyelids. Reconstruction of these full-thickness defects requires both the reconstruction of the lateral canthus and that of the adjacent eyelids and tarsal plates [50]. Replacement materials for these reconstructive cases may include autogenous tarsal flaps or grafts, hard palate mucosa, palmaris longus tendon, temporal parietal fascia, nasal mucosal tissues, dermal fascia, ear cartilage, cadaver sclera, and various animal, cadaver or artificial skin, dermis or fascial implants [51, 52]. Therefore, a combination of the techniques described above may be needed to reconstruct full-thickness lateral canthal defects (Fig. 4.13).

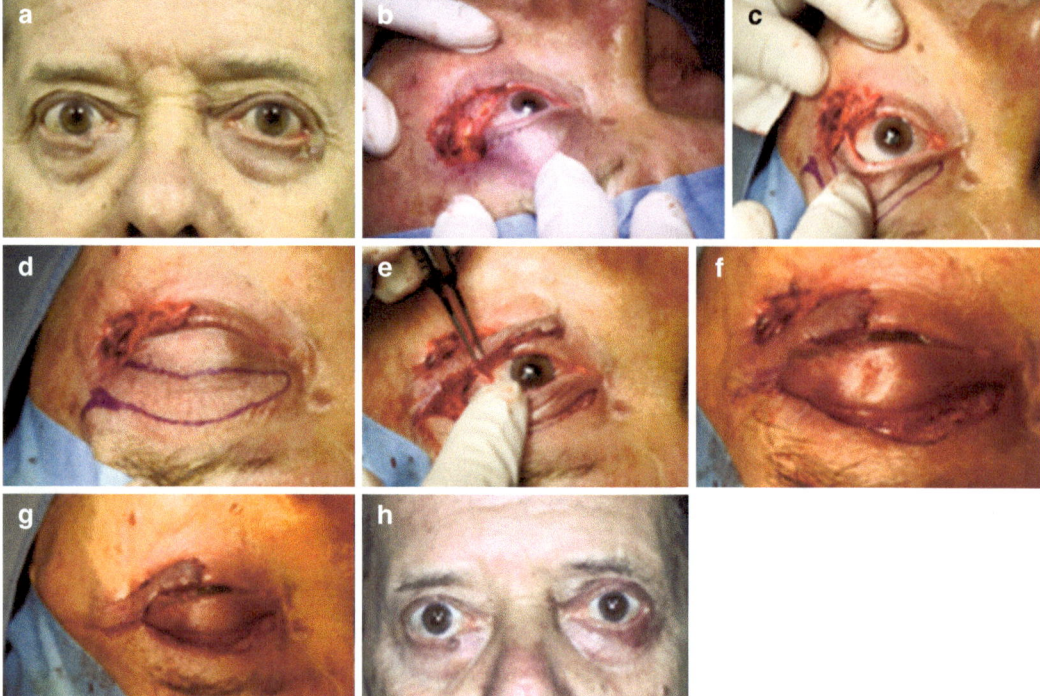

Fig. 4.13 (**a–h**) Lateral canthal defect repairing lateral-based upper-eyelid transposition flap

Postoperative Medications and Wound Care: Pattern of Follow-Up Visits and Evaluation

In general terms, for most eyelid procedures where a skin graft is not used, the postoperative management is similar.

- Management may be more complicated for dark skin patients due to the increased risk of hypertophic scars:
  - Antibiotic ointment to wound and in the eye (check first for allergies), double pad, tape.
  - Remove pad at home the next day and apply antibiotic ointment three times daily to wound.
  - When skin grafts are used, the pad should be left intact for a minimum of 48 h.
  - Follow-up in 1 week.

Complications of Eyelid Reconstruction

Upper Eyelid

The main complications of upper eyelid repair involve either the eyelid margin or the position of the eyelid [3].

Eyelid margin problems include:

- Notching
- Trichiasis
- Conjunctivalization

Complications relating to the upper eyelid position includes:

- Entropion
- Retraction and exposure
- Ptosis

Finally, unevenness of the posterior lamella such as after a posterior lamella or tarsal graft can result in reduced corneal lubrication and subsequent discomfort.

Lower Eyelid

Complications of lower eyelid repair can include [1]

Blurred vision or ocular irritation, secondary to:

- A suture
- Tissue irritation on the ocular surface
- Exposure keratopathy

Decreased orbicularis function with lagophthalmos
Swelling can cause mechanical ectropion
Excessive scarring can occur after reconstruction
Cicatricial ectropion

Medial Canthus

The predominant complications in this area include [35]:

- Cicatricial contracture, e.g., eyelid malposition
- Epiphora
- Web deformities

Lateral Canthus

Potential complications include [45]:

- Trichiasis
- Ocular surface irritation
- Ectropion
- Entropion

Full-Thickness Skin Graft Complications

The periocular region is a favorable FTSG recipient area by virtue of its high vascularity [53]. The usual donor sites for harvesting FTSG for the periocular area are upper eyelid, preauricular, postauricular, neck, clavicular, supraclavicular, and inner brachial area. Different sites yield different graft thickness.

Complications

Early complications seen in the first 2 weeks include [53]:

- Bleeding with hematoma formation beneath the graft
- Infection
- Seroma formation

These complications may prevent graft adherence to the underlying wound bed, prolong the ischemic phase, compromise the graft's vascular supply, and result in graft failure.

Late complications seen by 3 months are [53]:

- Cicatricial ectropion
- Graft hypertrophy and contracture

The long-term complications are mainly cosmetic or functional and result from color and texture mismatch, and hyper or hypopigmentation.

References

1. Holds JB. Lower eyelid reconstruction. Facial Plast Surg Clin N Am. 2016;24:183–91.
2. Czyz CN, Cahill KV, Foster JA, Michels KS, Clark CM, Rich NE. Reconstructive options for the medial canthus and eyelids following tumor excision. Saudi J Ophthalmol. 2011 Jan;25(1):67–74.
3. O'Donnell BA, Mannor GE. Oculoplastic surgery for upper eyelid reconstruction after cutaneous carcinoma. Int Ophthalmol Clin. 2009. Fall;49(4):157–72.

4. Fox SA, Beard C. Spontaneous lid repair. Am J Ophthalmol. 1964;58:947–52.
5. Mehta HK. Spontaneous reformation of lower eyelid. Br J Ophthalmol. 1981;65:202–8.
6. DaCosta J, Jones C. Laissez-Faire: how far can you go? Orbit. 2009;28:12–5.
7. Shankar J, Nair RG, Sullivan SC. Management of peri-ocular skin tumors by laissez-faire technique: analysis of functional and cosmetic results. Eye. 2002;16:50–3.
8. Colin JRO. Eye lid reconstruction & tumor management. In: Colin JRO, editor. A Manual of Systematic Eye Lid Surgery. Edinburgh: Churchill Livingstone; 1989.
9. Thaller VT, Then KY, Luhishi E. Spontaneous eyelid expansion after full thickness eyelid resection and direct closure. Br J Ophthalmol. 2001 Dec;85(12):1450–4.
10. Johnson TM, Brown MD, Sullivan MJ, et al. Immediate intraoperative tissue expansion. J Am Acad Dermatol. 1990;22:283–7.
11. Espinoza GM, Prost AM. Upper eyelid reconstruction. Facial Plast Surg Clin North Am. 2016 May;24(2):173–82.
12. Tenzel RR. Reconstruction of the central one half of an eyelid. Arch Ophthalmol. 1975;93:125–6.
13. Cutler NL, Beard C. A method for partial repair and total upper lid reconstruction. Am J Ophthalmol. 1955;39:1–7.
14. Weinstein GS, Anderson RL, Tse DT, et al. The use of a periosteal strip for eyelid reconstruction. Arch Ophthalmol. 1985;103:357–9.
15. Thaller VT, Then KY, Luhishi E. Spontaneous eyelid expansion after full-thickness eyelid resection and direct closure. Br J Ophthalmol. 2001;85:1450–4.
16. Leatherbarrow B. Eyelid reconstruction. In: Leatherbarrow B, editor. Oculoplastic surgery. London: Martin Dunitz; 2002. p. 117–39.
17. Hsuan J, Selva D. Early division of a modified Cutler-Beard flap with a free tarsal graft. Eye. 2004;18:714–7.
18. Dukic Y. Reconstruction of the upper eyelid with a pedicled bucket-handle brow flap. Face. 2009;6(3):165–7.
19. Jordan DR, Anderson RL, Nowinski TS. Tarsoconjunctival flap for upper eyelid reconstruction. Arch Ophthalmol. 1989;107:599–603.
20. Irvine F, McNab AA. A technique for reconstruction of upper lid marginal defects. Br J Ophthalmol. 2003;87:279–81.
21. Kakizaki H, Madge SN, Mannor G, Selva D, Malhotra R. Oculoplastic surgery for lower eyelid reconstruction after periocular cutaneous carcinoma. Int Ophthalmol Clin. 2009. Fall;49(4):143–55.
22. Mustarde JC. Repair and reconstruction in the orbital region. A practical guide. Edinburgh: Churchill Livingstone; 1980. p. 92–129.
23. Collin JRO. Eyelid reconstruction and tumor management. In: Collin JRO, editor. A Manual of Systemic Eyelid Surgery. 3rd ed. Philadelphia: Elsevier; 2006. p. 73–98.
24. Hughes WL. A new method for rebuilding a lower eyelid: report of a case. Arch Ophthalmol. 1937;17:1008–17.
25. Hughes WL. Total lower lid reconstruction: technical details. Trans Am Ophthalmol Soc. 1976;74:321–9.
26. McNab AA. Early division of the conjunctival pedicle in modified Hughes repair of the lower eyelid. Ophthalmic Surg Lasers. 1996;27:422–4.
27. Maloof A, Ng S, Leatherbarrow B. The maximal Hughes procedure. Ophthal Plast Reconstr Surg. 2001;17:96–102.
28. McNab AA, Martin P, Benger R, O'Donnell B, Kourt G. A prospective randomized study comparing division of the pedicle of modified Hughes flaps at two or four weeks. Ophthal Plast Reconstr Surg. 2001 Sep;17(5):317–9.
29. Leibovitch I, Selva D. Modified Hughes flap. Ophthalmology. 2004;111:2164–7.
30. Perry CB, Allen RC. Repair of 50-75% full-thickness lower eyelid defects: lateral stabilization as a guiding principle. Indian J Ophthalmol. 2016 Aug;64(8):563–7.
31. Leone CR Jr, Van Gemert JV. Lower lid reconstruction using tarsoconjunctival grafts and bipedicle skin-muscle flap. Arch Ophthalmol. 1989;107:758–60.
32. Hawes MJ, Grove AS Jr, Hink EM. Comparison of free tarsoconjunctival grafts and Hughes tarsoconjunctival grafts for lower eyelid reconstruction. Ophthal Plast Reconstr Surg. 2011;27:219–23.
33. Skippen B, Hamilton A, Evans S, Benger R. One-stage alternatives to the Hughes procedure for reconstruction of large lower eyelid defects: surgical techniques and outcomes. Ophthal Plast Reconstr Surg. 2016;32:145–9.
34. Katz TL, Pennington TE, Yohendran J, et al. One-step reconstruction of large lower eyelid defects: technique and outcomes. Clin Exp Ophthalmol. 2014;42:889–92.
35. Madge SN, Malhotra R, Thaller VT, Davis GJ, Kakizaki H, Mannor GE, Selva D. A systematic approach to the oculoplastic reconstruction of the eyelid medial canthal region after cancer excision. Int Ophthalmol Clin. 2009. Fall;49(4):173–94.
36. Chahal HS, Allen RC. Combination lateral rotational and glabellar flaps for medial canthal defects. JAMA Facial Plast Surg. 2016 Dec 1;18(6):491–2.
37. Kim JH, Kim JM, Park JW, Hwang JH, Kim KS, Lee SY. Reconstruction of the medial canthus using an ipsilateral paramedian forehead flap. Arch Plast Surg. 2013 Nov;40(6):742–7.
38. Ng S, Inkster CF, Leatherbarrow B. The rhomboid flap in medial canthal reconstruction. Br J Ophthalmol. 2001;85:556–9.
39. Custer PL. Trans-nasal flap for medial canthal reconstruction. Ophthalmic Surg. 1994;25:601–3.
40. Sullivan TJ, Bray LC. The bilobed flap in medial canthal reconstruction. Aust NZ J Ophthalmol. 1995;23:42–8.
41. McCord CD Jr, Wesley R. Reconstruction of the upper eyelid and medial canthus. In: McCord Jr CD, editor.

Oculoplastic and Orbit Surgery. 2nd ed. New York: Raven Press; 1987.

42. Jelks GW, Glat PM, Jelks EB, et al. Medial canthal reconstruction using a medially based upper eyelid myocutaneous flap. Plast Reconstr Surg. 2002;110:1636–43.

43. Li JH, Xing X, Liu HY, et al. Subcutaneous island pedicle flap. Variations and versatility for facial reconstruction. Ann Plast Surg. 2006;57:255–9.

44. Leibovitch I, Huilgol SC, Hsuan JD. Incidence of host site complications in periocular full thickness skin grafts. Br J Ophthalmol. 2005;89:219–22.

45. Andrews BT, Lin SJ, Rubin PA. Lateral canthal reconstruction after head-neck or periocular cutaneous malignancy: oculoplastic and facial plastic surgery techniques. Int Ophthalmol Clin. 2009. Fall;49(4):195–206.

46. Limberg AA. Mathematical principles of local plastic procedures on the surface of the human body. Leningrad: Government Publishing House for Medical Literature; 1946.

47. Fricke JCG. Die Bildung der Augenlider (Blepheroplastik) nach Zerstorungen und. Dadurch Hervorgebrachten Auswartswendungen Derselben. Hamburg: Perthes & Besser; 1829.

48. Game J, Morlet N. Lateral canthal fixation using an oblique vertically orientated asymmetric periosteal transposition flap. Clin Exp Ophthalmol. 2007;35:204–7.

49. Leone CR Jr. Lateral canthal reconstruction. Ophthalmology. 1987;94:238–41.

50. Jones IS, Cooper WC. Lateral canthal reconstruction. Trans Am Ophthalmol Soc. 1973;71:296–302.

51. Bachelor EP, Jobe RP. The absent lateral canthal tendon: reconstruction using a Y graft or palmaris longus tendon. Ann Plast Surg. 1980;5:362–8.

52. Acikel C, Celikoz B, Yildiz TF. Y-shape hard palate mucoperiosteal graft and V-Y advancement flap in the reconstruction of a combined defect involving lateral canthus and upper and lower eyelids. Ann Plast Surg. 2004 Jan;52(1):97–101.

53. Rathore DS, Chickadasarahilli S, Crossman R, Mehta P, Ahluwalia HS. Full thickness skin grafts in periocular reconstructions: long-term outcomes. Ophthal Plast Reconstr Surg. 2014 Nov-Dec;30(6):517–20.

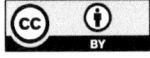

Sentinel Lymph Node Biopsy for Conjunctival and Ocular Adnexal Tumors

Sonal S. Chaugule and Bita Esmaeli

Sentinel lymph node biopsy (SLNB) is a method of detecting subclinical (microscopic) metastasis in regional lymph node at risk of metastasis and can be used to detect early metastasis from eyelid and conjunctival malignancies. Sentinel lymph node biopsy has been demonstrated to be technically feasible and have a reasonable positive yield for various eyelid and conjunctival cancers including melanoma, squamous cell carcinoma (SCC), sebaceous gland carcinoma (SGCa), and Merkel cell carcinoma (MCC); these cancers have various risks of regional lymph node metastasis (Table 5.1) [1–10].

The lymphatic drainage in the head and neck is complex and could be variable. However, commonly the lateral two-thirds of the upper eyelid, the lateral third of the lower eyelid, and the lateral half of the conjunctiva drain into the parotid (preauricular) lymph

Table 5.1 Rate of regional lymph node metastasis for eyelid tumors

Sr No	Type of tumor	Approximate rate of regional lymph node metastasis (%)
1	Eyelid and conjunctival melanoma	20–24
2	Squamous cell carcinoma	7–24
3	Sebaceous gland carcinoma	7–20
4	Merkel cell carcinoma	21

Data from references [1–10]

nodes, and the medial third of the upper eyelid, the medial two-thirds of the lower eyelid, and the medial half of the conjunctiva drain into the submandibular and deeper cervical nodes [11]. However, recent studies suggest that there is higher than expected preponderance of draining SLNs in the parotid and preauricular region even from the more medially located tumors [12].

SLNB is based on the concept of an orderly drainage of tumor cells through the lymphatic drainage system before dissemination in the bloodstream and involvement of other organs. The sentinel lymph nodes (SLNs) or first draining node(s) for a tumor can be identified by injecting tracer molecules into

S. S. Chaugule (✉)
Ophthalmic Plastic Surgery, Orbit and Ocular Oncology, PBMA's H V Desai Eye Hospital, Pune, India
e-mail: schaugule@eyecancercure.com

B. Esmaeli
Orbital Oncology and Ophthalmic Plastic Surgery Service, Department of Plastic Surgery, The University of Texas M. D. Anderson Cancer Center, Houston, TX, USA
e-mail: besmaeli@mdanderson.org

the tissue surrounding the tumor. Identification of SLN status provides the surgeon and the patient with valuable prognostic information [10]. Early detection and early management of micro-metastasis is believed to provide long-term survival benefits in oncological practices, and particularly in the recent era of availability of immune checkpoint inhibitors for metastatic melanoma and metastatic carcinomas and improved survival with these drugs, there is a more compelling reason to identify early metastatic disease in patients with biologically aggressive eyelid and conjunctival melanomas and carcinomas [13–16].

Patient Selection Criteria

Published studies and major reviews on SLNB in ocular and adnexal tumors have identified and described several risk factors for possible SLN involvement (Table 5.2) [2, 6, 7, 17–21].

Table 5.2 Risk factors for SLN involvement

Sr No	Type of tumor	Risk factor predicting SLN involvement
1	Conjunctival melanoma	Tumor thickness ≥2 mm Non-limbal location of conjunctival melanoma
1	Eyelid melanoma	Tumor thickness ≥1 mm and increasing Breslow depth Presence of >1 mitotic figure/HPF Presence of histopathologic ulceration
2	Sebaceous gland carcinoma	AJCC (7th edition) stage T2b or > size 10 mm in the greatest diameter
3	Squamous cell carcinoma	Tumors ≥2 cm (20 mm) wide Locally recurrent
4	Merkel cell carcinoma	Increasing diameter of the lesion Increasing thickness of the lesion Infiltrative growth pattern High mitotic rate

HPF High-power field
Data from references [2, 6, 7, 17–21]

Technique for Sentinel Lymph Node Biopsy [10]

1. *Preoperative lymphoscintigraphy* [22]
   (a) Topical anesthetic is applied on the eyelid surface.
   (b) 0.3–0.4 mCi of filtered technetium [Tc-99 m] sulfur colloid (0.2 ml volume) is injected in three to four spots around the eyelid lesion intradermally or subconjunctivally for conjunctival melanomas by an ophthalmic surgeon (precise injection of radioisotope into the area immediately surrounding the tumor is important to ensure the correct mapping of lymphatic channels).
   (c) Serial scanning is carried out every 15 min, once the first SLN is detected for visualization of all SLN.
   (d) Single-photon emission CT (SPECT-CT) is utilized to improve anatomic resolution and precise localization of SLN (Fig. 5.1a, b).
2. *Surgical procedure*
   (a) Ophthalmic surgeon: On the day of the planned primary surgical tumor resection, technetium-labeled sulfur colloid [Tc-99 m] is injected as described above in preoperative holding area approximately 90 min before the primary tumor resection; in some instances, if the preoperative SPECT/CT or lymphoscintigraphy took place the day before the planned surgery, there may not be a need for reinjection of technetium.
   (b) Head and neck or another oncologic surgeon: Intraoperatively, a handheld gamma probe is used to localize the SLNs (Figs. 5.2 and 5.3). *They are defined as lymph nodes that have radioactivity counts at least twice as high as the level of background radioactivity.*
   (c) The SLNs are then dissected and excised (Fig. 5.4).
   (d) The lymph node basin around the "hot" nodes is scanned again to look for any other SLNs that have high radioactive uptake. This is continued until little or no radioactivity is detectable in the draining lymph node basins.

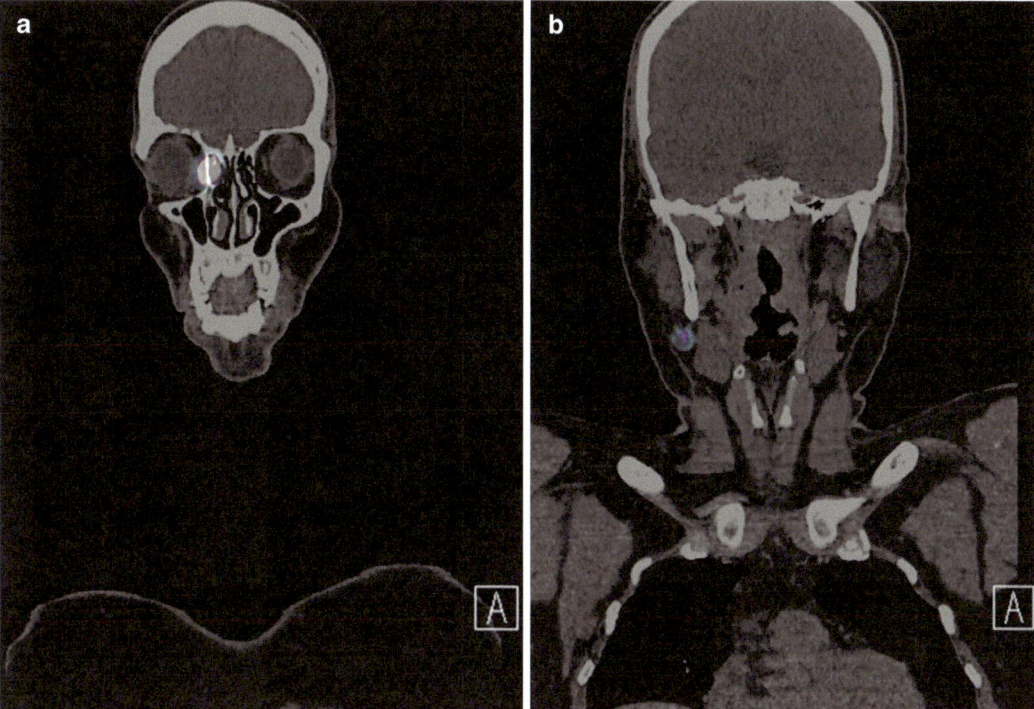

Fig. 5.1 Single-photon emission CT (SPECT-CT) image of primary eyelid sebaceous gland carcinoma (**a**) and of the sentinel lymph node (**b**)

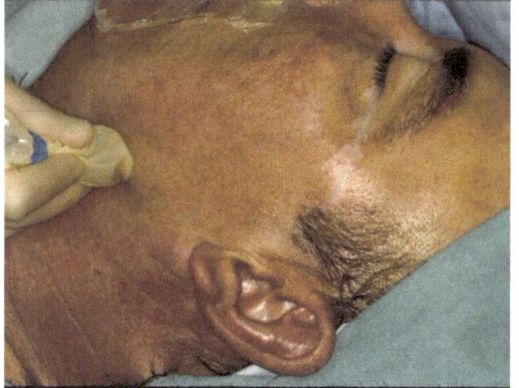

Fig. 5.2 Intraoperative use of handheld gamma probe to localize the sentinel lymph node

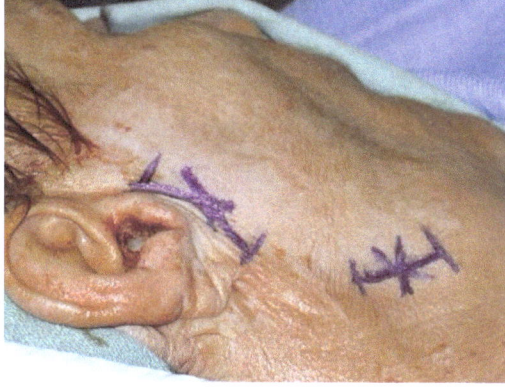

Fig. 5.3 Intraoperative surface markings after use of gamma probe

Histopathologic Evaluation of SLN

1. SLNs are serially sectioned using "bread-loaf" approach in 1–2-mm-thick sections, and the pathologist then examines the haematoxylin-eosin-stained sections for malignant cells.

2. If no malignant cells are found, additional sections are subjected to thorough immunohistochemical analysis.

3. Recommended immunohistochemical (IHC) markers:

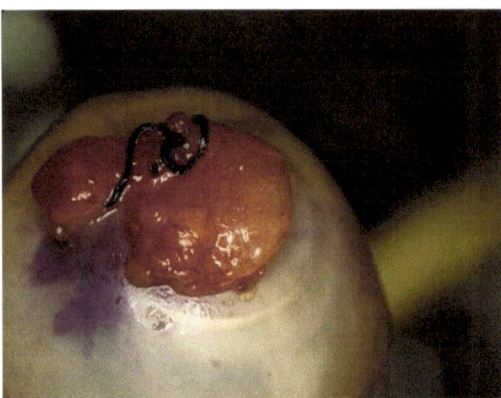

Fig. 5.4 Surgically excised lymph node

(a) Melanoma—antimelanocytic cocktail with HMB-45, anti-MART 1, and anti-tyrosinase [23, 24]
(b) Squamous carcinoma—anticytokeratin antibody cocktail with cytokeratin AE-1/AE-3 [25]
(c) Merkel cell carcinoma—antibodies to Cam5.3, chromogranin, and cytokeratin 20 [26, 27]
(d) Sebaceous gland carcinoma—anti-adipophilin and anti-perilipin antibodies [28–30]

SLN Positivity and False-Negative Results

A review of the published literature on SLNB for ocular adnexal tumors shows variable results of SLN positivity. Savar et al. in a relatively large series (n = 30) of SLNB in ocular adnexal melanoma report positivity rate of 17% [17]. In cases with sebaceous gland carcinoma classified higher than T2b and >10 mm in greatest diameter (n = 16); SLN positivity rate was 13% [10]. Both of these reports were generated from MD Anderson Cancer Center where a lot of the early feasibility studies for SLN biopsy for ocular adnexal cancers took place. A similar rate of 13% was also reported for squamous cell carcinoma (n = 8) by French colleagues [31]. Regarding Merkel cell carcinoma, studies report a SLN positivity rate of 27–48% for all anatomic location

[32–34]. The data on Merkel cell carcinoma of eyelid is insufficient to determine the positivity rate for SLN and prognosis, but there are definitely case reports and small case series of eyelid Merkel cell carcinoma with positive SLN biopsy results [10, 35, 36].

A case with histologically negative SLNs and subsequent development of nodal metastasis constitutes *a false-negative event*. The causes for false-negative events are cited as steep learning curve for SLNB for ocular adnexal as well as head and neck tumors, scarring from multiple prior surgeries at tumor site causing changes in lymphatic drainage routes, and in the event of in-transit metastasis that goes undetected on preoperative or intraoperative lymphatic mapping, as well as inaccurate detection of microscopic metastasis in the draining lymph nodes [10]. Our group at MD Anderson Cancer Center has performed SLN biopsy for ocular adnexal tumors since 2001; we have not encountered any cases of false-negative SLN biopsy results for the last 15 years suggesting the importance of experience with this technique.

However, barring the false-negative events that are rare in experienced hands, a negative SLNB result can be reassuring to the patient. And identification of microscopic metastasis in the draining lymph nodes could mean that the patient would benefit from earlier treatments for metastatic disease.

Further Considerations

Though there is a certain risk of metastasis to regional lymph nodes associated with different conjunctival and eyelid tumors, radical neck dissection and/or parotidectomy for all tumors or empiric radiation therapy for all does not seem to be justified given the relatively low yield, radiation-related complications, and lack of improvement in survival, as described by several published studies. The first Multicenter Selective Lymphadenectomy Trial (MSLT) -I confirmed the value of early nodal evaluation and treatment. This prospective, international, randomized trial showed that the pathologic status of the sentinel node or nodes was the most important prognostic factor and that patients who underwent sentinel-node biopsy had fewer recurrences of melanoma than patients who underwent wide excision and nodal observation. Among patients with intermediate-thickness melanomas (defined as 1.2–3.5 mm) and nodal metastases, early surgical treatment, guided by sentinel-node biopsy, was associated with increased melanoma-specific survival (survival until death from melanoma) [37–39]. These results provide support for the recommendation by several professional organizations that staging by means of sentinel-node biopsy should be performed when appropriate.

However, the subsequent management decision in patients with sentinel lymph node-positive metastasis, in the form of completion of lymph node dissection with or without radiation therapy or observation and imaging for clinically apparent disease before radical surgery, remains controversial.

In an effort to shed some light on this controversy, the most recent report by MSLT-II involving 1934 cases of cutaneous melanoma concludes that immediate completion of lymph node dissection in SLN-positive cases increased the rate of regional disease control, reduced the rate of regional nodal recurrence by nearly 70%, and provided prognostic information but did not improve melanoma-specific survival [40].

Thus, the subsequent management decision in sentinel lymph node metastasis needs to be taken at the surgeon's discretion and detailed discussion regarding disease control and survival for individual case with the patient and family.

In summary, SLNB technique is a relatively low-risk and minimally invasive procedure. It maintains a potential to offer important information to patients and surgeons in terms of accurate tumor staging and prognosis and potential for appropriate patients to receive additional surgery, radiation therapy, and/or systemic therapy for their microscopically metastatic nodal disease. The availability of immune checkpoint inhibitors for patients with metastatic melanoma and metastatic squamous carcinomas is an additional consideration making detection of early nodal metastasis more critical because of the potential for earlier treatment with this new class of drugs

that has revolutionized our expectations for the length and quality of life after diagnosis of metastatic melanoma [13–16].

References

1. Esmaeli B, Youssef A, Naderi A, et al. Margins of excision for cutaneous melanoma of the eyelid skin: the collaborative eyelid skin melanoma group report. Ophthal Plast Reconstr Surg. 2003;19:96–101.
2. Faustina M, Diba R, Ahmadi MA, et al. Patterns of regional and distant metastasis in patients with eyelid and periocular squamous cell carcinoma. Ophthalmology. 2004;111:1930–2.
3. Soysal HG, Markoç F. Invasive squamous cell carcinoma of the eyelids and periorbital region. Br J Ophthalmol. 2007;91:325–9.
4. Tryggvason G, Bayon R, Pagedar NA. Epidemiology of sebaceous carcinoma of the head and neck: implications for lymph node management. Head Neck. 2012;34:1765–8.
5. Shields JA, Demirci H, Marr BP, et al. Sebaceous carcinoma of the eyelids: personal experience with 60 cases. Ophthalmology. 2004;111:2151–7.
6. Ho VH, Ross MI, Prieto VG, et al. Sentinel lymph node biopsy for sebaceous cell carcinoma and melanoma of the ocular adnexa. Arch Otolaryngol Head Neck Surg. 2007;133:820–6.
7. Esmaeli B, Nasser QJ, Cruz H, et al. American Joint Committee on cancer T category for eyelid sebaceous carcinoma correlates with nodal metastasis and survival. Ophthalmology. 2012;119:1078–82.
8. Peters GB III, Meyer DR, Shields JA, et al. Management and prognosis of Merkel cell carcinoma of the eyelid. Ophthalmology. 2001;108:1575–9.
9. Pfeiffer ML, Ozgur OK, Myers JN, Peng A, Ning J, Zafereo ME, Thakar S, Thuro B, Prieto VG, Ross MI, Esmaeli B. Sentinel lymph node biopsy for ocular adnexal melanoma. Acta Ophthalmol. 2017;95(4):e323–8.
10. Pfeiffer ML, Savar A, Esmaeli B. Sentinel lymph node biopsy for eyelid and conjunctival tumors: what have we learned in the past decade? Ophthalmic Plast Reconstr Surg. 2013 Jan 1;29(1):57–62.
11. Dutton JJ. Atlas of Clinical and Surgical Orbital Anatomy. Philadelphia: WB Saunders Co; 1994. p. 84.
12. Nijhawan N, Ross MI, Diba R, Gutstein BF, Ahmadi MA, Esmaeli B. Experience with sentinel lymph node biopsy for eyelid and conjunctival malignancies at a cancer center. Ophthalmic Plast Reconstr Surg. 2004 Jul 1;20(4):291–5.
13. Ford J, Thuro BA, Thakar S, Hwu WJ, Richani K, Esmaeli B. Immune checkpoint inhibitors for treatment of metastatic melanoma of the orbit and ocular adnexa. Ophthal Plast Reconstr Surg. 2017;33(4):e82–5. e-Pub 9/2016. PMID: 27662198.

14. Schachter J, Ribas A, Long GV, Arance A, Grob JJ, Mortier L, Daud A, Carlino MS, McNeil C, Lotem M, Larkin J. Pembrolizumab versus ipilimumab for advanced melanoma: final overall survival results of a multicentre, randomised, open-label phase 3 study (KEYNOTE-006). Lancet. 2017; 390(10105):1853–62.

15. Kazandjian D, Suzman DL, Blumenthal G, Mushti S, He K, Libeg M, Keegan P, Pazdur R. FDA approval summary: nivolumab for the treatment of metastatic non-small cell lung cancer with progression on or after platinum-based chemotherapy. Oncologist. 2016 May 1;21(5):634–42.

16. Yun S, Vincelette ND, Green MR, Wahner Hendrickson AE, Abraham I. Targeting immune checkpoints in unresectable metastatic cutaneous melanoma: a systematic review and meta-analysis of anti-CTLA-4 and anti-PD-1 agents trials. Cancer Med. 2016 Jul 1;5(7):1481–91.

17. Savar A, Ross MI, Prieto VG, et al. Sentinel lymph node biopsy for ocular adnexal melanoma: experience in 30 patients. Ophthalmology. 2009;116:2217–23.

18. Paek SC, Griffith KA, Johnson TM, et al. The impact of factors beyond Breslow depth on predicting sentinel lymph node positivity in melanoma. Cancer. 2007;109:100–8.

19. Schwartz JL, Griffith KA, Lowe L, et al. Features predicting sentinel lymph node positivity in Merkel cell carcinoma. J Clin Oncol. 2011;29:1036–41.

20. Tuomaala S, Kivelä T. Metastatic pattern and survival in disseminated conjunctival melanoma: implications for sentinel lymph node biopsy. Ophthalmology. 2004;111:816–21.

21. Tuomaala S, Toivonen P, Al-Jamal R, et al. Prognostic significance of histopathology of primary conjunctival melanoma in Caucasians. Curr Eye Res. 2007;32:939–52.

22. Amato M, Esmaeli B, Ahmadi MA, et al. Feasibility of preoperative lymphoscintigraphy for identification of sentinel lymph nodes in patients with conjunctival and periocular skin malignancies. Ophthal Plast Reconstr Surg. 2003;19:102–6.

23. Prieto VG. Sentinel lymph nodes in cutaneous melanoma: handling, examination, and clinical repercussion. Arch Pathol Lab Med. 2010;134:1764–9.

24. Spanknebel K, Coit DG, Bieligk SC, et al. Characterization of micrometastatic disease in melanoma sentinel lymph nodes by enhanced pathology: recommendations for standardizing pathologic analysis. Am J Surg Pathol. 2005;29:305–17.

25. Trivedi NP, Ravindran HK, Sundram S, et al. Pathologic evaluation of sentinel lymph nodes in oral squamous cell carcinoma. Head Neck. 2010;32:1437–43.

26. Allen PJ, Busam K, Hill AD, et al. Immunohistochemical analysis of sentinel lymph nodes from patients with Merkel cell carcinoma. Cancer. 2001;92:1650–5.

27. Pulitzer MP, Amin BD, Busam KJ. Merkel cell carcinoma: review. Adv Anat Pathol. 2009;16:135–44.

28. Ansai S, Takeichi H, Arase S, et al. Sebaceous carcinoma: an immunohistochemical reappraisal. Am J Dermatopathol. 2011;33:579–87.

29. Izumi M, Mukai K, Nagai T, et al. Sebaceous carcinoma of the eyelids: thirty cases from Japan. Pathol Int. 2008;58:483–8.

30. Muthusamy K, Halbert G, Roberts F. Immunohistochemical staining for adipophilin, perilipin and TIP47. J Clin Pathol. 2006;59:1166–70.

31. Maalouf TJ, Dolivet G, Angioi KS, et al. Sentinel lymph node biopsy in patients with conjunctival and eyelid cancers: experience in 17 patients. Ophthal Plast Reconstr Surg. 2012;28:30–4.

32. Shnayder Y, Weed DT, Arnold DJ, et al. Management of the neck in Merkel cell carcinoma of the head and neck: University of Miami experience. Head Neck. 2008;30:1559–65.

33. Warner RE, Quinn MJ, Hruby G, et al. Management of Merkel cell carcinoma: the roles of lymphoscintigraphy, sentinel lymph node biopsy and adjuvant radiotherapy. Ann Surg Oncol. 2008;15:2509–18.

34. Maza S, Trefzer U, Hofmann M, et al. Impact of sentinel lymph node biopsy in patients with Merkel cell carcinoma: results of a prospective study and review of the literature. Eur J Nucl Med Mol Imaging. 2006;33:433–40.

35. Sniegowski MC, Warneke CL, Morrison WH, Nasser QJ, Frank SJ, Pfeiffer ML, El-Sawy T, Esmaeli B. Correlation of American Joint Committee on cancer T category for eyelid carcinoma with outcomes in patients with periocular Merkel cell carcinoma. Ophthal Plast Reconstr Surg. 2014;30(6):480–5.

36. Esmaeli B, Naderi A, Hidaji L, Blumenschein G, Prieto VG. Merkel cell carcinoma of the eyelid with a positive sentinel node. Arch Ophthalmol. 2002;120:650–2. PMID: 12003618.

37. Morton DL, Cochran AJ, Thompson JF, et al. Sentinel node biopsy for early stage melanoma: accuracy and morbidity in MSLT-I, an international multicenter trial. Ann Surg. 2005;242:302–11.

38. Morton DL, Thompson JF, Cochran AJ, et al. Sentinel-node biopsy or nodal observation in melanoma. N Engl J Med. 2006;355:1307–17.

39. Morton DL, Thompson JF, Cochran AJ, et al. Final trial report of sentinel-node biopsy versus nodal observation in melanoma. N Engl J Med. 2014;370:599–609.

40. Faries MB, Thompson JF, Cochran AJ, Andtbacka RH, Mozzillo N, Zager JS, Jahkola T, Bowles TL, Testori A, Beitsch PD, Hoekstra HJ. Completion dissection or observation for sentinel-node metastasis in melanoma. N Engl J Med. 2017 Jun 8;376(23):2211–22.

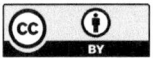

Part II

Conjunctival and Corneal Tumors

Overview and Classification of Conjunctival and Corneal Tumors

Raksha Rao and Carol L. Shields

Overview and Classification

Tumors affecting the conjunctiva and cornea include benign and malignant neoplasms arising from the conjunctival epithelium, conjunctival stroma, and structures within the stroma including the blood vessels, nerves, fat, and lymphoid tissue. Corneal tumors can arise specifically from the corneal epithelium and rarely does the stroma promote a tumor. Most corneal tumors are secondary to extension from an adjacent conjunctival tumor.

The first step in the management of a conjunctival tumor is to take a detailed history regarding the onset, previous precursors, rate of growth, and presence of symptoms such as pain or irritation. The second step is proper evaluation by external examination and slit lamp biomicroscopy. Tumor color, size, location, extension into the orbit or globe, and presence of related features like cysts, feeder, and intrinsic vessels, relationship to the limbus or fornix, and others should be recorded. In many instances, the clinician can differentiate malignant from benign tumors by history and examination. Following thorough clinical evaluation, ancillary testing with external photography,

anterior segment photography, anterior segment optical coherence tomography (AS-OCT), ultrasound biomicroscopy, and incisional or excisional biopsy are all important in achieving an accurate diagnosis. Treatment of conjunctival tumors requires a basic understanding of the biological behavior and the tumor response to currently available therapeutic modalities including surgery, chemotherapy, immunotherapy, and radiotherapy. In this chapter, some of the common benign and malignant tumors of the conjunctiva and their management are presented.

Conjunctival tumors are relatively infrequent [1–5]. An epidemiologic review of 125 patients with ocular cancers from the Singapore Cancer Registry found only 16 (13%) with a conjunctival tumor [3]. In a histopathology review of 2455 biopsied conjunctival lesions in adults at a tertiary referral center, Grossniklaus et al. identified a broad spectrum of lesions including inflammatory, degenerative, and pseudotumors (lesions simulating neoplasm) to represent 53% ($n = 1292$) of cases, while true tumors represented 47% ($n = 1163$) [4]. Among the tumors, the most common included acquired epithelial tumors (26%), pigmented tumors (13%), acquired subepithelial tumors (6%), and congenital tumors (2%) [4]. By contrast, in a clinical study from an ocular oncology tertiary referral center, pigmented (melanocytic) conjunctival tumors were found to be most common [5]. Shields et al. described 1643 conjunctival lesions, among which 872 (53%) were

R. Rao
Department of Orbit and Ophthalmic Oncology,
Narayana Nethralaya, Bangalore, India

C. L. Shields (✉)
Ocular Oncology Service, Wills Eye Hospital,
Thomas Jefferson University, Philadelphia, PA, USA

© The Author(s) 2019
S. S. Chaugule et al. (eds.), *Surgical Ophthalmic Oncology*,
https://doi.org/10.1007/978-3-030-18757-6_6

melanocytic tumors, including nevus, primary acquired melanosis, and melanoma [5]. Even in the pediatric population, melanocytic tumors are the most common tumor in a clinical practice as Shields et al. reviewed 262 children and noted the leading tumors included melanocytic (67%), choristomatous (10%), vascular (9%), and benign epithelial tumors (2%), as well as other miscellaneous lesions (10%) [6, 7].

Recent mega-data on over 5000 conjunctival tumors confirmed that melanocytic nevus was the most common conjunctival tumor (1163/5002, 23%) [8]. Other common tumors were primary acquired melanosis (623/5002, 12%), melanoma (612/5002, 12%), and squamous cell carcinoma (440/5002, 9%) [8]. A separate analysis of this mega-data on pediatric conjunctival tumors in 806 cases disclosed that melanocytic (492/806, 61%) followed by choristomatous tumors (65/806, 8%) were the most common tumors in this age group [9]. In the overall group, comparative analysis of patients with primary acquired melanosis versus melanoma in 1224 cases found those with melanoma more likely showing tarsal location (relative risk [RR] = 1.6), thickness >1 mm (RR = 2.8), presence of intralesional cysts (RR = 2.1), feeder vessels (RR = 2.3), intrinsic vessels (RR = 2.2), and hemorrhage (RR = 1.8) [8]. Comparative analysis of patients with conjunctival intraepithelial neoplasia versus squamous cell carcinoma in 715 cases found those with squamous cell carcinoma more likely showing greater diffuse involvement ($p < 0.0001$), median basal diameter ($p < 0.0001$) and thickness ($p < 0.0001$), location >1 mm from the limbus ($p = 0.0228$), brown pigmentation ($p = 0.0264$), and intrinsic vessels ($p = 0.0234$) [8]. Similarly, in children, nevus versus melanoma revealed melanoma more likely with greater tumor thickness ($p = 0.037$) and base (RR = 4.92), presence of tumor hemorrhage (RR = 25.3), and absence of intrinsic cysts (RR = 5.06), and lymphoid hyperplasia versus lymphoma revealed lymphoma more likely with larger mean basal dimension ($p = 0.002$) and diffuse in location vs nasal (RR = 16.5) [9].

Conjunctival tumors are classified based on the type of tissue that they arise from including conjunctival epithelium, melanocytes, blood vessels, nerves, adipose tissue, and lymphoid tissue. They can also be classified as melanocytic and non-melanocytic tumors, or as benign and malignant tumors. In the following paragraphs, we will discuss the various conjunctival tumors based on major grouping including choristomatous, epithelial, melanocytic, vascular, neural, xanthomatous, myxomatous, lipomatous, lymphoid, leukemic, caruncular, metastatic, and secondary tumors (Table 6.1).

Conjunctival Choristomas

Conjunctival choristoma is a tumor composed of tissues not normally present in the conjunctiva. A simple choristoma contains only one type of tissue, whereas a complex choristoma contains more than one type [10]. Choristomas form a minority of lesions in adults but are the second most common conjunctival tumors found in children after melanocytic tumors [5, 6]. Examples of choristomas include dermoid, osseous, lacrimal gland, respiratory, and complex choristomas. Most choristomas remain stable with little potential for malignant transformation.

Conjunctival Epithelial Tumors

Conjunctival epithelial tumors encompass a wide spectrum of conjunctival and corneal squamous cell proliferation including benign squamous papilloma, keratoacanthoma, hereditary benign intraepithelial dyskeratosis, dacryoadenoma, intraepithelial neoplasia, and malignant squamous cell carcinomas (SCC). Papillomas constitute approximately 1% of all lesions and are associated with human papillomavirus (HPV) in up to 81% of cases [11, 12]. In a large series of 5002 conjunctival tumors, there were only 77 (1.5%) childhood or adult papillomas [8]. Despite this small number, papillomas formed a majority of the benign conjunctival epithelial tumors (77/95, 81%) [8].

Ocular surface squamous neoplasia is an umbrella term for premalignant and malignant

Table 6.1 Classification of conjunctival tumors

Conjunctival tumors	Benign	Malignant
Choristomas	Dermoid	
	Dermolipoma	
	Simple and complex choristoma	
Epithelial tumors	Papilloma	Invasive squamous cell carcinoma (SCC)
	Keratoacanthoma	
	Hereditary benign intraepithelial dyskeratosis	
	Dacryoadenoma	
Melanocytic tumors	Nevus	Malignant melanoma
	Ocular melanocytosis	
	Complexion-associated melanosis	
	Primary acquired melanosis	
Vascular tumors	Pyogenic granuloma	Kaposi sarcoma
	Lymphangiectasia and lymphangioma	
	Varix	
	Cavernous hemangioma	
	Capillary hemangioma	
	Hemangiopericytoma	
	Glomus tumor	
Neural, xanthomatous, myxomatous, and lipomatous tumors	Neuroma and neurofibroma	
	Schwannoma	
	Fibrous histiocytoma	
	Lipoma	
	Myxoma	
	Juvenile xanthogranuloma	
Lymphoid and leukemic tumors	Benign reactive lymphoid hyperplasia	Lymphoid and plasmacytic tumors
		Leukemia
Caruncular tumors	Papilloma	SCC
	Nevus	Melanoma
	Lipoma	Sebaceous carcinoma
	Sebaceous hyperplasia and adenoma	Lymphoma
	Oncocytoma	Kaposi sarcoma
Metastatic tumors		Tumors metastasizing from primary tumors located in the breast, lungs, cutaneous melanoma, etc.
Secondary tumors		Tumors extending from the eyelid, orbit, intraocular structures, and paranasal sinuses

epithelial tumors on the eye, including conjunctival intraepithelial neoplasia (CIN) and invasive SCC. CIN is squamous neoplasia that extends through the entire thickness of the conjunctival epithelium but is confined to the epithelium, not invading beyond the basement membrane. On the other hand, invasive SCC has gross or microscopic invasion into the adjacent tissue.

Invasive conjunctival SCC typically presents in the elderly between 60 and 80 years of age. Younger patients with conjunctival SCC often have underlying disease that promotes a risk like immunodeficiency, allowing human papillomavirus (HPV) to proliferate, or xeroderma pigmentosa, with inability to repair DNA alterations. The exact pathogenesis of conjunctival SCC is not known but it most commonly occurs in areas with high ultraviolet light B rays exposure [13]. A close association with HPV infection has also been observed [13]. Patients with human immunodeficiency virus (HIV) and other immunodeficient diseases are reported to have recurrent and more aggressive tumors [13, 14]. There is also a relationship of conjunctival SCC with heavy cigarette smoking.

Clinically, conjunctival SCC typically manifests in the limbal area as a thin or thick placoid lesion with a gelatinous or papillomatous surface, occasionally forming a nodular mass. A clinical variant of this tumor, called diffuse conjunctival SCC, appears flat and gelatinous in a horizontal growth pattern with diffuse thickening of the conjunctiva and corneal surface. This can be mistaken as chronic conjunctivitis, leading to a delay in diagnosis and treatment. Invasive SCC is associated with feeder vessels, intrinsic vascularity, keratin formation, and sometimes surface inflammation. The tumor can extend into the sclera and globe or into the orbit in neglected cases. Rarely, metastasis to regional lymph nodes and distant sites can occur, particularly in immune-deficient patients. The mucoepidermoid variant of SCC tends to be more aggressive and has increased capacity for local invasion [15].

Conjunctival Melanocytic Tumors

The conjunctival melanocytic tumors include nevus, racial melanosis, primary acquired melanosis, and melanoma. Conjunctival nevus is the most common tumor in both children and adults [5–7, 16]. In a large clinical review of 5002 cases, nevus accounted for 45% ($n = 1163/2590$) of conjunctival melanocytic lesions and for 23% of all 5002 conjunctival lesions [8]. Although considered congenital, it frequently becomes clinically apparent in the first or second decade of life, especially if it is gaining pigment. The nevus evolves from a junctional to a compound and then to a subepithelial nevus with age, as the melanocytes migrate from the basal layer of the epithelium into the underlying stroma [17]. It can be pigmented or nonpigmented, and multiple clear intralesional cysts are commonly seen. Shields et al. described 410 consecutive cases of con-

junctival nevi and found that the most common location for a nevus was the bulbar conjunctiva (72%), followed by the caruncle (15%), semilunar fold (11%), fornix (1%), tarsus (1%), and cornea (1%). Malignant transformation occurs in less than 1% [16, 17].

Conjunctival primary acquired melanosis (PAM) refers to an acquired conjunctival pigmentation that is flat and noncystic, which does not resemble either a nevus or complexion-associated melanosis (CAM). PAM commonly presents in middle age and is usually unilateral. It can be focal or diffuse, and sometimes multifocal. Rarely, PAM can be nonpigmented. Progression to melanoma occurs when PAM demonstrates severe atypia, and this represents 13–48% of cases [18, 19].

Conjunctival melanoma arises either de novo or from a preexisting nevus or PAM. Melanoma arising from PAM accounts for 74% of cases, while those arising from a preexisting nevus and de novo account for 7% and 19% of cases, respectively [20]. The presentation is generally in middle-aged or elderly individuals and it appears as a pigmented or fleshy, elevated conjunctival mass with a lobulated surface. The most frequent location of melanoma is on the bulbar conjunctiva, although forniceal or palpebral conjunctiva is occasionally the site of origin [20]. Similar to nevus and PAM, conjunctival melanoma can be amelanotic and the diagnosis is confirmed on histopathology. Conjunctival melanoma is malignant and can metastasize to preauricular and submandibular lymph nodes, and carry potential for remote hematogenous spread to brain, liver, skin, and bone [17].

Conjunctival Lymphoid Tumors

Conjunctival lymphoma is a clonal proliferation of lymphoid tissue normally present in the conjunctiva. Lymphoid proliferation of the conjunctiva ranges from benign reactive lymphoid hyperplasia (BRLH) to malignant lymphoma. A lymphoid tumor occurring in the conjunctiva can be an isolated condition or a manifestation of generalized systemic disease. In the conjunctiva, the most commonly occurring lymphoma is B-cell non-Hodgkin lymphoma (NHL). Of the various subtypes, the most frequent includes extranodal marginal zone lymphoma (ENMZL), follicular lymphoma, diffuse large B-cell lymphoma, and mantle cell lymphoma [21]. Clinically, a lymphoid tumor presents as a diffuse, slightly elevated fleshy salmon-colored mass deep to the epithelium, frequently located in the forniceal or bulbar conjunctiva. A review of 117 patients with conjunctival lymphoma revealed that 31% eventually developed systemic lymphoma [22].

Caruncle Tumors

The caruncle is a composite structure that comprises both cutaneous elements such as hair follicles, sebaceous glands, and sweat glands, as also conjunctival tissue including accessory lacrimal gland tissue. Hence, the caruncle is a site for tumors of both skin and conjunctival origin. The common tumors of caruncle include papilloma (32%), melanocytic nevus (24%), inclusion cyst (7%), and oncocytoma (4%) [23]. Papilloma has a distinct frond-like vascular appearance arranged in hairpin loops. Caruncular nevus or melanoma is often pigmented and nodular. Oncocytoma originates from the accessory lacrimal gland ductal tissue and appears as a reddish blue solid or cystic mass. Sebaceous gland hyperplasia and sebaceous adenoma appear as a yellow mass.

Vascular, neural, fibrous, lipomatous, xanthomatous, metastatic, and secondary tumors of the conjunctiva are rare and together comprise approximately 10% of all conjunctival tumors [5]. For more information on those tumors, reference to major articles [1, 4–9] and textbooks [10, 17, 24–27] is advised.

References

1. Shields CL, Shields JA. Tumors of the conjunctiva and cornea. Surv Ophthalmol. 2004;49:3–24.
2. Marshall EC. Epidemiology of tumors affecting the visual system. Optom Clin. 1993;3(3):1–16.
3. Lee SB, Au Eong KG, Saw SM, et al. Eye cancer incidence in Singapore. Br J Ophthalmol. 2000;84:767–70.
4. Grossniklaus HE, Green WR, Luckenbach M, Chan CC. Conjunctival lesions in adults. A clinical and histopathologic review. Cornea. 1987;6:78–116.
5. Shields CL, Demirci H, Karatza E, Shields JA. Clinical survey of 1643 melanocytic and nonmelanocytic conjunctival tumors. Ophthalmology. 2004;111(9):1747–54.
6. Shields CL, Shields JA. Conjunctival tumors in children. Curr Opin Ophthalmol. 2007;18(5):351–60.
7. Zimmermann-Paiz MA, García de la Riva JC. Conjunctival tumors in children: histopathologic diagnosis in 165 cases. Arq Bras Oftalmol. 2015;78(6):337–9.
8. Shields CL, Alset AE, Boal NS, et al. Conjunctival tumors in 5002 cases. Comparative analysis of benign versus malignant counterparts. The 2016 James D. Allen lecture. Am J Ophthalmol. 2017;173:106–33.
9. Shields CL, Sioufi K, Alset AE, et al. Clinical features differentiating benign from malignant Conjunctival tumors in children. JAMA Ophthalmol. 2017 Mar 1;135(3):215–24.
10. Shields J, Shields C. Conjunctival and epibulbar choristomas. In: Shields J, Shields C, editors. Atlas of eyelid, conjunctival and orbital tumors. 3rd ed. Philadelphia: Lippincott/Wolters Kluwer; 2016. p. 251–66.
11. Sjö NC, von Buchwald C, Cassonnet P, et al. Human papilloma virus in normal conjunctival tissue and in conjunctival papilloma: types and frequencies in a large series. Br J Ophthalmol. 2007;91(8):1014–5.
12. Kaliki S, Arepalli S, Shields CL, et al. Conjunctival papilloma: features and outcomes based on age at initial examination. JAMA Ophthalmol. 2013;131(5):585–93.
13. Sun EC, Fears TR, Goedert JJ. Epidemiology of squamous cell conjunctival cancer. Cancer Epidemiol Biomark Prev. 1997;6:73–7.
14. Shields CL, Ramasubramanian A, Mellen PL, Shields JA. Conjunctival squamous cell carcinoma arising in immunosuppressed patients (organ transplant, human immunodeficiency virus infection). Ophthalmology. 2011;118:2133–7.
15. Lee GA, Hirst LW. Ocular surface squamous neoplasia. Surv Ophthalmol. 1995;39:429–50.
16. Shields CL, Fasiudden A, Mashayekhi A, et al. Conjunctival nevi: clinical features and natural course in 410 consecutive patients. Arch Ophthalmol. 2004;122:167–75.
17. Shields J, Shields C. Conjunctival melanocytic lesions. In: Shields J, Shields C, editors. Atlas of eyelid, conjunctival and orbital tumors. 3rd ed. Philadelphia: Lippincott/Wolters Kluwer; 2016. p. 307–48.
18. Shields JA, Shields CL, Mashayekhi A, et al. Primary acquired melanosis of the conjunctiva: risks for progression to melanoma in 311 eyes. The 2006 Lorenz E. Zimmerman lecture. Ophthalmology. 2008;115(3):511–9.
19. Folberg R, McLean IW, Zimmerman LE. Primary acquired melanosis of the conjunctiva. Hum Pathol. 1985;16(2):129–35.
20. Shields CL, Markowitz JS, Belinsky I, et al. Conjunctival melanoma: outcomes based on tumor

origin in 382 consecutive cases. Ophthalmology. 2011;118(2):389–95.e1-2.

21. Kirkegaard MM, Rasmussen PK, Coupland SE, et al. Conjunctival lymphoma–an international multicenter retrospective study. JAMA Ophthalmol. 2016;134(4):406–14.

22. Shields CL, Shields JA, Carvalho C, et al. Conjunctival lymphoid tumors: clinical analysis of 117 cases and relationship to systemic lymphoma. Ophthalmology. 2001;108(5):979–84.

23. Shields CL, Shields JA, White D, et al. Types and frequency of lesions of the caruncle. Am J Ophthalmol. 1986;102:771–8.

24. Shields J, Shields C. Vascular tumors and related lesions of the conjunctiva. In: Shields J, Shields C, editors. Atlas of eyelid, conjunctival and orbital tumors. 3rd ed. Philadelphia: Lippinoctt/Wolters Kluwer; 2016. p. 349–66.

25. Shields J, Shields C. Conjunctival neural, xanthomatous, fibrous, myxomatous, and lipomatous tumors. In: Shields J, Shields C, editors. Atlas of eyelid, conjunctival and orbital tumors. 3rd ed. Philadelphia: Lippinoctt/Wolters Kluwer; 2016. p. 367–78.

26. Shields J, Shields C. Conjunctival lymphoid, leukemic, and metastatic tumors. In: Shields J, Shields C, editors. Atlas of eyelid, conjunctival and orbital tumors. 3rd ed. Philadelphia: Lippinoctt/Wolters Kluwer; 2016. p. 379–92.

27. Shields J, Shields C. Caruncular tumors. In: Shields J, Shields C, editors. Atlas of eyelid, conjunctival and orbital tumors. 3rd ed. Philadelphia: Lippinoctt/Wolters Kluwer; 2016. p. 394–402.

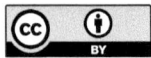

Surgical Techniques for Conjunctival and Corneal Tumors

Raksha Rao and Carol L. Shields

Surgical Management

A thorough examination with documentation of the clinical findings and systematic planning is a prerequisite to any surgery. Clinical examination by penlight and slit-lamp biomicroscopy helps determine the extent of the tumor. Careful inspection of the entire conjunctiva with lid eversion should be performed. Conjunctival nevus, primary acquired melanosis (PAM), or melanoma sometimes has amelanotic component which should be noted. A large drawing of the conjunctival tumor replicating the extent of the lesion in the eye is used in all cases in the office and at the time of surgery. The drawing should include the extent of corneal involvement and the surgical plan.

In general, management alternatives include surgical excision, topical or injection chemotherapy or immunotherapy, radiotherapy, chemotherapy, or targeted medications such as rituximab.

Tumors that come to surgical excision include malignant tumors and some symptomatic benign tumors. Complete excisional biopsy using the traditional "no-touch" technique is advised. The "no touch" technique involves tumor removal without directly touching the mass and only manipulating the surrounding normal tissue as well as the avoidance of balanced salt solution (BSS) for corneal wetting as this also can lead to tumor dissemination. So the entire procedure is performed under dry circumstances and without touching the tumor directly. This is especially important for conjunctival melanoma as it can easily seed into the subconjunctival space and demonstrate recurrence after surgery. Incisional surgery and frozen sections are not often used. However, there are certain exceptions in which incisional biopsy might be considered (Table 7.1).

For papillomas, excisional biopsy and cryotherapy using the "no touch" technique with or without adjuvant oral cimetidine and/or topical/injection interferon alfa-2b provides satisfactory tumor control [1]. For conjunctival intraepithelial neoplasia (CIN) and invasive squamous cell carcinoma (SCC), surgical excision can be performed especially if there is a need to quickly manage the patient, if there are dexterity problems in which the patient cannot place therapeutic eyedrops, or if there is concern about compliance. In such cases, complete surgical excision of SCC using the "no touch" technique is employed. However, with CIN and

Electronic supplementary material The online version of this chapter (https://doi.org/10.1007/978-3-030-18757-6_7) contains supplementary material, which is available to authorized users.

R. Rao (✉)
Department of Orbit and Ophthalmic Oncology, Narayana Nethralaya, Bangalore, India

C. L. Shields
Ocular Oncology Service, Wills Eye Hospital, Thomas Jefferson University, Philadelphia, PA, USA

Table 7.1 Indications for surgery or topical therapy for conjunctival tumors

Conjunctival tumor	Indication for excisional surgery	Indication for other treatments

CIN/SCC	Large, well-circumscribed tumor	Topical chemotherapy or immunotherapy
		  Small tumor
		  Large tumor for chemoreduction or immunoreduction before surgery
		  Diffuse tumor not amenable to surgery
		  Positive margins post-excision
		Plaque radiotherapy
		  Multiple recurrences
		  Scleroinvasive tumors
		Incisional surgery and possible exenteration
		  Tumor invasion into orbit

Nevus	Documented growth Atypical location (fornix, palpebral conjunctiva, cornea) Atypical age at presentation (middle age or later) Positive family history of conjunctival melanoma Patient insistence (cosmesis)	Observation Small, typical nevus
PAM	Lesion diameter ≥5 mm Documented progression of the lesion Thickness of the lesion Distinct nodule arising within the lesion (pigmented or non-pigmented) Nutrient vessels to the lesion Involvement of the cornea Involvement of palpebral conjunctiva Dysplastic nevus syndrome in the affected patient or close relatives Personal history of cutaneous or uveal melanoma	Observation Lesion diameter <5 mm
Melanoma	All cases except where exenteration is necessary	Incisional surgery and possible exenteration Orbital extension

SCC, topical chemotherapy (mitomycin-C and 5-flurouracil) and topical immunotherapy (topical or injection interferon alpha-2b) are alternatives to surgical resection for reliable patients, dexterous in placing eyedrops, for small tumors and for large tumors, especially important for the elderly or sickly patient not amenable to surgical procedures.

For malignancies that invade into the sclera, local plaque radiotherapy is performed to irradiate the invasive area and prevent intraocular growth. For SCC an apex dose of 4500 cGy is given and for melanoma the dose is 6000 cGy. Plaque radiotherapy is particularly useful for

those with multiple recurrences, in an effort to avoid orbital exenteration and other mutilating surgeries [2, 3].

Exenteration is reserved for advanced cases with clinical and radiological evidence of orbital invasion. In general, we use the eyelid sparing technique in which incision is made just outside the eyelash margin so that the posterior lamella is dissected up to the orbital rim, sparing the anterior lamella (skin and orbicularis muscle). The orbit is dissected and removed.

Special consideration is given to the management of conjunctival nevus and PAM. Conjunctival nevus can be managed by periodic observation with photographic documentation or surgical resection, depending on tumor size, symptoms, features, and parental concerns [4]. For most children with conjunctival nevus, observation is provided and the tumor is surgically removed when the patient is older, in the late teenage years. If growth is found, excision is advised. Prompt surgery for conjunctival nevus is considered in those presenting at atypical sites (fornix, palpebral conjunctiva, cornea), at an older age, in patients with family history of conjunctival or cutaneous melanoma, and in large nevus causing cosmetic blemish [4].

Newly discovered PAM which is flat and measures <5 mm in a patient without dysplastic nevus syndrome or cutaneous melanoma can be observed [5]. However, if the lesion shows growth, multifocality, or asymmetry compared to the opposite eye, or measuring ≥5 mm (>2 clock hours), surgery is indicated [5]. If PAM demonstrates even minimal nodulatity, melanoma is suspected and surgical removal is advised. Conjunctival melanoma is a surgical disease and all cases require careful removal of the entire lesion with negative margins [6].

Each tumor is managed in a slightly different way. Conjunctival choristoma is managed by superficial shaving or deeper excision with lamellar sclerectomy and keratectomy [7]. For papillomas, a meticulous "no touch" technique is employed and pedunculated tumors are excised at the base and additional interferon is considered [1]. CIN and SCC require wide excisional biopsy with 4 mm margins followed by cryotherapy to the resected edges [8]. Nevus is a benign growth and excisional biopsy is performed with 2 mm wide margins [4]. PAM and melanoma also require a 4 mm wide margin excisional biopsy and cryotherapy to the resected edges [5, 6, 9]. Lymphoid tumors are treated by excisional biopsy and cryotherapy for smaller tumors, and incisional biopsy followed by chemotherapy and radiotherapy for larger tumors [10, 11]. Caruncular tumors are always managed by complete surgical excision with an appropriate margin on the conjunctival edge [12, 13].

Surgical Techniques

Conjunctival tumor excision can be performed under local anesthesia. This is achieved by 5 mL of retrobulbar injection of a combination of 2% bupivacaine and 0.75% of mepivacaine with hyaluronidase into the retrobulbar space. The injection is given using a 1.25 inch 27G needle attached to a 5 mL syringe. A well-performed retrobulbar block eliminates pain sensation, prevents ocular motility, and does not produce any conjunctival chemosis. We specifically avoid subconjunctival anesthesia as this balloons the conjunctiva and blurs tumor margins. It is important to prevent chemosis to help identify the anatomical landmarks and tumor margins during the surgery. An eyelid speculum is applied and topical anesthesia used for the cornea. The surgery is always done under an operating microscope.

Surgical steps for benign and malignant tumors are similar, except for the need for wider surgical margins for malignant tumors, and a thin scleral base. Wide excision of the lesion (4 mm surgical margin) is the standard care of treatment for malignant conjunctival tumors including invasive SCC (Fig. 7.1a–i and Video 7.1) and malignant melanoma (Fig. 7.2a–l and Video 7.2). In contrast, a 1–2 mm surgical margin is adequate for conjunctival nevus (Fig. 7.3a–i and Video 7.3) and PAM (Fig. 7.4a–h and Video 7.4). The corneal component is identified and the site is gently patted – dry with a single movement without rubbing and with a dry cellulose sponge. Absolute alcohol (ethyl alcohol-ETOH) is applied directly to the affected cornea using a wexcel sponge for 10–20 s and then a second dry sponge absorbs the alcohol to prevent damage [14, 15]. This is done to devitalize the corneal tumor cells. The corneal tumor is removed off the cornea by gently scrolling the epithelium from center to limbus using a #57 Beaver scalpel and this is termed as alcohol keratoepitheliectomy. The plane of dissection is kept anterior to the Bowman's membrane so as to not cause corneal scarring. The scrolled tissue is left at the limbus in a dry fashion. Next, a 4 mm wide surgical margin around the conjunctival component is marked using a bipolar cautery. Minimum manipulation is

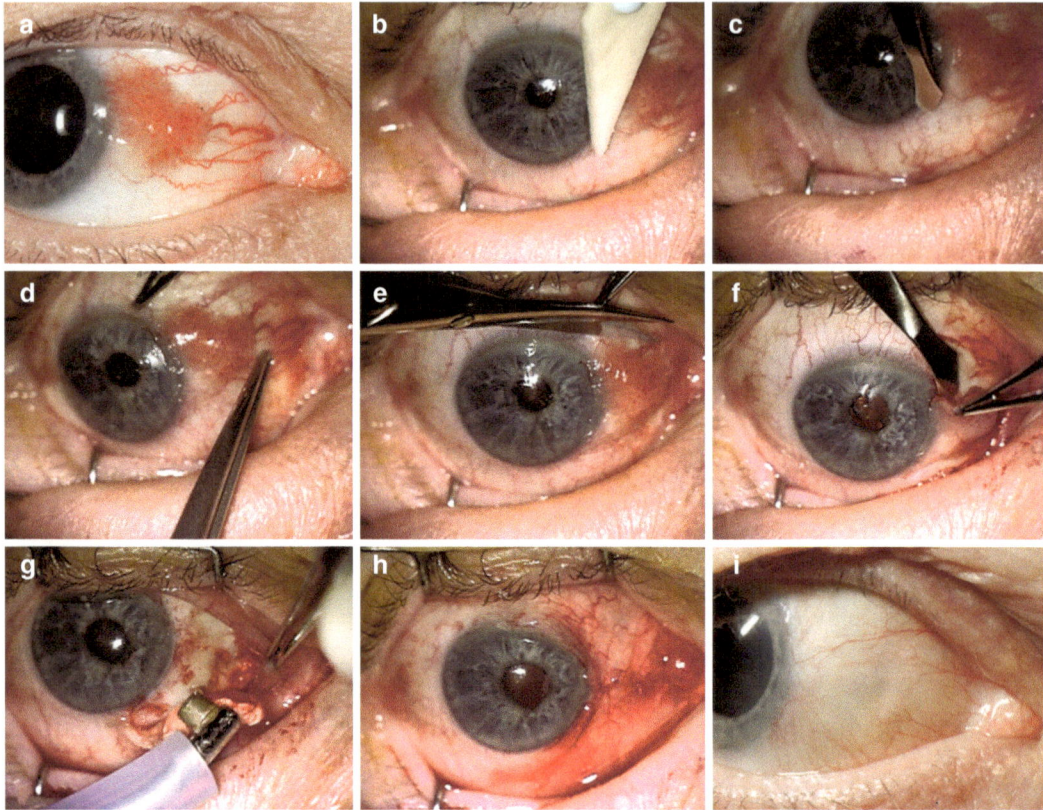

Fig. 7.1 Excision surgery for conjunctival squamous cell carcinoma. (**a**) Conjunctival squamous cell carcinoma of the left eye with prominent feeder and intrinsic vessels. (**b**) Corneal component of the tumor is identified and dried with a dry cellulose sponge, followed by application of absolute alcohol using a cotton-tipped applicator for 1 min. (**c**) Corneal tumor is excised off the cornea by gently scrolling away the epithelium using a #57 Beaver scalpel, with the plane of dissection maintained anterior to the Bowman's membrane. (**d**) Prominent feeder vessels are identified and cauterized to minimize bleeding. (**e**) The conjunctiva is incised with a 4-mm-wide surgical margin using a blunt-tipped conjunctival scissors. (**f**) At the limbus, limbectomy is done parallel to the limbus by sliding the blade back and forth, thus completely excising the tumor with a thin scleral base. (**g**) Double freeze-thaw cryotherapy is done to the resected edges of the conjunctiva by lifting the conjunctiva with forceps and freezing the underside of the conjunctiva to prevent accidental freezing of the sclera or the ciliary body. (**h**) Conjunctival closure is done using a 7-0 absorbable suture. (**i**) Minimal conjunctival scarring with no recurrence at 6 months follow-up

advised to prevent dispersion of the tumor cells. The peri-tumoral limbal conjunctiva is lifted using forceps, and a small incision placed in the conjunctiva at one end of the marked surgical margin using a blunt-tipped conjunctival scissors. A similar incision is placed at the other end of the marked margin. The conjunctiva is incised along the entire length of the surgical margin, allowing adequate normal tissue surrounding the tumor. Only normal conjunctiva is handled and the tumor is never touched. The tumor is then undermined from the tissues below with the help of the scis-

sors. Similar undermining of the Tenon's fascia is undertaken by gentle spreading of the scissors. In tumors where dissection is close to the insertion of the rectus muscles, the muscles may be hooked to avoid damage to the muscle fibers. Hemostasis is achieved with the use of bipolar cautery.

The scleral component of the tumor is removed using a clean #57 Beaver scalpel and a few underlying scleral fibers (5% thickness) are dissected with the mass to provide tumor-free basal margin [14, 15]. This is termed partial scleroconjunctivectomy. The sclerolimbectomy is done with the

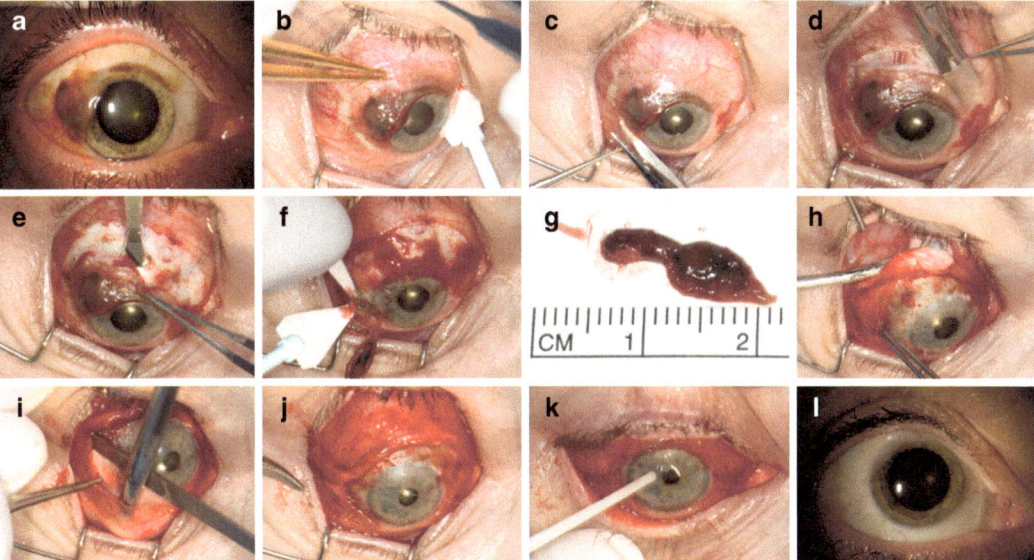

Fig. 7.2 Excision surgery for conjunctival melanoma. (**a**) Conjunctival melanoma of the right eye with dark pigmentation and prominent feeder vessels. (**b**) A 4-mm-wide surgical margin is delineated around the tumor using bipolar cautery, and the corneal component of the tumor is identified and dried with a dry cellulose sponge, followed by application of absolute alcohol using a cotton-tipped applicator for 1 min. (**c**) The limbal conjunctiva is lifted using a forceps, and a small incision placed in the conjunctiva at one end of the marked surgical margin using a blunt-tipped conjunctival scissors. (**d**) The conjunctiva is incised along the marked margin. (**e**) Corneal tumor is excised off the cornea by gently scrolling away the epithelium using a #57 Beaver scalpel, with the plane of dissection maintained anterior to the Bowman's membrane.

(**f**) At the limbus, limbectomy is done parallel to the limbus by sliding the blade back and forth, thus completely excising the tumor with a thin scleral base. (**g**) The excised tumor is placed on a cardboard and placed in 10% formalin for histopathology. (**h**) Double freeze-thaw cryotherapy is done to the resected edges of the conjunctiva by lifting the conjunctiva with forceps and freezing the underside of the conjunctiva to prevent accidental freezing of the sclera or the ciliary body. (**i**) Conjunctival relaxation is achieved by excising the intermuscular septum. (**j**) Conjunctival closure is done using a 7-0 absorbable suture. (**k**) Application of tissue glue on the ocular surface for patient comfort and better wound healing. (**l**) Minimal conjunctival and corneal scarring with no recurrence at 9 months follow-up

flat blade parallel to the limbus with the motion of the blade from the cornea toward the sclera, thus completely excising the tumor with a thin scleral base. Through all these steps of the surgery, use of BSS on the ocular surface is avoided, and this is the dry-technique of tumor excision. The tumor is labeled indicating all the margins on a cardboard bed, preserved in 10% formalin, and sent for histopathology ensuring the correct patient identity on the pathology form.

For further steps of the surgery, a fresh set of instruments is used to prevent any possible tumor seeding from the previous instruments. Episcleral hemostasis is achieved with bipolar cautery. Absolute alcohol is then applied over the bare sclera using a wexcel sponge to devitalize any remaining tumor cell on the scleral surface

then with a #57 beaver blade the episcleral debris is swept onto a wexcel sponge.

Double freeze-thaw cryotherapy is done to the resected conjunctiva edges. This is done by lifting the conjunctiva with Bishop-Harmon forceps and freezing the underside of the conjunctiva to prevent accidental freezing of the sclera or the ciliary body. A dense ice ball formation for 10 s is allowed before slow thawing is done. There is no BSS used for defrosting. The probe is shifted to an adjacent spot such that two adjacent frozen spots overlap slightly to prevent any untreated area. The entire margin is frozen in a freeze-defrost, freeze-defrost fashion (double freeze-thaw). Conjunctival closure is done in two layers with Tenon's fascia deep and conjunctiva superficial or with a superficial graft as described below.

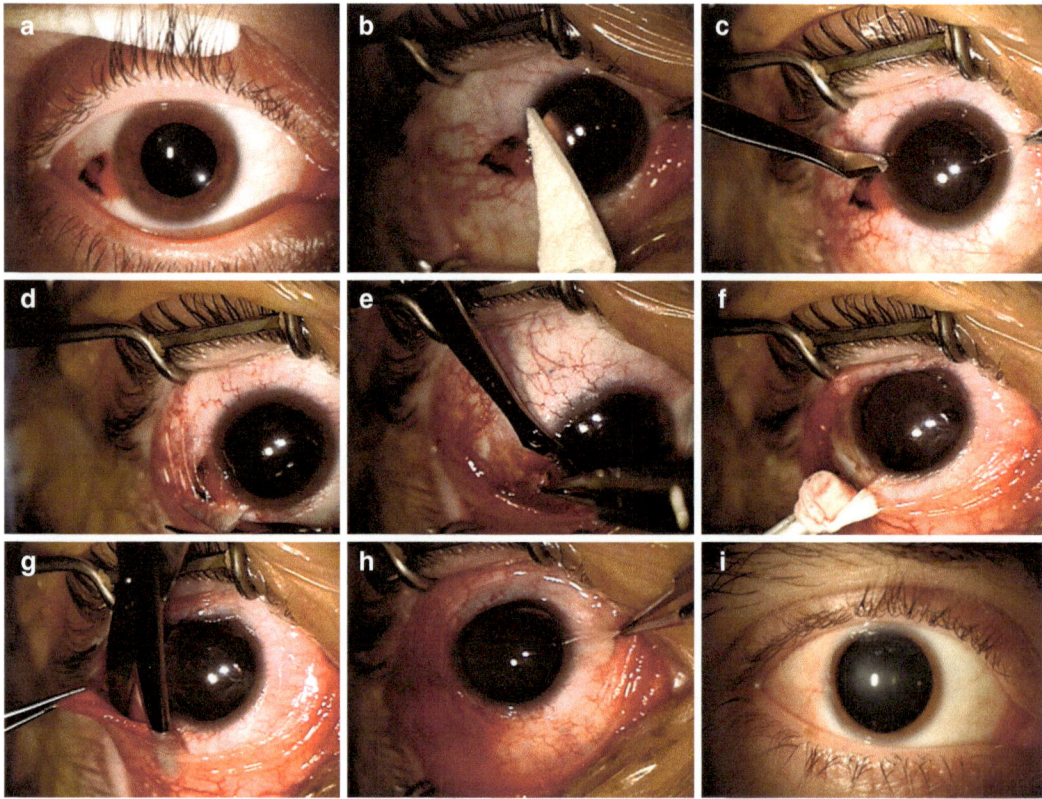

Fig. 7.3 Excision surgery for conjunctival nevus. (**a**) Conjunctival nevus of the right eye with melanotic and amelanotic components. (**b**) Corneal tumor is identified and dried with a dry cellulose sponge, followed by application of absolute alcohol using a cotton-tipped applicator for 1 min. (**c**) Corneal tumor is excised off the cornea by gently scrolling away the epithelium using a #57 Beaver scalpel, with the plane of dissection maintained anterior to the Bowman's membrane. (**d**) The conjunctiva is incised with a 2 mm wide surgical margin using a blunt-tipped conjunctival scissors. (**e**) At the limbus, limbectomy is done parallel to the limbus by sliding the blade back and forth, thus completely excising the tumor with a thin scleral base. (**f**) Double freeze-thaw cryotherapy is done to the resected edges of the conjunctiva by lifting the conjunctiva with forceps and freezing the underside of the conjunctiva to prevent accidental freezing of the sclera or the ciliary body. (**g**) Conjunctival relaxation is achieved by excising the intermuscular septum. (**h**) Conjunctival closure is done using a 7-0 absorbable suture. (**i**) Minimal conjunctival scarring with no recurrence at 5 months follow-up

Caruncular tumors can also be excised in a similar fashion. Medial rectus muscle hooking is necessary in larger tumors. However, unlike at other sites, it is not possible to obtain a 4 mm margin around the tumor of the caruncle.

Post-operative care involves patching of the eye for 2 days with cycloplegic drops and antibiotic-steroid ointment. Use of the ointment twice daily for 3 weeks is advised. Patient is generally seen in a month after the surgery by which time the pathology report is available and the patient can be counseled regarding the final histopathologic diagnosis. In invasive SCC, if the surgical margins are positive, topical immunotherapy (preferred over topical chemotherapy) is advised for 3 months. Radiotherapy in the form of surface plaque brachytherapy is gaining popularity for recurrent tumors and for tumors with deeper scleral invasion [2, 3]. For conjunctival melanoma, if the margins are positive, repeat surgery for clear margins is done. The patient can then be followed-up every 3 months for 1 year, every 6 months for 3 years, and yearly thereafter. The follow-up intervals can be extended for patients with benign tumors.

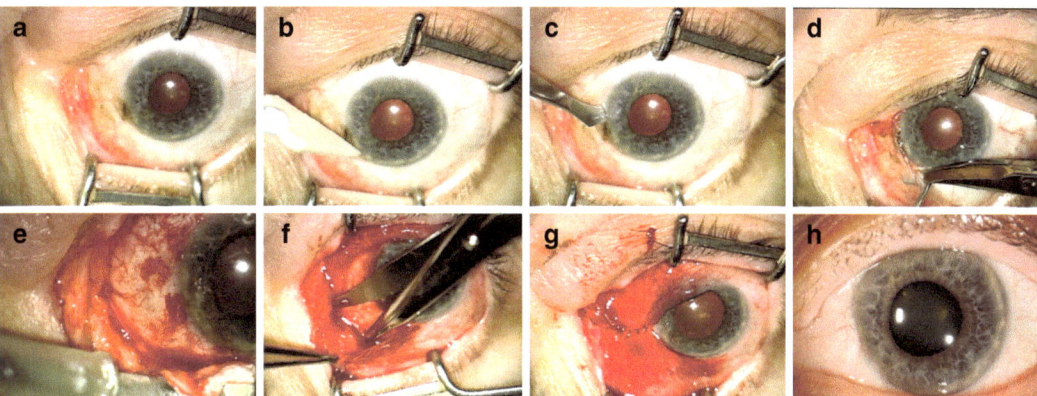

Fig. 7.4 Excision surgery for conjunctival primary acquired melanosis. (**a**) Conjunctival primary acquired melanosis of the left eye. (**b**) Corneal component of the tumor is identified and dried with a dry cellulose sponge, followed by application of absolute alcohol using a cotton-tipped applicator for 1 min. (**c**) Corneal tumor is excised off the cornea by gently scrolling away the epithelium using a #57 Beaver scalpel, with the plane of dissection maintained anterior to the Bowman's membrane. (**d**) The conjunctiva is incised with a 2-mm-wide surgical margin using a blunt-tipped conjunctival scissors. (**e**) Double freeze-thaw cryotherapy is done to the resected edges of the conjunctiva by lifting the conjunctiva with forceps and freezing the underside of the conjunctiva to prevent accidental freezing of the sclera or the ciliary body. (**f**) Conjunctival relaxation is achieved by excising the intermuscular septum. (**g**) Conjunctival closure is done using a 7-0 absorbable suture. (**h**) Minimal conjunctival scarring with no recurrence at 4-month follow-up

Ocular Surface Reconstruction

Conjunctival reconstruction is done by conjunctival advancement, rotational, and flap or with the use of amniotic membrane grafts (AMGs). Advancement flap involves sliding of the conjunctiva to cover the bare sclera. This is done by creating a peritomy at the limbus for 4–5 mm so that the conjunctiva can be mobilized over the defect. The conjunctiva is then closed with 7-0 Vicryl sutures in a running or an interrupted fashion in 2 layers (Tenon's fascia and conjunctiva). For larger conjunctival defects which cannot be closed by an advancement flap, a rotational flap or an AMG can be placed over the bare sclera. The rotational flap is derived generally from the superotemporal fornix and rotated into the defect. The AMG can be freeze-dried or frozen type and is anchored on the surface with the use of tissue glue alone, or by cardinal suturing it to the conjunctiva with 7-0 absorbable sutures. AMG is a source of stem cells and provides a surface over which conjunctivalization can take place [16, 17]. A recently popularized method for stem cell harvest is excision of a 2 × 2 mm area of the superior limbal tissue and cutting it into 8–10 pieces [18, 19]. These small limbal transplants are placed on the AMG, and fixed with tissue glue [18, 19]. This is known as the simple limbal epithelial transplantation (SLET).

Conjunctival Map Biopsy

Conjunctival map biopsies are performed for extensive conjunctival tumors or those that have invaded from adjacent structures, like sebaceous carcinoma. Sebaceous carcinoma has a tendency to exhibit diffuse involvement in the conjunctiva, known as the pagetoid spread (intraepithelial involvement). Small map biopsies are useful to determine the extent of the disease and to plan definitive treatment. The surgery is performed under local anesthesia using retrobulbar block as described above.

Routinely, 10–14 biopsies are taken depending on the suspected area of conjunctival involvement [20]. To gain good surgical access to the deeper fornix, the lids can be everted over a Desmarre's retractor or a simple Q-tip. The map biopsies must include both surface epithelium and tarsal tissue (or the stroma in the bulbar conjunctiva). Each biopsy is approximately 2 mm in basal diameter

[21, 22]. The areas of map biopsies includes superior tarsus ($n = 2$), inferior tarsus ($n = 2$), and all four quadrants on the bulbar conjunctiva ($n = 4$ or more) [21, 22]. If possible, central tarsus biopsy is avoided to prevent scarring that could lead to corneal erosion. If clinically limbal or corneal involvement is suspected, then limbal conjunctival biopsies ($n = 4$) are taken at superior, medial, inferior, and temporal limbus. Each of the specimens is carefully labeled and numbered on a large diagram for histopathologic study. The small map biopsy specimens should be submitted for permanent sections rather than frozen sections.

Once the permanent histopathologic results are obtained, then the definitive surgery can be undertaken after 3 weeks. The need for repeat map biopsies in a patient depends on the clinical findings during follow-up. Double freeze-thaw cryotherapy is done to most of the bulbar and palpebral conjunctiva to provide further assurance that microscopic intraepithelial involvement by the tumor is adequately treated [20].

In conclusion, a variety of benign and conjunctival tumors are seen in children and adults. A basic understanding of the biological behavior of the tumor is pertinent in planning its management. Not all conjunctival tumors require surgery. However, when a surgery is planned, the application of a protocol-based surgical technique can achieve a high cure rate. In addition, the use of adjunctive treatment including topical and locally injectable chemotherapy and immunotherapy, and surface application of plaque radiotherapy have rendered most conjunctival tumors eminently curable.

References

1. Kaliki S, Arepalli S, Shields CL, et al. Conjunctival papilloma: features and outcomes based on age at initial examination. JAMA Ophthalmol. 2013;131(5):585–93.
2. Walsh-Conway N, Conway RM. Plaque brachytherapy for the management of ocular surface malignancies with corneoscleral invasion. Clin Exp Ophthalmol. 2009;37(6):577–83.
3. Arepalli S, Kaliki S, Shields CL, Emrich J, Komarnicky L, Shields JA. Plaque radiotherapy in the management of scleral-invasive conjunctival squamous cell carcinoma: an analysis of 15 eyes. JAMA Ophthalmol. 2014;132(6):691–6.
4. Shields CL, Fasiudden A, Mashayekhi A, et al. Conjunctival nevi: clinical features and natural course in 410 consecutive patients. Arch Ophthalmol. 2004;122:167–75.
5. Shields JA, Shields CL, Mashayekhi A, et al. Primary acquired melanosis of the conjunctiva: risks for progression to melanoma in 311 eyes. The 2006 Lorenz E. Zimmerman lecture. Ophthalmology. 2008;115(3):511–9.
6. Shields CL, Markowitz JS, Belinsky I, et al. Conjunctival melanoma: outcomes based on tumor origin in 382 consecutive cases. Ophthalmology. 2011;118(2):389–95.e1-2.
7. Shields J, Shields C. Conjunctival and epibulbar choristomas. In: Shields J, Shields C, editors. Atlas of eyelid, conjunctival and orbital tumors. 3ed ed. Philadelphia: Lippinoctt, Wolters Kluwer; 2016. p. 251–66.
8. Lee GA, Hirst LW. Ocular surface squamous neoplasia. Surv Ophthalmol. 1995;39:429–50.
9. Folberg R, McLean IW, Zimmerman LE. Primary acquired melanosis of the conjunctiva. Hum Pathol. 1985;16(2):129–35.
10. Kirkegaard MM, Rasmussen PK, Coupland SE, et al. Conjunctival lymphoma—an international multicenter retrospective study. JAMA Ophthalmol. 2016;134(4):406–14.
11. Shields CL, Shields JA, Carvalho C, et al. Conjunctival lymphoid tumors: clinical analysis of 117 cases and relationship to systemic lymphoma. Ophthalmology. 2001;108(5):979–84.
12. Shields CL, Shields JA, White D, et al. Types and frequency of lesions of the caruncle. Am J Ophthalmol. 1986;102:771–8.
13. Shields J, Shields C. Caruncular tumos. In: Shields J, Shields C, editors. Atlas of eyelid, conjunctival and orbital tumors. 3ed ed. Philadelphia: Lippinoctt, Wolters Kluwer; 2016. p. 394–402.
14. Shields JA, Shields CL, De Potter P. Surgical management of circumscribed conjunctival melanomas. Ophthal Plast Reconstr Surg. 1998;14(3):208–15.
15. Shields JA, Shields CL, De Potter P. Surgical management of conjunctival tumors. The 1994 Lynn B. McMahan lecture. Arch Ophthalmol. 1997;115(6):808–15.
16. Tejwani S, Kolari RS, Sangwan VS, Rao GN. Role of amniotic membrane graft for ocular chemical and thermal injuries. Cornea. 2007;26(1):21–6.
17. Paridaens D, Beekhuis H, van Den Bosch W, et al. Amniotic membrane transplantation in the management of conjunctival malignant melanoma and primary acquired melanosis with atypia. Br J Ophthalmol. 2001;85(6):658–61.
18. Sangwan VS, Basu S, MacNeil S, Balasubramanian D. Simple limbal epithelial transplantation (SLET): a novel surgical technique for the treatment of unilateral limbal stem cell deficiency. Br J Ophthalmol. 2012;96(7):931–4.
19. Vazirani J, Basu S, Kenia H, et al. Unilateral partial limbal stem cell deficiency: contralateral versus ipsilateral autologous cultivated limbal epithelial transplantation. Am J Ophthalmol. 2014;157(3):584–90.e1-2.

20. Shields JA, Saktanasate J, Lally SE, et al. Sebaceous carcinoma of the ocular region: the 2014 Professor Winifred Mao lecture. Asia Pac J Ophthalmol (Phila). 2015;4(4):221–7.
21. Shields JA, Demirci H, Marr BP, Eagle RC Jr, Stefanyszyn M, Shields CL. Conjunctival epithelial involvement by eyelid sebaceous carcinoma. The 2003 J.Howard Stokes lecture. Ophthal Plast Reconstr Surg. 2005;21(2):92–6.
22. Putterman AM. Conjunctival map biopsy to determine pagetoid spread. Am J Ophthalmol. 1986;102(1):87–90.

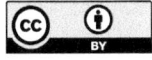

Overview of Intraocular Tumours

Ido Didi Fabian and Mandeep S. Sagoo

Intraocular tumours may be classified according to a wide range of variables, including their malignant potential, incidence, age of presentation, anatomical location within the eye, tissue from which the tumour arises, relation to systemic disease, and primary site of origin (i.e. a primary ocular tumour *versus* secondary deposit from a distant cancer).

Patients with intraocular tumours may present with acute vision-related symptoms, such as reduced visual acuity, visual field defects, flashing lights or floaters; however they can be asymptomatic, depending on the size and location of the tumour. A significant number of asymptomatic patients harbouring an intraocular tumour are diagnosed on routine eye examinations or as part of screening surveys for other diseases such as diabetic retinopathy.

The main benign and malignant intraocular tumours that will be discussed in this chapter are retinoblastoma, choroidal naevus, choroidal melanoma, choroidal osteoma, choroidal haemangioma, retinal capillary haemangioma, vasoproliferative tumour, sclerochoroidal calcification and intraocular lymphoma.

Retinoblastoma

Retinoblastoma is the most common intraocular malignancy of childhood, with a constant incidence worldwide of 1 in 15,000 to 1 in 20,000 live births [1]. In the majority of cases the tumour is initiated by a mutation in the *RB1* gene and mutations in both *RB1* alleles are a prerequisite for developing the cancer [2]. In heritable retinoblastoma, which in most cases affects both eyes, mutation in one *RB1* allele is constitutional, whereas a somatic mutation in the second allele initiates tumour growth in the sensory retinal cells. In non-heritable *RB1*-related retinoblastoma, both mutations are somatic, giving rise to unilateral, unifocal disease in the vast majority of cases. Retinoblastoma patients with the heritable form are also prone to developing additional non-ocular tumours [3] and are at risk of developing trilateral retinoblastoma [4].

Median age of diagnosis of unilateral retinoblastoma is 24 months and of bilateral retinoblastoma is 10 months [5]. A white pupillary reflex, also termed leucocoria (Fig. 8.1), is the most common presenting clinical sign, both in devel-

I. D. Fabian
Goldschleger Eye Institute, Sheba Medical Center, Tel-Aviv University, Tel-Aviv, Israel

International Centre for Eye Health, London School of Hygiene and Tropical Medicine, London, UK
e-mail: didi@didifabian.com

M. S. Sagoo (✉)
Ocular Oncology Service, Moorfields Eye Hospital and Retinoblastoma Service, Royal London Hospital, UCL Institute of Ophthalmology, London, UK
e-mail: mandeep.sagoo@nhs.net

© The Author(s) 2019
S. S. Chaugule et al. (eds.), *Surgical Ophthalmic Oncology*,
https://doi.org/10.1007/978-3-030-18757-6_8

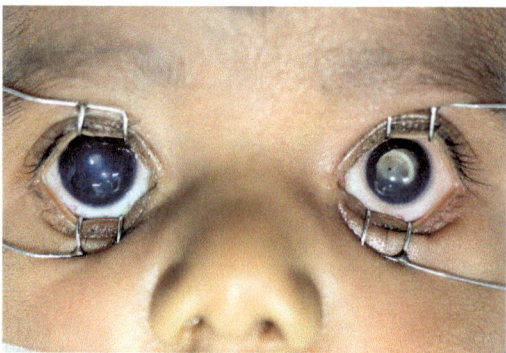

Fig. 8.1 Leucocoria, or white pupillary reflex

oping and developed countries [6–8]. Additional signs are strabismus, and less frequently, red eye, inflammation and additional non-specific signs [8]. Untreated, retinoblastoma will spread outside the globe, via the central nervous system, and haematogenously, inevitably leading to death. In developing countries, in which there is a lack of educational strategies and infrastructure is poor, retinoblastoma patients' survival rate is estimated to be 40% or less [1, 9]. In developed countries, while these were the rates in the early twentieth century, nowadays 5-year survival is estimated to be >95% [10].

Treatment strategies for retinoblastoma have evolved significantly throughout the years. Traditionally, retinoblastoma was treated by enucleation of the eye, a treatment modality still in use today in cases of advanced intraocular disease.

In the mid-twentieth century, external beam radiotherapy (EBRT) was developed and was found to be an effective conservative treatment modality for retinoblastoma. It soon replaced enucleation as the mainstay of treatment for most retinoblastoma cases [11, 12]. Unfortunately, after nearly half a century of extensive use of EBRT for retinoblastoma, it was recognized that radiation significantly increases the risk of developing a secondary cancer in survivors of hereditary retinoblastoma [13, 14]. As a result, radiotherapy was widely abandoned, replaced by chemotherapy as the primary treatment for intraocular retinoblastoma, and to date, is reserved only as a last resort, when all other

modalities have failed. Radiotherapy also forms a part of the protocol for treatment of Orbital RB. The use of systemic chemotherapy as a primary treatment modality for intraocular disease was initiated in the 1990s using potent chemotherapeutic agents, namely vincristine, etoposide and carboplatin (VEC). It was first given in combination with EBRT, resulting in 70% eyes salvaged [15], and following with additional focal therapy, used as an alternative to EBRT, and resulted with high eye salvage rate [16–18]. Soon after it was first introduced, the VEC regimen became the standard protocol for retinoblastoma in most centers.

In order to better predict outcomes of retinoblastoma patients treated with chemotherapy, the International Intraocular Retinoblastoma Classification (IIRC) was introduced in early 2000's [19]. Eyes manifesting the tumour were classified into five groups from A to E (Fig. 8.2) according to size, presence and extent of tumour seeds (vitreous or sub-retinal), and development of secondary complications (e.g. neovascular glaucoma).

In an attempt to avoid potential systemic complications of systemically delivered chemotherapy, new methods of delivery arose, namely, intra-arterial and intravitreal chemotherapy. The former method of delivery developed in Japan [20] and refined in the USA [21] is used in some centres as the primary modality for retinoblastoma, and the latter developed in Sweden [22, 23] and extensively used in Japan and Switzerland is used as adjuvant or salvage therapy [24, 25].

Choroidal Naevus

The commonest fundus tumour in adults is a benign choroidal naevus (Fig. 8.3), arising from melanocytes of the choroidal stroma, often discovered as an incidental finding and is rarely symptomatic. It is a flat or minimally elevated pigmented lesion, but infrequently can be a pale colour (amelanotic). Overlying changes such as drusen or retinal pigment epithelial changes imply chronicity. Approximately 5% of the white population has a choroidal naevus and the risk of

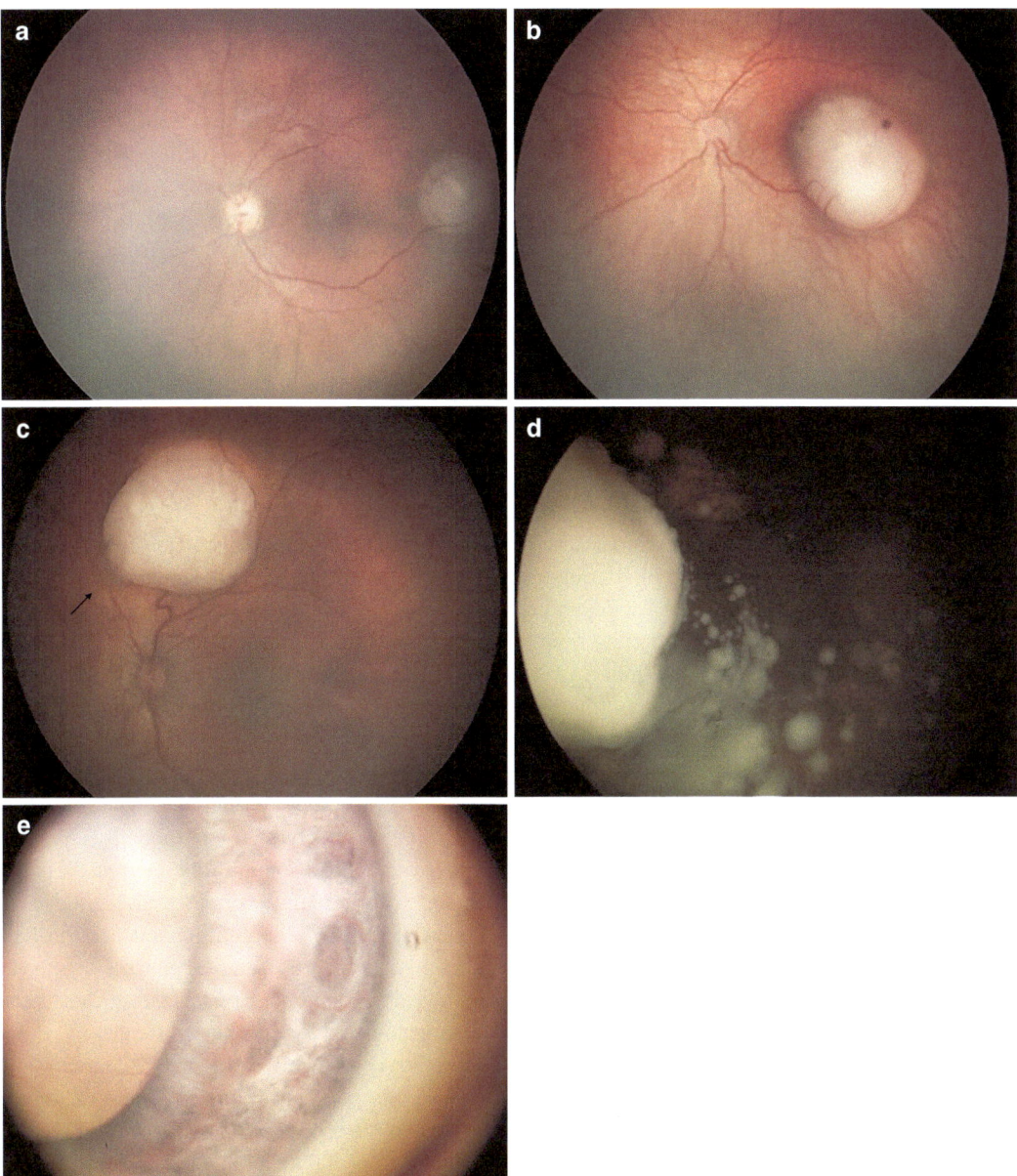

Fig. 8.2 Retinoblastoma tumour grouping according to the International Intraocular Retinoblastoma Classification. Group A: Tumour confined to the retina, >3 mm away from the macula (**a**); Group B: tumour confined to the retina, at the macular region (**b**); Group C: local seeding (arrow) (**c**); Group D: diffuse vitreous seeding (**d**); and Group E: iris neovascularization of the iris and a large tumour seen behind the crystalline lens (**e**)

malignant transformation is low (approximately 1:8000) [26].

A choroidal naevus does not usually warrant treatment, however leakage of fluid into the subretinal space, presence of visual symptoms, secretion of orange-pigmented lipofuscin and/ or growth, raise the suspicion for malignant transformation into choroidal malignant melanoma and need for intervention. Occasionally a naevus will cause symptoms without malignant transformation, such as the onset of choroidal neovascularization [27].

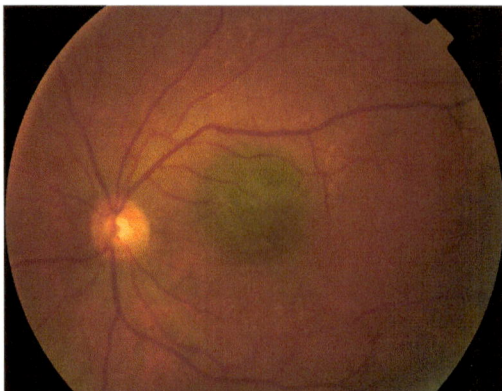

Fig. 8.3 A left eye choroidal naevus

Patients diagnosed from photographic diabetic retinopathy screening with a choroidal naevus should be referred to an ophthalmologist, retinal specialist or even an ocular oncologist depending on the level of suspicion for a complete evaluation. In future this may be changed into a virtual assessment process [28], but for now, the gold standard remains clinical examination, photographic and ultrasonographic documentation.

Uveal Melanoma

Uveal melanoma is the most common primary intraocular malignancy in adults, occurring in approximately 6 individuals per million population annually [29]. Of these, 5% originate from the iris, 10% from the ciliary body, and the majority, 85%, are choroidal (Fig. 8.4). Uveal melanoma mainly affects light-skinned individuals, though it can occur less frequently in dark-skinned. There is a slight male preponderance. It is considered to be a sporadic event, although associated with dysplastic naevus syndrome and ocular melanocytosis.

An undiagnosed or untreated choroidal melanoma will eventually not only threaten vision, but also the integrity of the globe and even risk life. Early detection of a choroidal melanoma is of paramount importance, as tumour size directly correlates with chances of metastatic spread [30].

Common symptoms related to choroidal melanoma include blurred vision, floaters and photopsia. However, patients can be asymptomatic, and the lesion picked up on a routine eye check. Compared to choroidal naevus a choroidal melanoma is an active cancer that grows in size (albeit slowly) and leaks subretinal fluid, and therefore more commonly causes visual symptoms.

Examination reveals a dome-shaped or 'collar stud' mass, located in the choroid, usually pigmented, but can occasionally be partly or entirely non-pigmented (amelanotic). Retinal detachment and lipofuscin orange pigment deposition are common features. Less frequently, they can cause severe glaucoma, cataract, and even extra-ocular extension into the orbit. Such tumours generally carry a worse prognosis.

Historically, uveal melanoma was treated by primary enucleation. However with advances in radiation delivery, most centers now use radiotherapy by proton beam or plaque brachytherapy if tumour size allows, with high local tumour control rates and more than 90% eyes salvaged [31]. In spite of treatment, vision is often compromised or lost due to radiation damage to the retina and optic nerve. Additional modalities, used less frequently, include surgical resection, by means of transscleral local resection or endoresection. Deciding on which treatment modality should be employed depends on multiple factors, including tumour size, visual acuity of the affected eye and contralateral eye, age and general health of the patient, and the presence of metastases.

Uveal melanoma metastasizes via haematogenous spread primarily to the liver, and is believed to occur early in the course of the disease, despite successful treatment of the eye [32]. In a retrospective analysis by Shields et al. of more than 8000 patients, 33% and 25% of ciliary body and choroidal melanoma patients, respectively, were diagnosed with metastatic spread at 10 years [30]. Iris melanoma had a more favourable prognosis. Size of the primary tumour at time of detection was important in determining the chances for secondary spread: at 10 years, metastasis were diagnosed in 12% of small melanoma (elevation ≤3.0 mm), 26% of medium melanoma (elevation 3.1–8.0 mm) and 49% of large melanoma (elevation >8.0 mm). Metastatic spread at the time of presentation with the intraocular tumour is unusual, but sys-

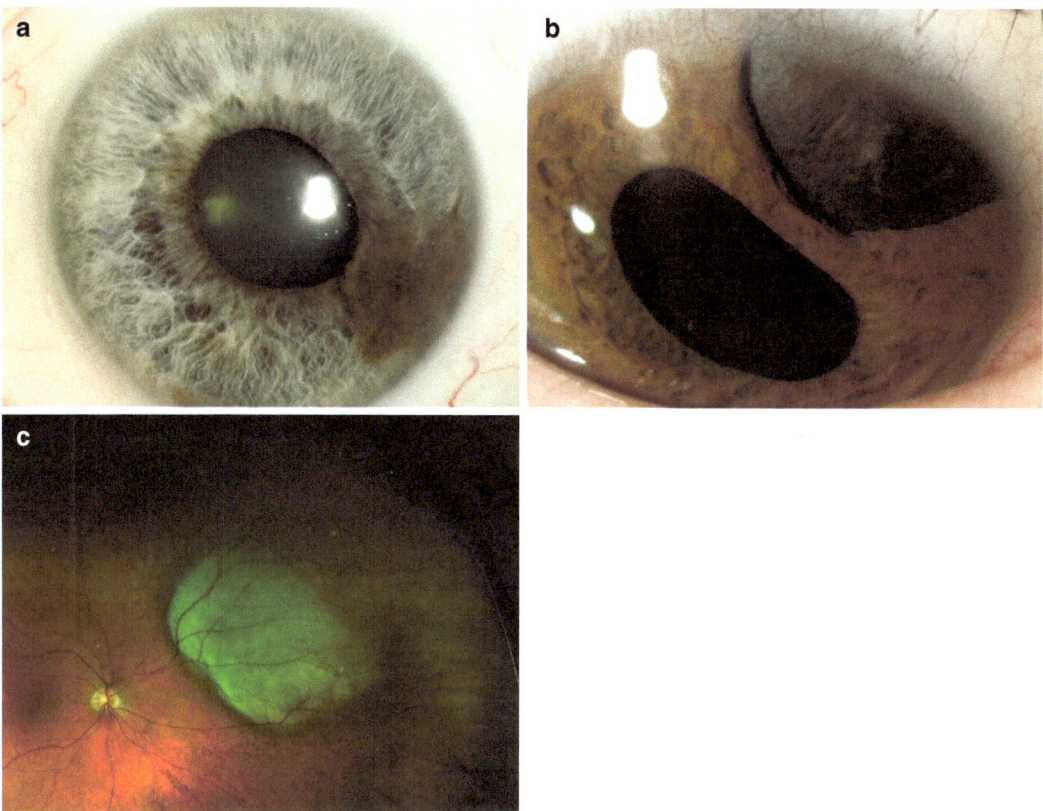

Fig. 8.4 Uveal melanoma in the iris (**a**), ciliary body with iris root erosion (**b**) and choroid (**c**)

temic screening is advised for detection of liver involvement, even years after treatment of the primary intraocular tumour. Despite the improvements in treatment of the primary tumour, a corresponding decrease in metastatic death has not been documented and stands overall at a 5 year survival of 20–30% and a 10 year survival estimate of 50% [33, 34]. To date, metastatic uveal melanoma is a major challenge for physicians to treat although many new targeted immune modulatory treatments are now available such as PD1 inhibitors and MEK inhibitors in addition to targeted hepatic chemotherapy.

Ocular Metastasis

Secondary deposits from distant malignancies occur in the eye; particularly in the choroid due to its vascular nature [35]. The commonest primary cancers to metastasize to the eye are lung cancer in males and breast cancer in females. In approximately 2/3 of cases the primary site of the cancer is already known, but in the other 1/3 will prompt examination and imaging of the rest of the body. If no primary cancer is found, then biopsy of the eye tumour may be required. Choroidal metastases present as yellow creamy subretinal deposits that grow rapidly (Fig. 8.5). They tend to leak fluid in large amounts, as compared to primary ocular malignancies.

Treatment involves controlling the primary tumour site, but also local treatment to the eye with EBRT, visudyne photodynamic therapy (PDT) or plaque radiotherapy to try to preserve as much vision as possible. Patients with poor systemic status usually warrant observation only and systemically treatment-naïve patients that were newly diagnosed might benefit from systemic therapy (e.g. chemotherapy) to have a positive effect on the ocular deposits.

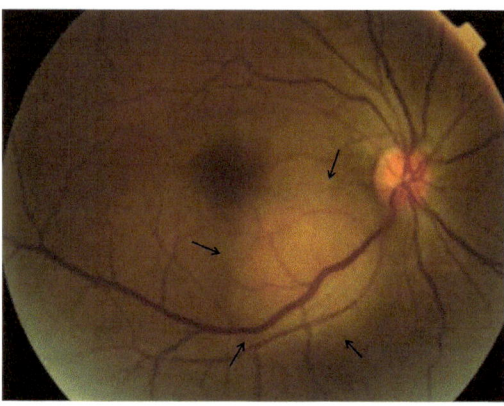

Fig. 8.5 A right eye pale choroidal metastasis (arrows)

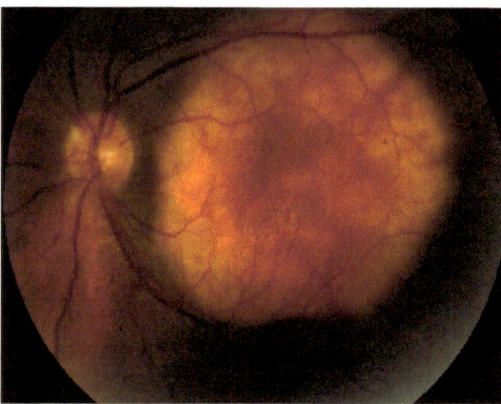

Fig. 8.6 A left eye choroidal osteoma in the macular region

Choroidal Osteoma

Choroidal osteoma (Fig. 8.6) is a benign intraocular tumour composed of mature bone that typically replaces the full thickness of the choroid, and hence is a choristoma (abnormal tissue growth not indigenous to that anatomical location). The tumour classically manifests as an orange-yellow plaque deep to the retina in the juxtapapillary or macular region. It typically occurs as a unilateral condition found in healthy young females in the second or third decades of life. Patients with a choroidal osteoma may be asymptomatic. When symptoms are present they include mild to severe visual blurring, metamorphopsia, and visual field defects corresponding to the location of the tumour. Clinical complications

of a choroidal osteoma include enlargement of its basal diameter, leakage of subretinal fluid and development of subretinal neovascularization with or without haemorrhage [36]. Management options include observation, when no complications occur, or the use of intravitreal anti-VEGF or laser for treatment of neovascular membrane and subretinal fluid.

Choroidal Haemangioma

Choroidal haemangiomas are benign, vascular hamartomas, classified as circumscribed or diffuse. The circumscribed form (Fig. 8.7) occurs sporadically, while the diffuse one is related to Sturge-Weber syndrome, a rare non-hereditary neuro-oculo-cutaneous syndrome presenting at childhood [37].

Circumscribed choroidal haemangiomas commonly occur between the second and fourth decades of life, are usually asymptomatic, but may be associated with visual symptoms, including decreased vision, metamorphopsia, floaters and photopsia. On clinical examination, circumscribed choroidal haemangiomas appear as orange-coloured masses with indistinct borders. Ultrasonography usually demonstrates a dome shaped choroidal lesion with high internal echogenicity. Leakage of fluid into the subretinal space overlying the choroidal lesion is a common manifestation, and depending on location, might result with visual loss. Management options for circumscribed choroidal haemangiomas include monitoring asymptomatic cases, use of oral beta blockers, laser photocoagulation, and visudyne PDT and for resistant or large tumours – EBRT or brachytherapy. Resolution of SRF is achieved in most cases; however visual prognosis depends mainly on tumour location (i.e. involvement of macula).

Retinal Capillary Haemangioma

Retinal capillary haemangioma (RCH) is a benign retinal vascular tumour (Fig. 8.8). RCH may occur sporadically or in association with von Hippel Lindau (VHL) disease, a genetic disorder,

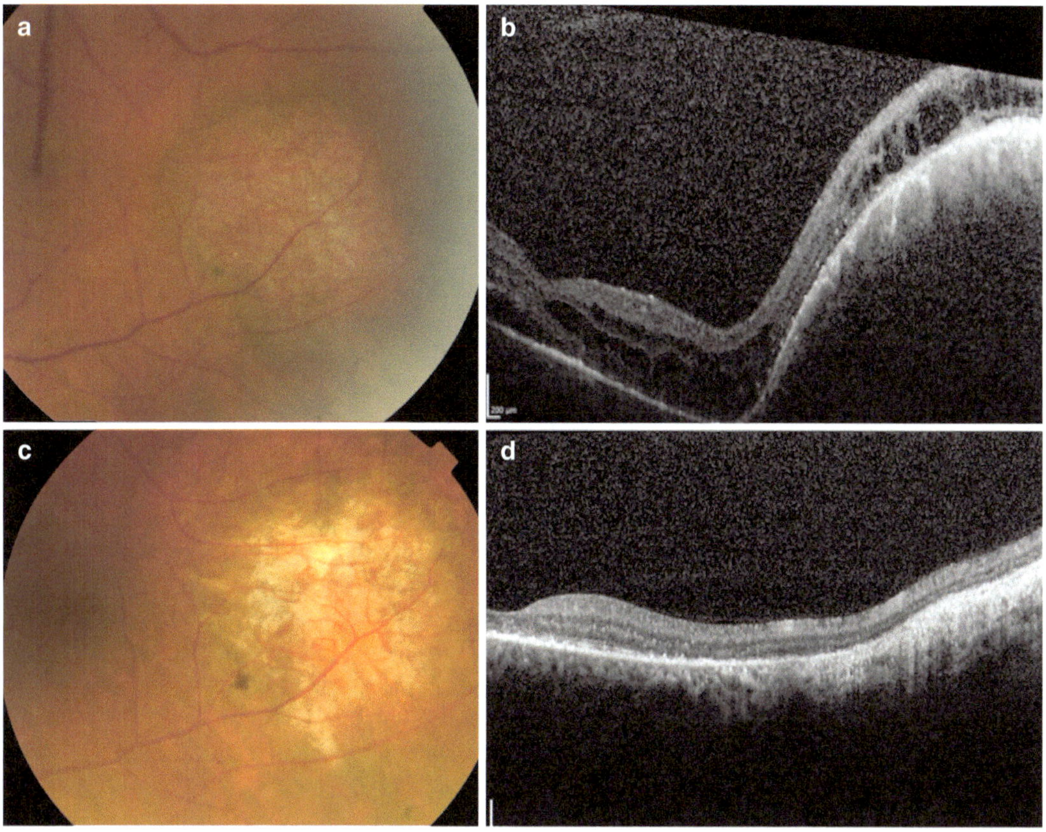

Fig. 8.7 A left eye choroidal haemangioma (**a**), with overlying sub- and intra-retinal fluid, as shown on OCT (**b**). After treatment with photodynamic therapy, the lesion formed into a scar (**c**) and fluid resolved (**d**)

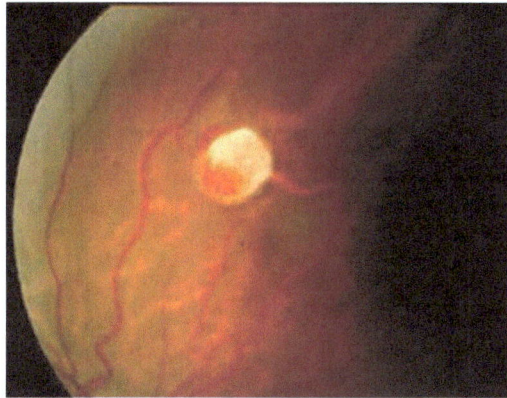

Fig. 8.8 A right eye retinal capillary haemangioma with feeding and draining vessels

which may involve the adrenal glands, kidneys, cardiovascular system, spine and central nervous system [38].

The mean age of diagnosis of RCH in VHL patients is 25 years old. Common symptoms include vision deterioration and photopsia, but some patients may be asymptomatic and diagnosed indecently in a routine eye examinations or as part of screening test for families with VHL. On clinical examination and more evident on fluorescein angiography, a prominent feeding vessel and a draining vein are commonly seen entering and exiting the tumour. Most RCH are located in the temporal periphery and cause intra- and subretinal leakage. Treatment options include observation for small tumours, laser photocoagulation of the tumour and/or feeding artery, cryotherapy, visudyne PDT and plaque radiotherapy. In advanced cases, complicated with retinal detachment, vitreoretinal surgery is a valid option. Regular screening of the body is also recommended.

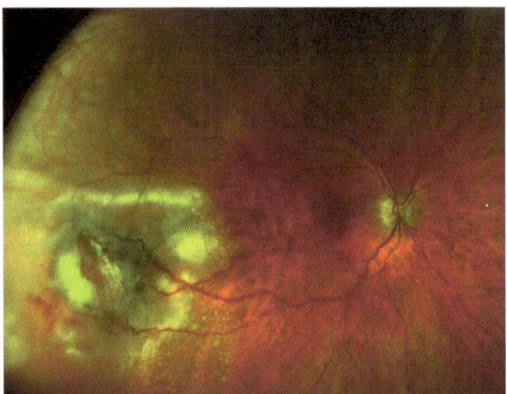

Fig. 8.9 A right eye vasoproliferative tumour with surrounding exudation

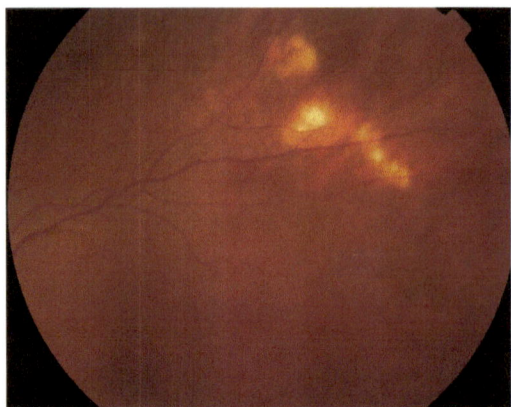

Fig. 8.10 Typical appearance of a left eye sclerochoroidal calcifications located along the superotemporal arcade

Vasoproliferative Tumour

Similar to RCH, a vasoproliferative tumour (VPT) is a benign vascular retinal lesion, present at the third–fourth decades of life. VPTs appear as isolated lesions (Fig. 8.9), but may develop secondary to a pre-existing ocular disorder, in which case multiple lesions are commonly found [39]. VPTs are usually present in the peripheral retina and show significant leakage of fluid. They can be distinguished from RCHs by the absence of large dilated feeder and drainage vessels that commonly occur with RCHs. Macular pucker is a common feature, causing visual deterioration. Treatment options used for RCH are also used for VPT, and decisions as to the best management step depend on tumour size, location, related clinical complications (e.g. exudation, epiretinal membrane) and association to other ocular disorders.

Sclerochoroidal Calcification

Sclerochoroidal calcification is a rare benign condition that classically manifests as multiple discrete yellow lesions, often discovered as an incidental finding in asymptomatic older white individuals (Fig. 8.10). This condition may be idiopathic, secondary to hypercalcemia, or syndrome-associated [40]. The clinical appearance is typical and recognizable by indirect ophthalmoscopy as an elevated mass with overlying

retinal pigment epithelial atrophy. Diagnostic evaluation using ultrasonography can confirm the presence of intrinsic calcification. The lesions are commonly bilateral and located in the superotemporal quadrant along the arcades, and are frequently multiple, features that help differentiating them from choroidal osteoma.

Patients diagnosed with sclerochoroidal calcifications require no ocular intervention unless vision loss occurs from the development of a choroidal neovascular membrane. They should undergo systemic workup to screen for abnormalities in calcium and phosphate metabolism.

Primary Intraocular Lymphoma

Primary intraocular vitreoretinal lymphoma, or PIOL (Fig. 8.11), is an intraocular malignancy that is a subset of primary central system lymphoma (PCNSL). Approximately one-third of PIOL patients will have concurrent PCNSL at presentation, and up to 90% will develop PCNSL within 1–2 years [41]. PIOL is bilateral in up to 85% of cases, although initially it may seem unilateral. Posterior segment findings of PIOL include the presence of vitreous cells in the majority of cases. Another sign is the development of creamy lesions with orange–yellow infiltrates that are deep to the retina. Imaging studies, including fluorescein angiography, OCT and ultrasonography, and tissue (vitreous/retina/choroid) biopsy are usually required for

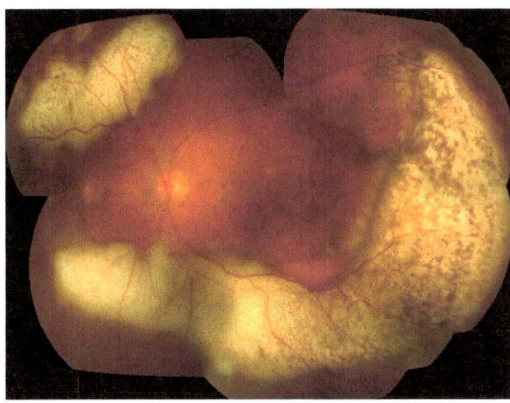

Fig. 8.11 Primary intraocular lymphoma in the left eye showing diffuse subretinal creamy deposits

diagnosis. Treatment of PIOL includes systemic chemotherapy and eyes and brain radiotherapy. Intravitreal chemotherapy with methotrexate and/or rituximab is used to control the ocular disease. Mortality rate in PIOL patients may be as high as 80% at 3 years.

Conclusion

There are many different types of intraocular tumours. Pattern recognition with suitable ancillary testing can assist in the diagnosis and subsequent management of the majority of tumour types.

References

1. Kivelä T. The epidemiological challenge of the most frequent eye cancer: retinoblastoma, an issue of birth and death. Br J Ophthalmol. 2009;93(9):1129–31. https://doi.org/10.1136/bjo.2008.150292.
2. Knudson a G. Mutation and cancer: statistical study of retinoblastoma. Proc Natl Acad Sci U S A. 1971;68(4):820–3. https://doi.org/10.1073/pnas.68.4.820.
3. Eng C, Li FP, Abramson DH, et al. Mortality from second tumors among long-term survivors of retinoblastoma. J Natl Cancer Inst. 1993;85(14):1121–8. https://doi.org/10.1093/jnci/85.14.1121.
4. de Jong MC, Kors WA, de Graaf P, Castelijns JA, Moll AC, Kivelä T. The incidence of trilateral retinoblastoma: a systematic review and meta-analysis. Am J Ophthalmol. 2015; https://doi.org/10.1016/j.ajo.2015.09.009.
5. MacCarthy A, Birch JM, Draper GJ, et al. Retinoblastoma in Great Britain 1963–2002. Br J Ophthalmol. 2009;93(1):33–7. https://doi.org/10.1136/bjo.2008.139618.
6. Bowman RJC, Mafwiri M, Luthert P, Luande J, Wood M. Outcome of retinoblastoma in East Africa. Pediatr Blood Cancer. 2008;50(1):160–2. https://doi.org/10.1002/pbc.21080.
7. Menon BS, Alagaratnam J, Juraida E, Mohamed M, Ibrahim H, Naing NN. Late presentation of retinoblastoma in Malaysia. Pediatr Blood Cancer. 2009;52(2):215–7. https://doi.org/10.1002/pbc.21791.
8. Abramson DH, Frank CM, Susman M, Whalen MP, Dunkel IJ, Boyd NW. Presenting signs of retinoblastoma. J Pediatr. 1998;132(3 Pt 1):505–8. https://doi.org/10.1016/S0022-3476(98)70028-9.
9. Dimaras H, Kimani K, Dimba E a O, et al. Retinoblastoma. Lancet. 2012;379(9824):1436–40. https://doi.org/10.1016/S0140-6736(11)61137-9.
10. Shields CL, Meadows AT, Leahey AM, Shields JA. Continuing challenges in the management of retinoblastoma with chemotherapy. Retina. 2004;24(6):849–62. http://www.ncbi.nlm.nih.gov/pubmed/15579981. Accessed 13 Oct 2015.
11. Stallard HB. Irradiation of retinoblastoma (glioma retinae). Lancet (London, England). 1952;1(6717):1046–9. http://www.ncbi.nlm.nih.gov/pubmed/14928558. Accessed 15 Oct 2015.
12. Reese AB, Merriam GR, Martin HE. Treatment of bilateral retinoblastoma by irradiation and surgery; report on 15-year results. Am J Ophthalmol. 1949;32(2):175–90. http://www.ncbi.nlm.nih.gov/pubmed/18111333. Accessed 15 Oct 2015.
13. Fletcher O, Easton D, Anderson K, Gilham C, Jay M, Peto J. Lifetime risks of common cancers among retinoblastoma survivors. J Natl Cancer Inst. 2004;96(5):357–63. http://www.ncbi.nlm.nih.gov/pubmed/14996857. Accessed 16 Oct 2015.
14. Kleinerman RA, Tucker MA, Tarone RE, et al. Risk of new cancers after radiotherapy in long-term survivors of retinoblastoma: an extended follow-up. J Clin Oncol. 2005;23(10):2272–9. https://doi.org/10.1200/JCO.2005.05.054.
15. Kingston JE, Hungerford JL, Madreperla SA, Plowman PN. Results of combined chemotherapy and radiotherapy for advanced intraocular retinoblastoma. Arch Ophthalmol (Chicago, Ill 1960). 1996;114(11):1339–43. http://www.ncbi.nlm.nih.gov/pubmed/8906024. Accessed 20 Oct 2015.
16. Gallie BL, Budning A, DeBoer G, et al. Chemotherapy with focal therapy can cure intraocular retinoblastoma without radiotherapy. Arch Ophthalmol (Chicago, Ill 1960). 1996;114(11):1321–8. http://www.ncbi.nlm.nih.gov/pubmed/8906022. Accessed 20 Oct 2015.
17. Murphree AL, Villablanca JG, Deegan WF, et al. Chemotherapy plus local treatment in the management of intraocular retinoblastoma. Arch Ophthalmol (Chicago, Ill 1960). 1996;114(11):1348–56. http://www.ncbi.nlm.nih.gov/pubmed/8906025. Accessed 20 Oct 2015.

18. Shields CL, De Potter P, Himelstein BP, Shields JA, Meadows AT, Maris JM. Chemoreduction in the initial management of intraocular retinoblastoma. Arch Ophthalmol (Chicago, Ill 1960). 1996;114(11):1330–8. http://www.ncbi.nlm.nih.gov/pubmed/8906023. Accessed 20 Oct 2015.

19. Linn Murphree A. Intraocular retinoblastoma: the case for a new group classification. Ophthalmol Clin N Am. 2005;18(1):41–53, viii. https://doi.org/10.1016/j.ohc.2004.11.003.

20. Yamane T, Kaneko A, Mohri M. The technique of ophthalmic arterial infusion therapy for patients with intraocular retinoblastoma. Int J Clin Oncol. 2004;9(2):69–73. https://doi.org/10.1007/s10147-004-0392-6.

21. Abramson DH, Dunkel IJ, Brodie SE, Kim JW, Gobin YP. A phase I/II study of direct intraarterial (ophthalmic artery) chemotherapy with melphalan for intraocular retinoblastoma initial results. Ophthalmology. 2008;115(8):1398–404, 1404.e1. https://doi.org/10.1016/j.ophtha.2007.12.014.

22. LA E, ROSENGREN BH. Present therapeutic resources in retinoblastoma. Acta Ophthalmol. 1961;39:569–76. http://www.ncbi.nlm.nih.gov/pubmed/13890561. Accessed 8 Nov 2015.

23. Seregard S, Kock E, af Trampe E. Intravitreal chemotherapy for recurrent retinoblastoma in an only eye. Br J Ophthalmol. 1995;79(2):194–5. http://www.pubmedcentral.nih.gov/articlerender.fcgi?artid=505058&tool=pmcentrez&rendertype=abstract. Accessed 8 Nov 2015.

24. Kaneko A, Suzuki S. Eye-preservation treatment of retinoblastoma with vitreous seeding. Jpn J Clin Oncol. 2003;33(12):601–7. http://www.ncbi.nlm.nih.gov/pubmed/14769836. Accessed 8 Nov 2015.

25. Munier FL, Gaillard M-C, Balmer A, et al. Intravitreal chemotherapy for vitreous disease in retinoblastoma revisited: from prohibition to conditional indications. Br J Ophthalmol. 2012;96(8):1078–83. https://doi.org/10.1136/bjophthalmol-2011-301450.

26. Shields CL, Furuta M, Berman EL, et al. Choroidal nevus transformation into melanoma: analysis of 2514 consecutive cases. Arch Ophthalmol (Chicago, Ill 1960). 2009;127(8):981–7. https://doi.org/10.1001/archophthalmol.2009.151.

27. Papastefanou VP, Nogueira V, Hay G, et al. Choroidal naevi complicated by choroidal neovascular membrane and outer retinal tubulation. Br J Ophthalmol. 2013;97(8):1014–9. https://doi.org/10.1136/bjophthalmol-2013-303234.

28. Balaskas K, Gray J, Blows P, et al. Management of choroidal naevomelanocytic lesions: feasibility and safety of a virtual clinic model. Br J Ophthalmol. 2015; https://doi.org/10.1136/bjophthalmol-2015-307168.

29. Egan KM, Seddon JM, Glynn RJ, Gragoudas ES, Albert DM. Epidemiologic aspects of uveal melanoma. Surv Ophthalmol. 1988;32(4):239–51. http://www.ncbi.nlm.nih.gov/pubmed/3279559. Accessed 30 Mar 2015.

30. Shields CL, Furuta M, Thangappan A, et al. Metastasis of uveal melanoma millimeter-by-millimeter in 8033 consecutive eyes. Arch Ophthalmol. 2009;127(8):989–98. https://doi.org/10.1001/archophthalmol.2009.208.

31. Wilson MW, Hungerford JL. Comparison of episcleral plaque and proton beam radiation therapy for the treatment of choroidal melanoma. Ophthalmology. 1999;106(8):1579–87. https://doi.org/10.1016/S0161-6420(99)90456-6.

32. Eskelin S, Pyrhönen S, Summanen P, Hahka-Kemppinen M, Kivelä T. Tumor doubling times in metastatic malignant melanoma of the uvea: tumor progression before and after treatment. Ophthalmology. 2000;107(8):1443–9. https://doi.org/10.1016/S0161-6420(00)00182-2.

33. Burr JM, Mitry E, Rachet B, Coleman MP. Survival from uveal melanoma in England and Wales 1986 to 2001. Ophthalmic Epidemiol. 14(1):3–8. https://doi.org/10.1080/09286580600977281.

34. Singh AD, Turell ME, Topham AK. Uveal melanoma: trends in incidence, treatment, and survival. Ophthalmology. 2011;118(9):1881–5. https://doi.org/10.1016/j.ophtha.2011.01.040.

35. Arepalli S, Kaliki S, Shields CL. Choroidal metastases: origin, features, and therapy. Indian J Ophthalmol. 2015;63(2):122–7. https://doi.org/10.4103/0301-4738.154380.

36. Aylward GW, Chang TS, Pautler SE, Gass JD. A long-term follow-up of choroidal osteoma. Arch Ophthalmol (Chicago, Ill 1960). 1998;116(10):1337–41. http://www.ncbi.nlm.nih.gov/pubmed/9790633. Accessed 1 Dec 2015.

37. Tsipursky MS, Golchet PR, Jampol LM. Photodynamic therapy of choroidal hemangioma in sturge-weber syndrome, with a review of treatments for diffuse and circumscribed choroidal hemangiomas. Surv Ophthalmol. 2011;56(1):68–85. https://doi.org/10.1016/j.survophthal.2010.08.002.

38. Haddad NMN, Cavallerano JD, Silva PS. Von hippel-lindau disease: a genetic and clinical review. Semin Ophthalmol. 2013;28(5–6):377–86. https://doi.org/10.3109/08820538.2013.825281.

39. Shields CL, Shields JA, Barrett J, De Potter P. Vasoproliferative tumors of the ocular fundus. Classification and clinical manifestations in 103 patients. Arch Ophthalmol (Chicago, Ill 1960). 1995;113(5):615–23. http://www.ncbi.nlm.nih.gov/pubmed/7748132. Accessed 1 Dec 2015.

40. Shields CL, Hasanreisoglu M, Saktanasate J, Shields PW, Seibel I, Shields JA. Sclerochoroidal calcification: clinical features, outcomes, and relationship with hypercalcemia and parathyroid adenoma in 179 eyes. Retina. 2015;35(3):547–54. https://doi.org/10.1097/IAE.0000000000000450.

41. Sagoo MS, Mehta H, Swampillai AJ, et al. Primary intraocular lymphoma. Surv Ophthalmol. 2014;59:503–16. https://doi.org/10.1016/j.survophthal.2013.12.001.

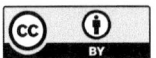

Localised Therapy and Biopsies of Intraocular Tumors

Dan S. Gombos

The majority of intraocular neoplasms are amenable to a variety of treatment options depending on the underlying pathology and location within the globe. Increasingly the role of diagnostic and prognostic biopsies has become an integral part of the management of these lesions. Enucleation and radiation therapy are important treatment modalities that are discussed elsewhere in this textbook. This chapter will review focal modalities including cryotherapy and laser treatment as well as incisional and excisional biopsy techniques.

Cryotherapy

There are many tumors amenable to cryotherapy including retinoblastoma, retinal capillary hemangioblastoma, and vasoproliferative tumors of the retina [1, 2]. Generally, anterior tumors less than 3 mm in height are preferred for this approach. Multiple applications may be necessary to ensure complete tumor regression. The

technique can be performed on an outpatient basis with a local block or alternatively under general anesthesia for children. Using indirect ophthalmoscopy and scleral depression the tumor is visualized and cryotherapy is administered trans-scleraly. The surgeon visualizes the uptake of ice through the entire extent of the tumor followed by thawing. Generally, 2–3 freeze-thaw cycles are administered per session depending on the thickness of the tumor. Care is also taken not to freeze the overlying vitreous. Complications can include serous and rhegmatogenous retinal detachment, vitreous hemorrhage and periocular edema. It is recommended not to administer cryotherapy to retinoblastoma foci associated with significant calcification due to the risk of retinal tear [3].

There are various cryotherapy models that are available, some with greater length and curvature. While the technique is best suited for anterior tumors, following a conjunctival cut down, access and administration to posterior segment lesions is possible.

Laser Therapy

Laser therapy plays a significant role in the treatment of various tumors managed by ocular oncologists. It can be administered as a primary or adjuvant modality and is used for both malignant and benign neoplasms including

Electronic supplementary material The online version of this chapter (https://doi.org/10.1007/978-3-030-18757-6_9) contains supplementary material, which is available to authorized users.

D. S. Gombos (✉)
Section of Ophthalmology, Department of Head & Neck Surgery, MD Anderson Cancer Center, Houston, TX, USA
e-mail: dgombos@mdanderson.org

uveal melanoma, choroidal metastasis, retinoblastoma, circumscribed choroidal hemangioma, and retinal capillary hemangiomas. There are different types of lasers each with distinct indications. These include traditional photocoagulation, thermotherapy, and photodynamic therapy.

Thermotherapy

Thermotherapy is generally used to manage uveal tumors as well as retinoblastoma. Small lesions can be lasered as a primary modality. Alternatively, it can be administered in an adjuvant setting after primary radiation or chemotherapy [4–6]. The laser is painful and requires either retrobulbar or (for pediatric patients) general anesthetic. The technique utilizes an 810 nm laser administered via slit lamp or indirect attachment. Principles of therapy include continuous large spot application directly to the tumor. The clinician begins at a low energy setting and gradually increases power at small intervals until a gray uptake is appreciated. A dense white appearance and application directly to retinal vessels should be avoided. Concomitant administration of indocyanine green (ICG) can be used for amelanotic lesions such as retinoblastoma and select choroidal metastases [7]. Complications to therapy include retinal and vitreous hemorrhage, vascular occlusion, serous and rhegmatogenous retinal detachment. It is preferred to avoid direct laser over areas with calcification for retinoblastoma foci. In general, this technique requires multiple applications until an acceptable endpoint with flattening of the tumor is achieved.

Photocoagulation

Photocoagulation administers therapy at higher temperatures than thermotherapy. It is commonly used for retinal tumors including capillary hemangiomas and in select cases as an adjuvant for retinoblastoma. Historically it was used to manage small uveal melanomas however, this has largely been abandoned. Laser can be administered with various wavelengths. A common one is 532 nm. For retinal capillary hemangioblastomas, topical anesthesia is administered and laser applied via slit lamp or indirect attachment. Spots are applied circumferentially avoiding draining vessels. Subsequently, laser is administered to the surface of the lesion. Settings employ a low power, long interval approach. Multiple sessions may be necessary to achieve complete regression [8, 9]. Complications include hemorrhage, vascular occlusion, retinal exudation, and detachment. Treating retinoblastoma lesions with this modality requires care to avoid retinal perforation, tear, and rupture of the tumor leading to seeding. Clinicians should avoid direct application to areas of calcification and maintain low power settings with a gray endpoint.

Photodynamic Therapy

Photodynamic therapy was initially introduced for the management of macular degeneration. It includes the intravenous infusion of a photosensitizing agent, verteporfin, followed by laser administration. Subsequent studies demonstrated efficacy in the management of circumscribed choroidal hemangiomas [10, 11]. Recent reports have expanded its indication to include choroidal metastatic tumors [12]. Treatment involves topical anesthesia and administration of the photosensitizing agent intravenously. Similar to macular degeneration treatment is applied with a large spot over the entire neoplasm. If the lesion is too large to be encompassed with one spot, multiple spots can be applied with minimal overlap. Full fluence (50 J/cm^2 600 mW/cm^2 689 nm light over 83 seconds) as well as half fluence (25 J/cm^2 600 mW/cm^2 689 nm light over 83 seconds) has been described. One or two sessions are effective in inducing tumor regression. Following laser, patients should be instructed to avoid sunlight due to the photosensitizing agent.

Intraocular Biopsy

Historically many clinicians deferred intraocular biopsy for concern of extraocular extension. The last two decades has seen a significant shift toward increased use of this technique. Biopsies may be excisional with the intent of tumor resection or incisional with the desire of tumor sampling. Incisional biopsies can be performed for diagnostic or prognostic purposes. Except under unique circumstances, the biopsy of an eye thought to be harboring retinoblastoma is contraindicated. The techniques differ for tumors in the anterior versus posterior segment.

Posterior Segment Incisional Biopsy

Indications of incisional biopsy are for histopathologic diagnosis or prognostic testing for diseases such as uveal melanoma. Posterior segment lesions can be approached with either an ab interno or ab externo approach. External approaches are preferred for tumors anterior to the equator. Internal approaches work best for those located more posteriorly.

An Interno

Internal approaches involve sampling the eye from the pars plana through the vitreous into the retina and underlying choroid. This can be achieved with a use of an indirect ophthalmoscope and a 25- or 27-gauge needle [13, 14]. The patient is placed under general anesthesia and a conjunctival peritomy is performed. The muscles are isolated in standard fashion and indirect ophthalmoscopy is used to visualize the tumor. The biopsy is obtained from the same quadrant were the tumor is located. The needle is inserted between 3 and 4 mm posterior to the limbus and is visualized through its introduction into the eye toward the center of the tumor. The sample is aspirated under direct visualization and the needle removed through the pars plana. Cryotherapy can be administered at the biopsy site to lower the risk of extraocular extension. The same approach can be used with a traditional three-port vitrectomy. Some surgeons prefer a two-port approach (excluding the infusion line) using a small gauge vitrector. It should be noted that biopsies requiring histopathologic assessment often require more tissue than those for prognostic testing alone. Complications include vitreous hemorrhage and retinal detachment (Video 9.1).

Ab Externo

For tumors anterior to the equator, an external approach is sometimes preferred and allows for larger volume tissue sampling. Following a peritomy and isolation of the extraocular muscles, the tumor is identified with a combination of transillumination and indirect ophthalmoscopy. The biopsy is directed toward thickest portion of the tumor. A 90% thickness scleral flap measuring approximately 4×4 mm is constructed and hinged over the center of the neoplasm. Toward the base of the flap, the remaining fibers of the sclera are pierced with a blade, removing a uveal sample approximately one by one millimeters in size. Judicious application of cautery and use of systemic hypotension are helpful in minimizing bleeding. The wound is closed with nylon or silk suture. If lymphoma the tissue should be placed in liquid media (RPMI).

Vitrectomy

Primary intraocular lymphoma often presents as a vitritis. Vitrectomy is critical in obtaining accurate diagnosis. In these cases, a three-port vitrectomy is used with a low rate of cutting on the vitrector. As much vitreous debris as possible should be removed. An initial undiluted core sample is sent to the pathologist as well as the cassette. The pathologist should be informed in advance of the possible diagnosis of intraocular lymphoma so that the specimen can be properly analyzed with ThinPrep and flow cytometry [15].

Biopsy of Anterior Segment Tumors

Similar to the posterior segment, the anterior segment can be biopsied via an internal or external approach. For fine-needle aspirations, a 27-gauge or smaller-gauge needle is inserted through the limbus under direct microscopic visualization into the tumor. The surgeon or assistant performs the aspiration. Following removal of the needle, the anterior chamber may need to be reinflated with BSS. Post biopsy hyphema can occur and is often self-limited. Alternatively, an external approach can be used in which a keratome is inserted slightly behind the limbus in the quadrant of the tumor allowing the iris to present at the wound. Using forceps and iris scissors a small piece of tumor is excised and the iris positioned back into the anterior chamber. The wound is then closed with interrupted nylon suture in traditional fashion.

Excisional Biopsy of Intraocular Neoplasm

Posterior scleral-uvectomy was once a common technique within the field of ocular oncology. Its use has diminished significantly in part due to its technical difficulties and numerous complications. It is more common for this approach to be used for smaller irido-ciliary neoplasms.

The patient is placed under general anesthesia preferably under hypotensive conditions. Following a peritomy and isolation of the extraocular muscles, the margins of the tumor are demarcated with an adjacent circumferential 2–3 mm margin. A nearly full-thickness scleral flap is constructed hinged toward the fornix. Cautery is applied to the peripheral edges and the tumor is then incised with a knife and circumferentially excised with scissors. As the tumor is expressed, it is gently separated from the retina. The sclera is then reapproximated with interrupted nylon suture and the eye reinflated with BSS. Some surgeons combine this approach with a posterior vitrectomy. Following excision adjuvant radiotherapy in the form of a plaque may be necessary. Common complications include hypotony, retinal detachment, and vitreous hemorrhage. Incomplete excision and expulsive hemorrhage are also possible [16, 17].

Excisional Biopsy of Iris Tumors

The complete excision of an iris tumor is similar to the approach used for extracapsular cataract surgery. The patient is given general or local (retrobulbar) anesthesia. An incision is made into the anterior chamber in the same quadrant as the neoplasm. Corneal scleral scissors are used to extend the wound 1–2 mm beyond the margins of the tumor. Using iris forceps and scissors a wedge of the iris is excised and the lesion removed from the anterior segment. Care is made to avoid extension into the ciliary body region. Localized hemorrhage can occur. The wound is reapproximated with interrupted nylon suture and the anterior chamber inflated with BSS. Due to the associated defect of the iris, some surgeons suture the edges of the lesion with a nonabsorbable (prolene) suture to reconstruct the pupil. Adjuvant radiotherapy may be necessary if the margins are positive on histopathology. Complications include hyphema, incomplete excision, photophobia and polyopia.

Conclusion

Focal therapies such as laser and cryotherapy are important treatment options in the management of many intraocular neoplasms such as retinoblastoma and uveal melanoma. Similarly, excisional and incisional biopsy techniques have become increasingly important, as the role of prognostic testing for uveal melanoma has become standard of care. It is imperative that the ocular oncologist understand the advantages and complications of each technique to provide an individualized approach for tumor management.

Acknowledgments We are grateful to Vikas Khetan MD, Shri Bhagwan Mahavir Vitreoretinal Services, Sankara Nethralaya, Chennai, India, for his contribution as the expert reviewer for this section.

The video-9.1 Intraocular tumor biopsy was contributed by Pukhraj Rishi. MD, FRSC, FRSCEd, Shri Bhagwan Mahavir Vitreoretinal Services, Sankara Nethralaya, Chennai, India.

References

1. Shields JA, Parsons H, Shields CL, Giblin ME. The role of cryotherapy in the management of retinoblastoma. Am J Ophthalmol. 1989;108(3):260–4.
2. Kim H, Yi JH, Kwon HJ, et al. Therapeutic outcomes of retinal hemangioblastomas. Retina. 2014;34(12):2479–86.
3. Anagnoste SR, Scott IU, Murray TG, et al. Rhegmatogenous retinal detachment in retinoblastoma patients undergoing chemoreduction and cryotherapy. Am J Ophthalmol. 2000;129(6):817–9.
4. Shields CL, Santos MC, Diniz W, et al. Thermotherapy for retinoblastoma. Arch Ophthalmol. 1999;117(7):885–93.
5. Journée-de Korver JG, Keunen JE. Thermotherapy in the management of choroidal melanoma. Prog Retin Eye Res. 2002;21(3):303–17.
6. Ardjomand N, Kucharczyk M, Langmann G. Transpupillary thermotherapy for choroidal metastases. Ophthalmologica. 2001;215(3):241–4.
7. Puri P, Gupta M, Rundle PA, Rennie IG. Indocyanine green augmented transpupillary thermotherapy in the management of choroidal metastasis from breast carcinoma. Eye (Lond). 2001;15(Pt 4):515–8.
8. Singh AD, Shields CL, Shields JA. von Hippel-Lindau disease. Surv Ophthalmol. 2001;46(2):117–42.
9. Schmidt D, Natt E, Neumann HP. Long-term results of laser treatment for retinal angiomatosis in von Hippel-Lindau disease. Eur J Med Res. 2000;5(2):47–58.
10. Cerman E, Çekiç O. Clinical use of photodynamic therapy in ocular tumors. Surv Ophthalmol. 2015;60(6):557–74.
11. Blasi MA, Tiberti AC, Scupola A, et al. Photodynamic therapy with verteporfin for symptomatic circumscribed choroidal hemangioma: five-year outcomes. Ophthalmology. 2010;117(8):1630–7.
12. Ghodasra DH, Demirci H. Photodynamic therapy for choroidal metastasis. Am J Ophthalmol. 2016;161:104–9.
13. Augsburger JJ, Shields JA. Fine needle aspiration biopsy of solid intraocular tumors: indications, instrumentation and techniques. Ophthalmic Surg. 1984;15(1):34–40.
14. Augsburger JJ, Corrêa ZM, Schneider S, et al. Diagnostic transvitreal fine-needle aspiration biopsy of small melanocytic choroidal tumors in nevus versus melanoma category. Trans Am Ophthalmol Soc. 2002;100:225–32.
15. Raparia K, Chang CC, Chévez-Barrios P. Intraocular lymphoma: diagnostic approach and immunophenotypic findings in vitrectomy specimens. Arch Pathol Lab Med. 2009;133(8):1233–7.
16. Damato B, Foulds WS. Indications for trans-scleral local resection of uveal melanoma. Br J Ophthalmol. 1996;80(11):1029–30.
17. Damato BE, Paul J, Foulds WS. Risk factors for residual and recurrent uveal melanoma after trans-scleral local resection. Br J Ophthalmol. 1996;80(2):102–8.

Suggested Videos

https://www.youtube.com/watch?v=QeG_mqfqKMA
https://eyetube.net/video/23-25g-chandelier-assisted-biopsy-of-choroidal-mass
https://www.aao.org/clinical-video/choroidal-tumor-biopsy

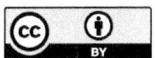

Part IV

Orbital Tumors

Zeynel A. Karcioglu

Incidence of Orbital Tumors

Primary Tumors of Orbit

Although the incidence of different orbital tumors varies considerably among large series, it is plausible to group the orbital space-occupying lesions as 60% benign and 40% malignant pathologies in adults.

The frequency of malignancy is about 20% among young patients within the age range of 1–18 years. The incidence of malignant tumors upsurges with aging chiefly because of the higher prevalence of lymphomas and metastatic tumors [1–9].

Another approach to classification is to divide the orbital tumors as cystic or partially cystic, versus solid lesions; in adults this ratio is about 30% and 70% respectively. The percentage of cystic lesions is higher in younger age groups primarily because of the common occurrence of dermoid and other congenital hamartomas (vascular and others) and rarely as a result of cystic degeneration within some solid tumors such as meningioma and schwannoma in children [10–11].

The most common diagnoses in all age groups are vascular hamartomatous lesions [infantile hemangioma, cavernous malformations, and venolymphatic malformations] representing approximately 15–20% of all orbital masses. Lymphoproliferative lesions and lacrimal fossa masses represent between 10% and 15%, while non-specific orbital inflammatory lesions, optic nerve tumors [glioma and meningioma], and secondary masses from regional tumors all represent between 5% and 10%. Metastatic tumors from a systemic primary disease may represent approximately 5% of orbital disease. Mesenchymal lesions such as schwannoma, rhabdomyosarcoma, osteogenic tumors, etc. are encountered much less frequently, usually below 2–3% in large series.

The most frequently encountered primary orbital tumors in adults are lymphoproliferative lesions and cavernous malformations. In children, the most common orbital tumors tend to be cystic and benign including dermoid cysts and vascular lesions [infantile hemangioma, venolymphatic malformations]. Less common malignancies include rhabdomyosarcoma, histiocytic tumors, Burkitt's lymphoma, neuroblastoma, Ewing sarcoma, Wilms tumor, and leukemia [12–13].

Metastatic Tumors of Orbit

The prevalence of metastatic neoplasms to orbit has increased in recent decades, due to increased numbers of cancer patients in general, viral epidemics, higher levels of UV and chemical exposures. Further, improved treatments have

Z. A. Karcioglu (✉)
Department of Ophthalmology,
University of Virginia, Charlottesville, VA, USA
e-mail: zak8g@virginia.edu

© The Author(s) 2019
S. S. Chaugule et al. (eds.), *Surgical Ophthalmic Oncology*,
https://doi.org/10.1007/978-3-030-18757-6_10

led to an upsurge in the median survival of these patients, which may increase the risk of developing metastatic lesions throughout the body, including the orbit. An improved level of awareness for orbital metastases has increased detection of these lesions across all disciplines of medicine.

Recent cumulative data indicates that the most commonly affected regions of the orbit with metastatic tumors are lateral (40%), superior (30%), medial (20%), and inferior (10%) quadrants [14]. Another report claims that the anterior orbit, adjacent to lymphatic rich conjunctiva and eyelids, is most commonly involved with metastatic tumors [15].

Some malignancies show distinct tissue selectivity in metastatic disease, for instance, prostate cancer tends toward bone, breast to orbital fat, and carcinoid tumor to muscle. These tendencies can aid in diagnostic planning.

In about 25% of the cases, there may be no history of systemic cancer at the time of orbital tumor presentation. Similar to primary tumors of the orbit, most common presenting signs and symptoms include rapidly developing proptosis and associated eyelid and conjunctiva anomalies, pain, diplopia, and rarely isolated optic neuropathy and enophthalmos. Because of the rapid growth of the malignant neoplasm, the motility disturbance may be out of proportion to the degree of proptosis. Enophthalmos is rare and typically seen in sclerotic carcinomas or after radiation therapy of a preceding orbital mass. Isolated metastases to the eyelid and periocular skin and eyelids are rare [16–17].

Most commonly encountered secondary and metastatic tumors in adult orbit are squamous cell carcinoma (SCC) of paranasal sinuses, meningiomas from CNS and breast, lung and prostate cancers respectively [14].

General Considerations in Orbital Tumor Patient

During the patient assessment process, it is vital to establish a good rapport with the patient and the family, which will fortify their trust with the surgeon. It is further critical that the patient's problem be discussed in detail at every step of management as cancer is usually a serious issue with high morbidity and mortality. If possible, the images of MRI or CT revealing a space-occupying mass in the orbit should be shared with the patient and the family; the obvious difference between the tumor containing orbit and the normal one is usually very informative and convincing for the patient. Furthermore, the reasons for surgery, the expected benefits, and especially potential complications should be discussed in an open manner. If the case is inoperable, alternative management plans should be debated. It is most important that the patient and the family, not the surgeon, decide whether to proceed with surgery. It should be carefully explained that the orbital problem may be part of a systemic disease and that better understanding of the orbital pathology may eventually help to arrive at an effective systemic treatment.

Clinical Evaluation of Orbital Tumor Patient

The evaluation of the orbit begins with a thorough history and physical examination. Detailed systemic and ocular inquiries offer many useful clues. The family history should specify any cancer, craniofacial abnormalities, and other systemic familial diseases such as neurofibromatosis. A history of previous hospitalizations, head and neck injuries, and surgeries should be investigated. A list of the patient's medications and allergies should be obtained and a tendency toward bleeding should specifically be elicited. Anticoagulants and chemicals which may affect bleeding should be noted and appropriately addressed by cessation at an appropriate interval prior to surgery or managed in conjunction with an internist/hematologist.

Special emphasis on the duration and speed of progression of the symptoms should be heard in the patient's own words. Symptoms such as displacement of the eye(s), pain, tenderness, diplopia, pulsation, change in the degree of proptosis with position or Valsalva maneuver, and disturbance of visual acuity and/or visual fields are typically elicited [18–19].

A complete ophthalmic examination including assessment of visual acuity, visual field, extraocular motility, anterior and posterior segments, sensory capacity and cranial is essential. Periorbital/orbital changes such as proptosis, abnormal eyelid configuration, skin lesions, edema, chemosis, and the appearance of conjunctival vessels should be carefully evaluated and photographs should be obtained if possible. Apposition and motility abnormalities of the eyelids and the status of lacrimal drainage system (LDS) are additional key points to be checked during the examination.

Diminished or changing visual acuity, color vision, abnormal visual fields, and pupillary abnormalities are important to note. Motility dysfunction and diplopia should be carefully assessed and quantified if possible by Hess screen and/or alternating prism cover test throughout the course of illness. Intraocular pressure should be elevated. Slit lamp examination can discern chemosis, congested tortuous vessels. Dilated indirect ophthalmoscopy may reveal optic disc edema or pallor, retinal detachment, choroidal folds, scleral indentation, vascular engorgement or shunt vessels [19–21].

Fig. 10.1 Checking the position of the globes with Hertel's exophthalmometer (**a**, **b**); "Worm's eye view" examination of proptosis of the left eye secondary to a large space occupying lesion in the orbit; (**c**) Axial CT image showing left eye proptosis (**d**)

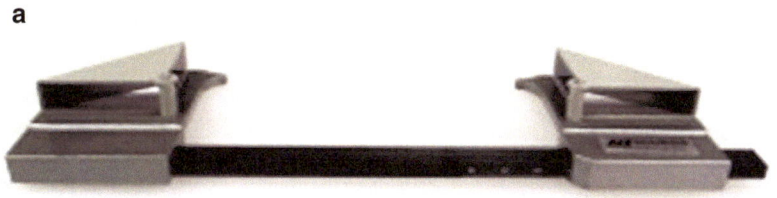

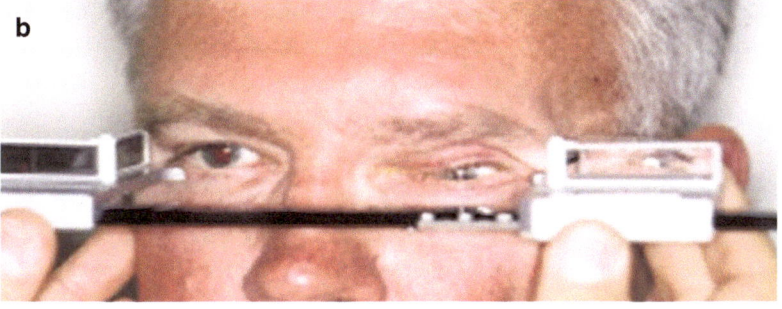

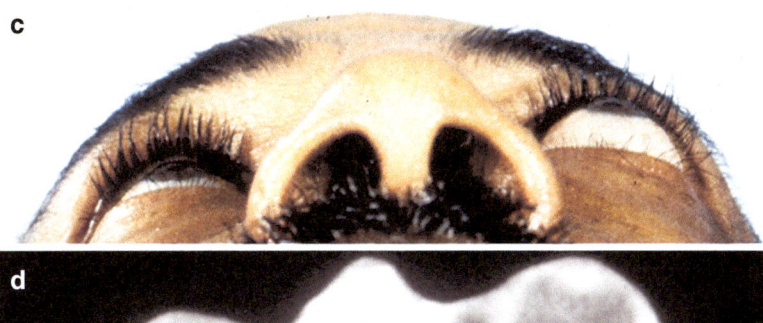

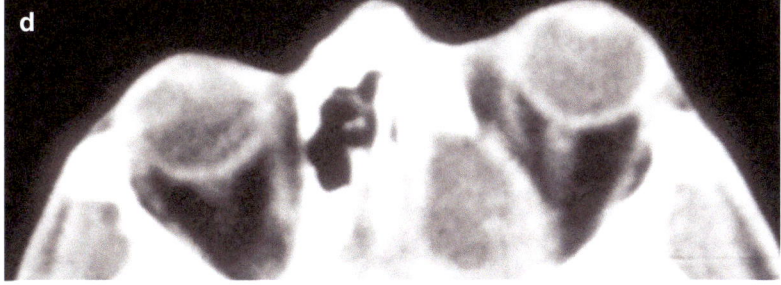

Bilateral or unilateral displacement of the eye (proptosis) is an important clinical manifestation of orbital space-occupying lesions. In addition to axial proptosis, one should note the displacement of the eye in planes other than the antero-posterior direction, vertical and lateral globe dystopia should be documented. The degree of displacement, compared to the fellow eye is generally quantified in millimeters with exophthalmometry (typically with Hertel Exophthalmometer) (Fig. 10.1). If an exophthalmometer is not available, the relative protrusion can be observed by simply standing behind a seated patient and gazing downward from the forehead to assess the displacement of one globe compared to the other. Alternatively, this can be noted by having the patient elevate the head and looking from below the nose or "worm's-eye" view. The displacement (proptosis) of the eye is estimated based on the distance (in millimeters) in an anterior-posterior plane between the anterior surface of the cornea and the anterior margin malar eminence. This distance normally varies from 16.5 to 21.5 mm in Caucasian men and 15.5–20 mm in Caucasian women. In African American adults, the measurements are increased by approximately 2 mm in both sexes (Fig. 10.2) [22–24].

External examination for orbital pathology must include the changes of the eyelids, conjunctiva, and periorbital skin and the underlying soft tissues. Regional lymph nodes should be examined. Edema, discoloration, and tenderness of these tissues may provide information regarding the orbital process. Edema of the eyelids without erythema or other inflammatory signs may be associated with vascular and neurogenic tumors, presumably secondary to long-standing venous stasis. Edema with inflammatory signs such as hyperemia and/or tenderness is commonly associated with thyroid eye disease (particularly if in association with eyelid retraction) and orbital inflammatory syndromes (infectious and non-infectious, specific and nonspecific). Ecchymosis should not be confused with hyperemia (Fig. 10.3). The former is often seen in metastatic neuroblastoma but may also be encountered with amyloidosis, plasmacytoma, and leukemic infiltrates. A typical feature of ecchymosis, secondary to neuroblastoma, is its changing appearance from day to day [25].

Xanthelasmas on the periorbital skin should also be noted, since they may be a part of orbital xanthogranuloma or systemic disease (Fig. 10.4) [26–27].

Lesions palpable in the anterior orbit can be evaluated for mobility and the solid versus cystic

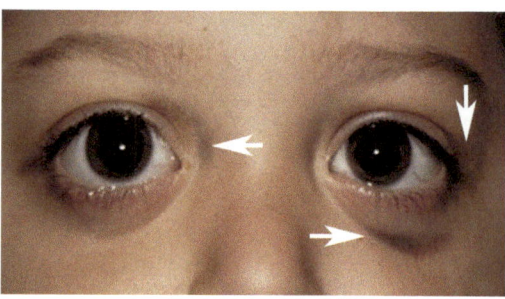

Fig. 10.3 Bilateral ecchymosis in a patient with metastatic neuroblastoma. (From Karcioglu [8], with permission)

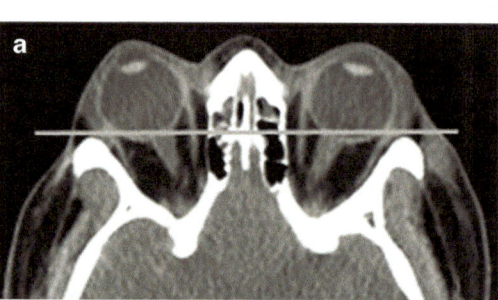

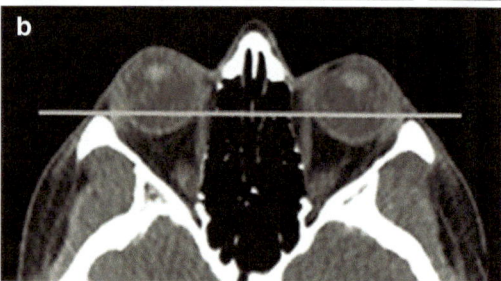

Fig. 10.2 (**a**, **b**) Normal anatomy of orbits in white and black women in CT. (From Karcioglu [8], with permission)

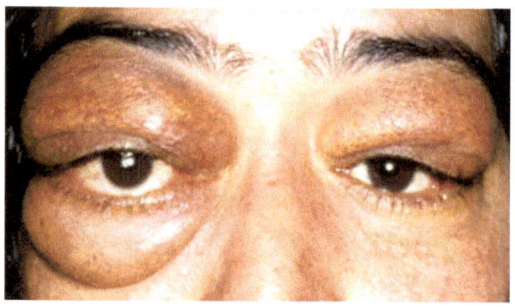

Fig. 10.4 Bilateral upper lid xanthelasmas in the patient. (From Karcioglu [8], with permission)

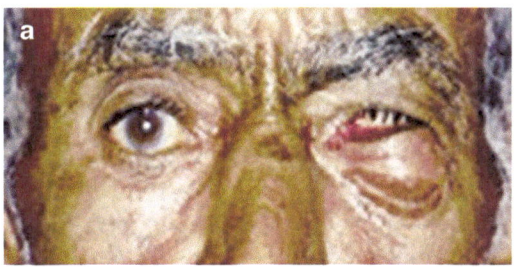
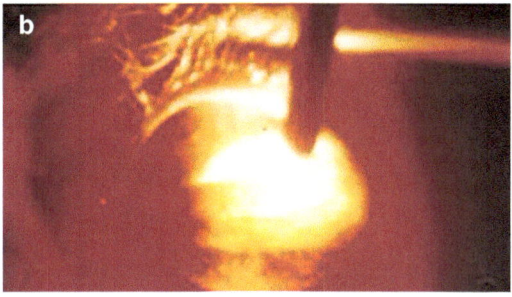

Fig. 10.5 (**a**, **b**) Transillumination of cystic basal cell carcinoma in inferior orbit displacing the globe superiorly. (From Karcioglu [8], with permission)

nature of the mass and its relationship to orbital bones and to other underlying tissues. Some anterior cystic masses can be transilluminated over the skin (Fig. 10.5).

Retropulsion is the degree of posterior freedom of movement of the globe which can be tested by the examiner's hand, pushing over patient's closed lids without creating too much discomfort. Tactile examination is also helpful to reveal pulsations of the globe secondary to arteriovenous communications and occasionally crepitations in an emphysematous orbit. Auscultation of the orbit may rarely detect a bruit, secondary to A-V malformations or carotid-cavernous fistula but it is of vital importance to recognize this sign clinically. Attention should also be paid to regional lymph nodes for enlargement and tenderness. Certain types of clinical laboratory tests may also be helpful throughout the diagnosis and management of the tumor patient (Table 10.1).

Imaging in Orbital Tumor Patient

Whereas many pathologic processes intrinsic to the globe may be easily evaluated under direct visualization, radiological imaging is of greater value in the evaluation of orbital and intracranial processes. In current practice, imaging including CT and MRI is the gold standard for diagnosis

Table 10.1 Laboratory tests for orbital tumor patient

Tests to screen for cancer or precancerous conditions
Tumor marker tests measure the presence, levels, or activity of specific proteins or genes in tissue and blood that may be signs of cancer
Tests for cancer gene mutations
For example, searching for BRCA1 and BRCA2 mutations that play a role in the development of breast, ovarian, and other cancers
Tests to screen for immune status of the patient
Tests for antibody deficiency: IgG, IgA and IgM levels in blood
Tests for evaluation of cellular (T-cell) immunity
Tests for evaluation of neutrophil function
Tests for evaluation of complement: hemolytic complement assay or CH50
Tests to determine HIV/AIDS, HPV, EB and other virus positivity when indicated
Pre-operative and post-operative tests to assure a safe surgical course
Complete blood count (CBC) and clotting studies including prothrombin time (PT), activated partial thromboplastin time (aPTT), and thrombin time (TT), to assess blood clotting function of the patient
Tests to diagnose cancer at the time of biopsy
Frozen-section, histopathology, immunohistochemistry, Immunophenotyping
Flow-cytometry, DNA sequencing and antibody/gene microarray, PCR, quantitative PCR
Tests to make a management plan
Confirmation of tumor type and staging for chemo and radiation treatments
Tests to determine the dissemination of cancer; sentinel node biopsy; LP cytology; BM biopsy
Tumor marker tests to measure the presence, levels, or activity of specific proteins or genes in tissue and blood that may indicate the presence of cancer. A tumor that shows greater than normal level of a certain tumor marker may respond to treatment with a drug targeting that specific marker
Tests to monitor the patient during treatment and look for adverse effects of the treatment
Urinalysis; CBC; blood chemistry; tests detect metabolites, electrolytes, fats, and proteins, and enzymes including blood urea nitrogen (BUN) and creatinine and many others
Tests to determine whether the tumor is responding to treatment and tests to monitor recurrence
Clinical Laboratory tests can be useful for orbital tumor patient for numerous purposes. Although many of these tests are only available in major medical and research centers, the spectrum of laboratory capabilities is important to appreciate

and management [28–31] (Tables 10.2, 10.3, 10.4, 10.5, 10.6 and 10.7).

CT and MRI, independently or together, provide a wealth of information on orbital lesions. Each has

Table 10.2 Imaging protocols for CT and MRI

Routine imaging protocol for orbit and brain CT
The standard orbital CT protocol calls for the acquisition of 0.625 mm axial source images which are then reconstructed as overlapping 1.25 mm slices and also converted into soft tissue and bone algorithms. Additionally, overlapping 1.5 mm sagittal and coronal reformatted images are routinely generated
Routine imaging protocol for orbit and brain MRI
Generally speaking, T1-weighted images provide the best overall anatomic detail. Several tissues demonstrate high T1 signal: fat, subacute blood, and often melanin. Tissues with high fluid content (such as edema) demonstrate high T2 intensity. Fat-suppressed sequences are typically performed in the orbit to allow for differentiation of hyperintense structures from the underlying normal fat, for instance, in contrast-enhanced sequences. Diffusion weighted images (DWI) and the apparent diffusion coefficient (ADC) help to evaluate ischemic tissues and cellular tumors like lymphomas, which can be bright on DWI and dark on ADC. Today MRI is most commonly performed with 1.5 T units using either head or surface coils
MRA and MRV
Magnetic resonance angiography and venography may be added to conventional MRI protocols when differential diagnosis includes cavernous carotid fistula, arterial dissection, vascular malformations or other vascular anomalies

Data from ICRP statement on tissue reactions. International Committee on Radiological Protection [33]; Belden and Zinreich [34]; Sepahdari et al. [35] and Lee et al. [36]

Table 10.3 Advantages and disadvantages of CT and MRI

	Advantages	Disadvantages
CT	Low cost	Ionizing radiation
	Availability and fast scanning time	Contrast reaction
	Good detail of bone anatomy	Beam-hardening and other artifacts
MRI	Superior detail of anatomy	Incompatible with a number of metallic implantable medical devices and foreign bodies
	No ionizing radiation	Motion and other artifacts
		High cost, longer scanning times

Table 10.4 MRI features of well-delineated orbital lesions (appearance and signal with respect to vitreous)

	Orbital lesions	T1-weighted image	T2-weighted image	Enhancement with Gd-DTPA[a]	Comments
1	Lymphoproliferative disorders	Homogenous	Homogenous	Homogenous	Oval, lobulated, molding to other structures
		Iso-/ hyperintense	Iso-/ hypointense		
2	Cavernous malformation	Homogenous	Homogenous	Heterogenous early, homogenous late	Well delineated round frequently intraconal
		Iso-/ hyperintense	Iso-/ hyperintense	++++	
3	Orbital metastasis	Homo-/ heterogenous	Homo-/ heterogenous	Homogenous/ rarely cystic	May be associated with sinus, lymphatic or intracranial lesions
		Iso-/ hyperintense	Iso-/ hyperintense	+/++	
4	Peripheral nerve tumors (schwannoma, neurofibroma)	Heterogenous	Heterogenous	Heterogenous (in malignant change)	Central enhancement, focal cystic change
		Hypo/ isointense	Hyperintense, "target-sign"	+/+++	
5	Rhabdomyosarcoma	Homogenous	Homogenous	Homogenous	About 15% intraconal, other intra & extraconal
		Hypo-/ isointense	Hyperintense	++++	

Table 10.4 (continued)

	Orbital lesions	T1-weighted image	T2-weighted image	Enhancement with Gd-DTPA[a]	Comments
6	Solitary fibrous tumor (SFT)	Heterogenous	Heterogenous	Heterogenous	Can be dark on T1 and T2 sequences
		Iso-/ hyperintense	Iso-/hypo intense	++	
7	Optic nerve sheath meningioma	Homogenous	Homogenous	Homo-/ heterogenous	"Tram track" calcification, distension posterior to globe
		Isointense	Iso-/ hyperintense	++++ with fat suppression	

[a] Gd-DTPA – gadolinium-diethylenetriaminepentaacetic acid

Table 10.5 MRI features of infiltrating orbital lesions (appearance and signal with respect to vitreous)

	Orbital lesions	T1-weighted image	T2-weighted image	Enhancement with Gd-DTPA[a]	Comments
1	Langerhans-cell and non L-cell Histiocytosis	Homogenous (benign or malignant)	Homogenous(benign), heterogenous (malignant)	High T2 (hypercellular)	Bone involvement on CT
		Iso-/ hyperintense		Low T2 (less cells, more collagen)	
2	Capillary hemangioma	Homo-/ heterogenous	Homo-/heterogenous	Homogenous	Delineated without capsule T2 flow voids occasionally
		Hypo-/ isointense	Iso-/hyperintense	++++	
3	Orbital metastasis	Homo-/ heterogenous	Homo-/heterogenous	Homo/ heterogenous	Bony infiltration on CT, located anywhere in orbit
		Hyperintense	Hypointense	+/++++	
4	Orbital inflammatory syndrome	Homogenous	Homogenous	Homogenous; but may be variable	
		Iso-/ hyperintense	Iso-/hypointense		
5	Neurofibromatosis	Heterogenous	Heterogenous	Heterogenous	Can be nodular, infiltrating, cystic or solid
		Iso-/ hyperintense	Iso-/hyperintense	+/+++	

[a] Gd-DTPA, gadolinium-diethylenetriaminepentaacetic acid

a role. CT has advantages in the examination of bony or other high-density lesions. Positron emission tomography (PET) CT is useful for the detection of suspicious lesions throughout the body, in the context of a potentially metastatic orbital tumor.

MRI is advantageous for delineating soft tissue processes, in that different sequences can highlight differences in cellular content of lesions and the local surrounding tissues. Special sequences such as diffusion-weighted MRI, MRI arteriography, and MRI venography can also be particularly helpful for specific suspected diagnoses. Time-resolved sequences such as TRICKS or TWIST can also be useful for vascular lesions.

Ultrasonography (US) which can be done quickly in the clinic at a low cost is uniquely suitable to reveal dynamic changes such as compressibility and internal reflectivity, as well as the cystic nature of lesions. Doppler imaging can provide information regarding vascular flow characteristics within a lesion. This modality is typically applicable primarily for anteriorly located lesions. The information US provides can also be additive to other types of imaging [32].

The most irreplaceable benefit of orbital imaging is not only to provide insight into the differential diagnosis of the tumor but also to reveal the exact localization of the pathology in the orbit. This anatomical precision allows the ophthalmologist to appropriately plan for potential surgery, whether incisional or excisional. Such improvements in preop-

Table 10.6 MRI features of lacrimal fossa lesions (appearance and signal with respect to vitreous)

	Orbital lesions	T1-weighted image	T2-weighted image	Enhancement with Gd-DTPA[a]	Comments
1	Lympho-proliferative disorder	Homogenous	Homogenous	Homogenous	Diffusion-weighted imaging may help to detect malignancy
		Hyperintense	Hypointense	+++	
2	Pleomorphic adenoma (benign mixed tumor)	Homogenous	Homogenous	Homogenous (small)	Scalloping of orbital bone
		Hypo-/isointense	Iso-/hyperintense	Heterogenous (large)	
				+++	
3	Adenoid cystic carcinoma	Heterogenous	Heterogenous	Homo-/ heterogenous	Haphazard infiltration
		Hyperintense	Hypointense		Bony destruction with Ca ++ on CT
4	Dacryoadenitis	Homogenous	Homogenous	Homogenous	On CT hypo/iso to muscle
		Hypo-/isointense	Iso-/hyperintense	Variable, not very helpful	
5	Dacryops	Homogenous	Homogenous	Minimal, homogenous	Cyst with fluid density on contrast enhanced CT
		Iso-/hyperintense	Hypo-/isointense		

[a] Gd-DTPA, gadolinium-diethylenetriaminepentaacetic acid

Table 10.7 MRI features of cystic orbital lesions (appearance and signal with respect to vitreous)

	Orbital lesions	T1-weighted image	T2-weighted image	Enhancement with Gd-DTPA[a]	Comments
1	Dermoid cyst	Heterogenous	Heterogenous	Homogenous	Perilesional inflammation if ruptured; bone remodeling on CT occasionally
		Hypointense	Hypo-/hyperintense	+++	
2	Epithelial cyst	Homogenous	Homogenous	Homogenous (small)	DDx choriostoma, congenital cyst, colobomatous cyst
		Iso-/hyperintense	Iso-/hypointense	Heterogenous (large)	
				+++	
3	Hydatid cyst	Homogenous	Homogenous	Homo-/ heterogenous	Multiple cysts, may be calcified
		Isointense	Isointense		
4	Mucocele	Homo-/heterogenous	Homo-/heterogenous	Homogenous	High protein content; high signal in T1
		Hypo-/isointense	Iso-/hypo-/ hyperintense	Variable, not very helpful	
5	Lymphangioma	Heterogenous	Heterogenous	Minimal, homogenous	Fluid-fluid level on CT and MRI
		Iso/hyperintense	Hyperintense		
6	Cholesterol granuloma	Heterogenous	Heterogenous	Heterogenous	Fat suppression
		Hyperintense	Hyperintense	Central hyper, rim hypointense	Remains high signal

[a] Gd-DTPA, gadolinium-diethylenetriaminepentaacetic acid

erative data availability have led to less invasive approaches such as anterior orbitotomies through conjunctival and skin incisions, rather than wider lateral approaches where the location is less well understood preoperatively [33–36].

Summary

As in any medical diagnostic process, the data obtained in the assessment is assembled into a plan for the patient. The history will guide the examination, and the findings will in turn guide the selection of ancillary procedures and often imaging. Often the differential diagnosis at this point can be narrow, and reasonably so. Based on the requirements of differentiating these diagnostic possibilities and their respective treatment modalities, a management plan is selected. It is often the case in orbital disease that a tissue sample would be required, and the critical decision will be related to whether this tissue sample is obtained in fine needle aspirate, open incisional biopsy, excisional biopsy, or en bloc resection. This decision will be based on the characteristics of the lesion, the considerations for diagnosis and treatment beyond, as well as the wishes of the patient and the capabilities of the treating team.

Acknowledgments We are grateful to Dr. Daniel Rootman, Assistant Professor, Orbital and Ophthalmic Plastic Surgery, Doheny Eye Institute, University of California, Los Angeles, for his contribution as the expert reviewer for this section.

References

1. Shields JA, Shields CL, Scartozzi R. Survey of 1264 patients with orbital tumors and simulating lesions: the 2002 montgomery lecture, part 1. Ophthalmology. 2004;111(5):997–1008.
2. Goldberg SH, Cantore WA. Tumors of the orbit. Curr Opin Ophthalmol. 1997;8(5):51–6.
3. Carroll GS, Haik BG, Fleming JC, et al. Peripheral nerve tumors of the orbit. Radiol Clin N Am. 1999;37(1):195–202.
4. Yan J, Wu Z. Cavernous hemangioma of the orbit: analysis of 214 cases. Orbit. 2004;23(1):33–40.
5. Honavar SG, Manjandavida FP. Recent advances in orbital tumors—a review of publications from 2014–2016. Asia-Pac J Ophthalmol. 2017;6:153–8.
6. Perry JD, Singh AD. Clinical ophthalmic oncology: orbital tumors. 2nd ed. Berlin Heidelberg: Springer; 2014.
7. Andreasen S, Esmaeli B, Holstein SL, et al. An update on tumors of the lacrimal gland. Asia Pac J Ophthalmol (Phila). 2017;6(2):159–72.
8. Karcioglu ZA. Orbital tumors: diagnosis and treatment. 2nd ed. New York: Springer; 2015.
9. Bonavolontà G, Strianese D, Grassi P, et al. An analysis of 2480 space-occupying lesions of the orbit from 1976 to 2011. Ophthal Plast Reconstr Surg. 2013;29(2):79–86.
10. Pahwa S, Sharma S, Das CJ, et al. Intraorbital cystic lesions: an imaging spectrum. Curr Probl Diagn Radiol. 2015;44(5):437–48.
11. Narayan D, Rajak S, Patel S, Selva D. Cystic change in primary pediatric optic nerve sheath meningioma. Orbit. 2016;35(4):236–8.
12. Zwaann J, Karcioglu ZA. Benign pediatric tumors. In: Karcioglu ZA, editor. Orbital tumors: diagnosis and treatment. New York: Springer; 2015. p. 337–48.
13. Karcioglu ZA, Hadjistilianou D. Malignant pediatric tumors. In: Karcioglu ZA, editor. Orbital tumors: diagnosis and treatment. New York: Springer; 2015. p. 349–60.
14. Ahmad SM, Esmaeli B. Metastatic tumors of the orbit and ocular adnexa. Curr Opin Ophthalmol. 2007;18:405–13.
15. Shields JA, Shields CL, Brotman HK, et al. Cancer metastatic to the orbit: the 2000 Robert M. Curts lecture. Ophthal Plast Reconstr Surg. 2001;17:346–54.
16. Hartstein ME, Beisman B, Kincaid MC. Cutaneous malignant melanoma metastatic to the eyelid. Ophthalmic Surg Lasers. 1998;29:993–5.
17. Zografos L, Ducrey N, Beati D, et al. Metastatic melanoma in the eye and orbit. Ophthalmology. 2003;110:2245–56.
18. Tailor TD, Gupta D, Dalley RW, et al. Orbital neoplasms in adults: clinical, radiologic, and pathologic review. Radiographics. 2013;33(6):1739–58.
19. Karcioglu ZA, Jenkins TL. Clinical evaluation of the orbit. In: Karcioglu ZA, editor. Orbital tumors: diagnosis and treatment. New York: Springer; 2015. p. 43–53.
20. Nassr MA, Morris CL, Netland PA, Karcioglu ZA. Intraocular pressure change in orbital disease. Surv Ophthalmol. 2009;54(5):519–44.
21. De La Paz MA, Boniuk M. Fundus manifestations of orbital disease and treatment of orbital disease. Surv Ophthalmol. 1995;40(1):3–21.
22. Hertel E, Simonsz HJ. A simple exophthalmometer. Strabismus. 2008;16(2):89–91.
23. Burde R, Savino P, Trobe J. Proptosis and adnexal masses. In: Clinical decisions in neuro-ophthalmology. 2nd ed. St. Louis: CV Mosby; 1992. p. 379–416.
24. Barretto RL, Mathog RH. Orbital measurement in black and white populations. Laryngoscope. 1999;109(7. Pt 1):1051–4.
25. Smith SJ, Diehl NN, Smith BD, Mohney BG. Incidence, ocular manifestations, and survival in children with neuroblastoma: a population-based study. Am J Ophthalmol. 2010;149(4):677–82; e2.
26. Vick VL, Wilson MW, Fleming JC, Haik BG. Orbital and eyelid manifestations of xanthogranulomatous diseases. Orbit. 2006;25(3):221–5.
27. Karcioglu ZA, Sharara N, Boles T, Nasr A. Orbital xanthogranuloma: clinical morphologic features in eight patients. Ophthalmic Plast Reconstr Surg. 2003;19:372–81.
28. Müller-Forell WS. Computed tomograpy. In: Müller-Forell WS, editor. Imaging of orbital and visual pathway pathology. Berlin: Springer; 2010.
29. Yousem DM, Grossman RI. Orbit. In: Yousem DM, Grossman RI, editors. The requisites. *Neuroradiology*. Philadelphia: Mosby/Elsevier; 2010. p. 1–20, 321–355.

30. Gandhi RA, Nair AG. Role of imaging in the management of neuro-ophthalmic disorders. Indian J Ophthalmol. 2011;59:111–6.

31. Fetkenhour DR, Shields CL, Chao AN, et al. Orbital cavitary rhabdomyosarcoma masquerading as lymphangioma. Arch Ophthalmol. 2001;119: 1208–10.

32. Nasr AM, Abou Chacra GI. Ultrasonography in orbital differential diagnosis. In: Karcioglu ZA, editor. Orbital tumors: diagnosis and treatment. New York: Springer; 2015. p. 69–81.

33. ICRP statement on tissue reactions. International Committee on Radiological Protection, 2011.

34. Belden CJ, Zinreich SJ. Orbital imaging techniques. Semin Ultrasound CT MR. 1997;18:413–22.

35. Sepahdari AR, Kapur R, Aakalu VK, et al. Diffusion-weighted imaging of malignant ocular masses: results and directions for further study. AJNR Am J Neuroradiol. 2012;33(2):314–9.

36. Lee AG, Johnson MC, Policeni BA, Smoker WR. Imaging for neuro-ophthalmic and orbital disease—a review. Clin Exp Ophthalmol. 2009;37:30–53.

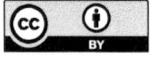

Surgical Techniques for Orbital Tumors

Zeynel A. Karcioglu

Anesthesia in Orbital Tumor Patient

Many mid and deep orbital surgeries in adults and virtually all procedures in children are performed under general anesthesia; however, anterior orbit explorations and/or simple biopsies in adults can be performed with local anesthesia and intravenous sedation [1].

The administration of regional anesthetics, even when general anesthesia is used, containing epinephrine about 5–15 min prior to incision into the soft tissues of the surgical field contributes to vasoconstriction significantly. If nasal or sinus involvement is anticipated during the orbital exploration, it may be helpful to use a vasoconstrictive nasal spray and pack the nose with half-inch gauze-strip, soaked in Neosynephrine or another vasoconstrictive agent [2].

All local anesthetic solutions are prepared as weak hydrochloride salts to extend their shelf lives and to stabilize added vasoconstrictors. However, this weak acid assembly delays their onset of action and makes them painful on injection. Lidocaine (1% or 2%) is the most

widely used local anesthetic and produces the least amount of pain on injection. Anesthetics commonly utilized can be generally ordered on a scale from least to most painful for injection: lidocaine 1%, procaine 2%, bupivacaine 0.5%, and etidocaine 1%. Pain during injection varies with pH of solution, osmolality, lipid solubility, temperature, the speed of injection, size of needle, as well as other environmental and emotional patient-related factors [3, 4].

Addition of epinephrine (1:100,000, 1:200,000, 1:400,000) for vasoconstriction decreases the absorption rate, prolongs the action, but increases the pain of local anesthetics at injection. At the incision site, lidocaine with epinephrine is usually injected subcutaneously into deeper soft tissues. The use of a long-acting local anesthetic, administration of an IV steroid to minimize inflammation and utilization of a nonsteroidal anti-inflammatory drug on a regular basis will minimize the need for postoperative opioids, and this works well in ASA I and II patients.

The effect of local anesthetics begins approximately 5 and 4 min after injection without and with epinephrine respectively. The duration of the effect ranges from 1 to 2 h. The maximum recommended dose is 4.4 mg/kg without epinephrine and 7.0 mg/kg with epinephrine. Lidocaine, like all other local anesthetics, may lead to systemic toxicity with increased BP and heart rate, arrhythmias, dysrhythmias, and CNS signs and symptoms of drowsiness, seizures, and

Electronic supplementary material The online version of this chapter (https://doi.org/10.1007/978-3-030-18757-6_11) contains supplementary material, which is available to authorized users.

Z. A. Karcioglu (✉)
Department of Ophthalmology, University of Virginia, Charlottesville, VA, USA
e-mail: zak8g@virginia.edu

headaches. In patients who use nonselective beta blocker (B1, B2), the administration of a vaso-constrictor will act solely at the a1 site, producing vasoconstriction. Epinephrine may not be used with patients who are on tricyclic antidepressants or MAO inhibitors. On the other hand, patients who are on the newer SSRIs such as Prozac may be given epinephrine.

Small doses of local anesthetics injected into the orbit and periorbital tissues may rarely produce serious adverse reactions similar to systemic toxicity such as confusion, convulsions, respiratory arrest, and cardiovascular changes. These reactions may be due to unintended intra-arterial injection of the local anesthetic with retrograde flow to the cerebral circulation. Patients receiving these blocks should be under constant observation. Resuscitative equipment and personnel for treating adverse reactions should be immediately available [5, 6].

General Surgical Principles in Orbital Tumor Patient

The details of the lesions in individual compartments of the orbit should be ascertained together with the below listed general concepts of orbital surgery. The anatomic distributions of tumors in orbital compartments are not perfectly defined; however some lesions do have a tendency toward one region or another. These include, in the upper-outer quadrant (lacrimal gland fossa), dermoid cyst, lacrimal gland tumors, and lymphoma; in the upper-inner quadrant (lacrimal gland fossa), dermoid cyst, lacrimal gland tumors, and lymphoma; in the upper-inner quadrant, commonly mucocele; in the inferior orbit, basal cell carcinoma medially, and inflammatory or squamous lesions from perinasal sinuses centrally; in the lateral and posterior orbit, commonly cavernous malformations and nonspecific inflammatory disease; and, in the posterior and apical orbit, meningioma, cavernous malformations, Schwannoma, and inflammatory lesions (Tables 11.1 and 11.2). Understanding these tendencies may assist in planning the approach, as well as in preparing for the gross appearance of the lesion and the tactile characteristics of the capsule and/or internal contents of the mass.

The best position for orbital surgery is reverse Trendelenburg, which reduces arterial flow to the orbit and promoted venous return to the heart. The head should be positioned according to the planned orbitotomy. It is best to prep both sides allowing intra-operative comparison to opposite orbit for assessment of symmetry. If tissue harvesting from other sites (thigh, retro auricular area, fellow eyelid, etc.) will be performed, graft sites should also be prepared and covered with sterile towels. If the use of a microscope or endoscope is planned, the OR team and anesthesiologist should be notified beforehand. Refer to Fig. 11.1 for an example of hand-held instrument tray for common orbital surgeries.

Incisions

Skin incisions of the eyelids and the periorbital area should ideally follow the relaxed skin tension lines (RSTLs) and are best placed in natural creases or other hidden locations such as the conjunctival fornix or the eyelid caruncle (Fig. 11.2) [7]. Prior to injection with local anesthetics, the incision line should be marked with a surgical pen. The skin incisions can be made with a Bard-Parker 15-C or a 3 mm, 30° sharp, disposable blade (e.g., Super Blade®). Ideally, the incision should cut only the skin, not the underlying subcutaneous tissues, as dissection can carry forward in a stepwise, layer-by-layer manner. In general, the skin incisions are made perpendicular to the skin surface; however, if an eyebrow incision is needed, the incision may be made at a 45° angle following the angulation of the hair follicles in a beveled manner to allow for hair growth through the incision after healing.

The lazy-S incision, starting in the mid-eyelid crease is particularly useful to gain access to superior and lateral orbital space. Other surgeons convincingly claim that the transconjunctival inferior approach provides quicker surgical access to the intraconal zone with a low incidence of complications and a better aesthetic outcome than lateral orbitotomy. (Personal communication with Dr. Santosh Hanovar, ISOO Meeting 2019). Conjunctival incisions allow direct admission to the primarily inferior compartments of the

Table 11.1   Space-occupying lesions of the orbit in anatomical compartments

Location of commonly encountered lesions	Proptosis	Associated findings	Surgical approach
Benign lacrimal fossa lesions (pleomorphic adenoma, cysts such as dermoid)	Inferior/nasal	Choroidal folds; disproportionally preserved EOM to lesion size	Lacrimal gland fossa exposure through lid-crease or brow incision
Malignant lacrimal fossa lesions (adenocarcinoma, adenoid cystic carcinoma)	Inferior/nasal	Pain; sensory deficit; poor motility; lymphadenopathy	Same approach may need to expand superiorly or laterally depending on the extent of tumor
Superior/inferior medial lesions (cysts such as dermoid, mucocele, LDS tumors, SCC from ethmoid cells)	Inferior/temporal	Usually w/o choroidal folds; associated trauma, sinusitis, pain; horizontal or diffuse EOM limitation	Transcutaneous (Lynch incision) or transcaruncular medial orbitotomy
Anterior lesions (lymphoma, cysts like dermoid, epithelial)	Mild proptosis away from the site of lesion	Lid/conjunctival involvement	Anterior orbit exposure according to the location of lesion
Benign muscle cone lesions (cavernous malformation, schwannoma)	Axial	Posterior choroidal folds; vein congestion; early disk edema; optic nerve dysfunction	Lateral orbitotomy
Extraconal and intraconal lesions (vascular hamartomas; rhabdomyosarcoma)	Massive without rule	Lid/conjunctival involvement; optic nerve dysfunction w or w/o disc edema; amblyopia	Lateral orbitotomy modified according to the location and size of lesion
Infiltrating lesions (orbital inflammatory syndromes; metastatic carcinoma)	Uneven/"frozen" proptosis; enophthalmos; severe motility dysfunction	Abnormal motility in all gazes; ON dysfunction, lymph nodes	Location oriented approach; core needle biopsy or FNAB or FACT
Inferior lesions (SCC from maxillary sinus, inflammatory lesions)	Superior/axial	Pain and/or sensory deficit in lower periorbital area; motility dysfunction	Inferior trans-conjunctival or subciliary skin approach w or w/o lateral crus incision ("swinging lid")
Posterior orbit, apical lesions (meningioma, glioma, paraganglioma)	Minimal axial, late proptosis	Optic nerve dysfunction; mild axial proptosis	Lateral orbitotomy; deep transorbital approach
Entire orbit such as solid/cystic teratoma	Massive proptosis	Distortion of orbital anatomy; axial displacement of globe with marked chemosis	Usually requires exenteration; globe may be saved in rare cases

Table 11.2   Orbital inflammations that may cause space-occupying lesions in the orbit

Infections	Nonspecific orbital inflammatory syndrome (NSOIS)	Specific inflammations	Vasculitides	Connective tissue disorders
Tuberculosis	Anterior	Sarcoidosis	Wegener's granulomatosis	Lupus erythematosus
Mucormycosis	Myositis	Sjögren's syndrome	Polyarteritis nodosa	Dermatomyositis
Viral Dacryoadenitis	Dacryoadenitis	Sclerosing orbital inflammation	Churg-Strauss syndrome	Rheumatoid arthritis
Echinococcosis, Cysticercosis	Tolosa hunt	HLA B27 related	Behçet's disease	Psoriatic
Allergic Aspergillosis	Diffuse	IgG4-related	Kimura's disease	Scleroderma

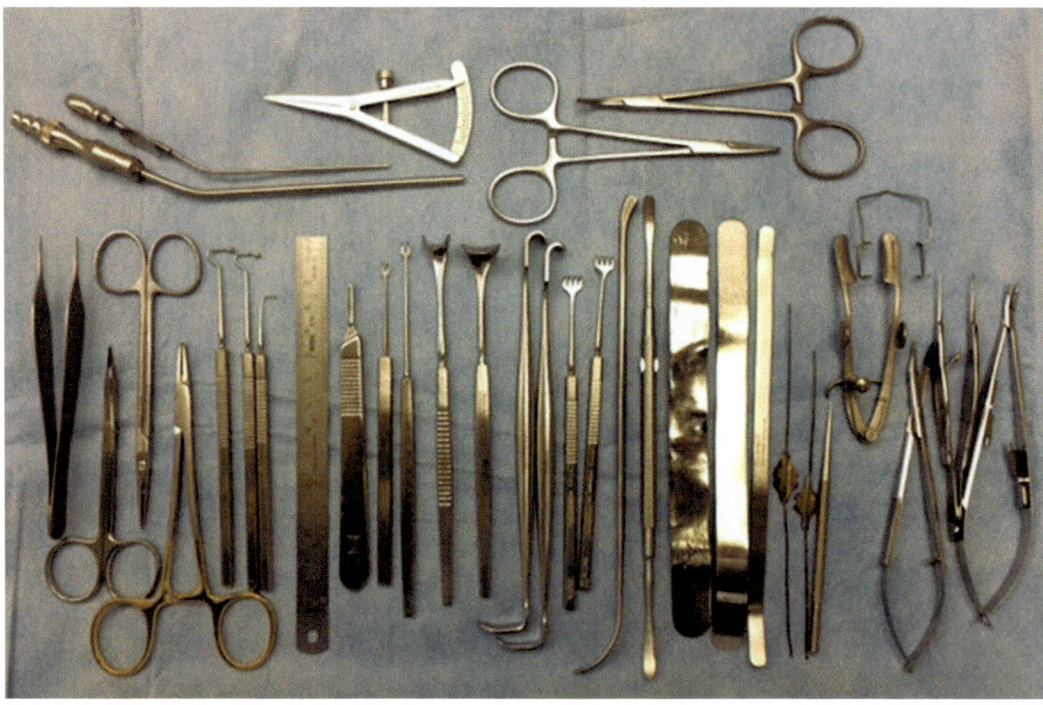

Fig. 11.1 A typical tray containing commonly used hand-held instruments for orbital tumor surgery. Rarely utilized instruments such as rongeurs, Kerrison punch, mallet, chisel, and gouge are not included. Larger surgical apparatus like reciprocating saw, rotary drill, Bovie and bipolar cauterizes, cryo instruments and tips, and dermatomes are not depicted as well

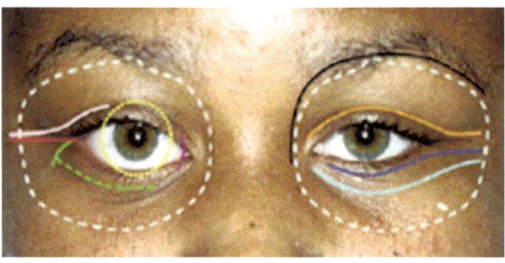

Fig. 11.2 Skin and conjunctival incisions for orbit surgery. The dotted white circle roughly corresponds to the bony margin of the orbit. Black: sub-brow incision in continuity with lynch incision; orange: lid. Crease incision; purple: caruncular incision; red: lateral canthal incision; Blue: sub-ciliary incision; green: lateral crus incision ("swinging"), "Lid incision"; turquoise: lower lid incision; yellow: perilimbal incision; Pink: lazy-s incision within the lid crease of upper lid. (From Karcioglu [29], with permission)

orbit with minimal external scaring. The addition of a lateral inferior cantholysis, converting to a swinging eyelid incision, can enhance access to the lateral orbit and midface. Any quadrant of the orbit can be approached through a segmental con-

junctival peritomy overlying the area. The intraconal space may easily be approached through perilimbal incisions through the sub-Tenon's space. For the extraconal space one should use forniceal incisions, which are particularly useful medially and inferiorly [8].

The medial conjunctival approach (through the caruncle) allows ample access to the ethmoid/medial wall area of the orbit. Furthermore, the caruncular incision provides excellent access to the medial and posterior orbit [9, 10]. These conjunctival incisions can be combined to allow for an extended orbital exposure of the floor and medial wall.

The most commonly used medial and superior medial skin incisions include modifications of the Lynch approach and the sub-brow incision. Although the classic Lynch incision can leave visible scarring, it may be quite advantageous in some cases to provide access to the lacrimal drainage system (LDS), the ethmoid sinuses, and the nasal cavity.

Superior and superior lateral fornix incisions are not ordinarily used, to avoid traumatizing the palpebral portion of the lacrimal gland and the ductules.

Innovative techniques to enhance the surgical exposure of the posterior orbit and apex have been proposed by many plastic and craniofacial surgeons and neurosurgeons [11, 12]. However, most of these approaches require elaborate procedures and experienced surgical teams and should not be attempted in ordinary ophthalmic surgery settings.

Bone incisions (osteotomies) may offer certain advantages but again these techniques are rarely needed to be utilized for orbital biopsy and only in experienced hands. In orbital tumor surgery, the bone is removed for two main reasons: first, the removal of the marginal bone to provide a wider surgical field, such as in lateral orbitotomy. Secondly, the bone may need to be removed to control a malignancy advancing into the bone, such as adenoid cystic carcinoma of the lacrimal gland.

Surgical Field

During orbital exploration, magnification and lighting are very important. A great majority of cases can be done under 3- to 5-power surgical loupes. A headlight combined with surgical loupes provides the best illumination.

Exposure for Exploration

The orbit is a small anatomical chamber crowded with vital tissues that are suspended within a septal network that compartmentalizes the orbital structures and orbital fat. It may be quite inhospitable to the surgeon particularly when the additional volume is added to this tight space by a tumor and secondary edema.

From whatever direction, the orbital exploration commits the surgeon to a deep, three-dimensional field with poor visibility.

Furthermore, changes in the anatomic relationships between structures because of the orbit's conal shape add to the difficulty of the pursuit of the tumor. Therefore, adequate exposure of the surgical field is of utmost importance. The optimization of the exposure begins with the proper selection of initial incision and is maintained with precise positioning of the surgical retractors and placement of traction sutures. Continuous maneuvering employed during orbital exploration to gain ideal exposure often takes more time than the actual biopsy or removal of the tumor.

Proper placement of the patient's head, positioning of the surgeon and assistants, as well as optimum lighting and magnification are the key elements of success in orbital surgery. Patience is an important virtue in orbital dissection, to maintain a bloodless surgical field and adequate exposure of the pathology and the surrounding structures. Because of unanticipated shifting of the orbital fat, the surgeon should be familiar with continuous interruptions of the visibility. The fat can be retracted from the field and often the use of small neurosurgical patties keeps the retracted fat under control; however, the fat moves like water and small variations in position are translated into great perturbations in visualization. All surgical maneuvers should be done with minimum trauma, typically with blunt rather than sharp dissection.

Most of the retraction requirements throughout the procedure are accomplished with the use of hand-held retractors. A wide range of retractors, including Desmarres, Semm, Ragnell, and malleable ribbon retractors (3/8–1 in. width), are used. In addition, rakes (Peck or Follet), muscle hooks (Graf or Jameson), and skin hooks (Joseph or Freer) function well for different levels of tissue retraction (Fig. 11.1).

Another method of improving the surgical visibility is to utilize sutures to pull tissues away from the field. One common application is to use 4–0 silk for eyelid retraction. It is also advisable to pass a marking suture under the extraocular muscles (EOM) to ensure that they can be identified during the later stages of the procedure. In particular, medial and inferior recti muscles should be anchored with sutures during orbital explorations of corresponding sites. Traction sutures may also be applied to the stumps of disinserted EOMs. A good example is the capture of the stump of the medial rectus during medial orbitotomy through the conjunctival approach. It is best to run a 5-0 Vicryl or Mersilene suture at the stump of the medial rectus muscle and cuff both ends of the suture with silicone tubing to avoid corneal and conjunctival damage during retraction of the globe (Fig. 11.3) (also see Videos 11.1 and 11.2).

Sutures may also be used to retract bone. For example, the zygomatic arch is attached to the temporalis fascia/muscle can be hinged laterally and posteriorly by traction sutures passed through pre-drilled holes in the bone. With this approach, the closure is quicker and the arch fits in its original position well, healing better and faster.

At all times, the orbital surgeon should maintain a mental correlation between the imaging of the lesion and its actual position within the orbit and should approach the lesion through appropriate planes of tissue. The importance of the definition of the plane of entry is aptly emphasized by Rootman, Stewart, and Goldberg: "Instead of entering directly into the pathologically involved tissue planes, the surgeon should begin the dissection in the more easily distracted and pliable normal tissues adjacent to the lesion" [13].

This approach allows the distinct advantage of comparing the normal tissues and the abnormal areas in order to permit the ready identification of the pathology.

Hemostasis

In case of bleeding the first thing to do is to determine if the hemorrhage experienced in the surgical field is due to a damaged blood vessel or to generalized oozing of blood. This can usually be accomplished by alternating suction and gentle pressure over a neurosurgical patty. Usually, a negligible amount of time allows vasoconstriction and subsequent clotting to occur in most cases of small unnamed vessels.

If brisk bleeding is experienced, the culprit blood vessel should be identified, isolated, and cauterized with an insulated bipolar cautery. If the bleeding is due to generalized oozing, it is beneficial to apply thrombin-soaked Gelfoam™ or surgical cottonoids. Neurosurgical cotton paddies are preferable because they are easier to identify and remove once the oozing has stopped. Powdered Avitene® can also be packed into the surgical field or delivered by syringe in cases with persistent oozing; Avitene® should be irrigated gently at the end of the procedure (Fig. 11.4).

As mentioned earlier, hemostasis should be initiated by hypotensive anesthesia, as well as by injection of epinephrine-containing local

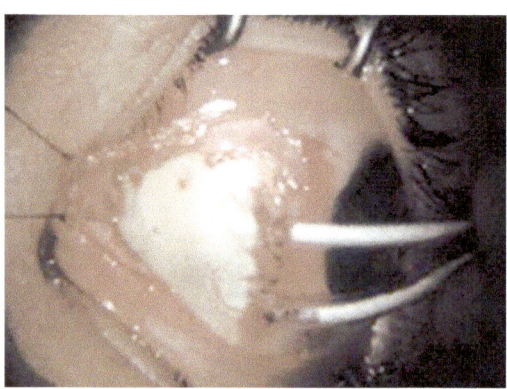

Fig. 11.3 Silicone tubing cuffed over traction suture to protect underlying cornea and conjunctiva during the course of medial orbitotomy. (From Karcioglu [29], with permission)

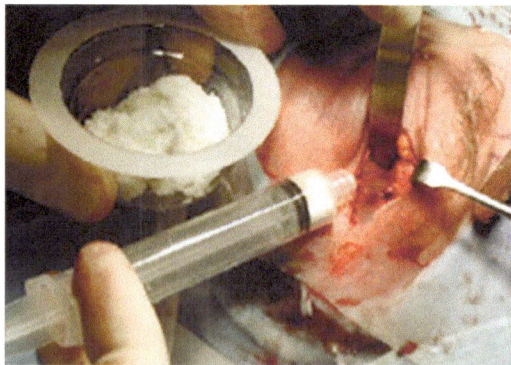

Fig. 11.4 Application of Avitene® to control oozing blood in the surgical field. (From Karcioglu [29], with permission)

Table 11.3 Hemostasis in orbital surgery

Pre-surgical
Reverse Trendelenburg position on the operating table
Hypotensive general anesthesia
Application or injection of chemical vasoconstrictors (epinephrine, cocaine, etc.)
Surgical
Application of strip gauze and/or neurosurgical paddies soaked with chemical vasoconstrictors and/or coagulators (Avitene®)
Thrombin-soaked gelatin sponge (Gelfoam®)
Oxidized regenerated cellulose (Surgicel®)
Bone wax for oozing in osteotomies
Cautery application (bipolar, unipolar, fine-tipped disposable)
Pressure by hand or hand-held instruments
Post-surgical
Gentle extubation at the end of the procedure without "bucking"
Application of pressure bandage over the orbit with head bandage with gauze
Immediate application of crushed ice on orbit in OR in plastic bag or surgical glove
Application of ice for 24–48 h after surgery

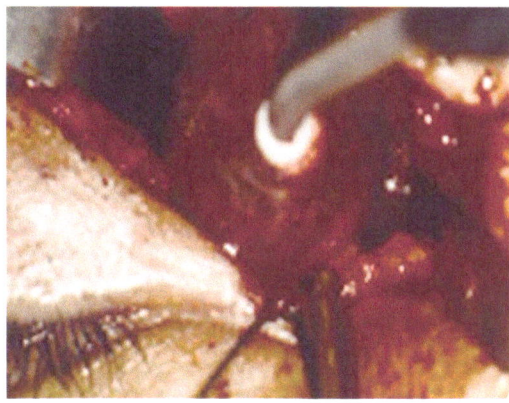

Fig. 11.5 Cryoprobe attached to tumor, is being used as a handle during extraction of tumor. (From Karcioglu [29], with permission)

anesthetics. Intraoperative bleeding can be controlled with bipolar or unipolar coagulators; the fine-needle tip (Colorado tip®) is preferred. Furthermore, vascular ties, clips, and chemical adjuncts can be used to maintain hemostasis (Table 11.3).

Orbital Biopsy

Orbital biopsy is a very important procedure, and in fact more than half of tumor-related surgeries are performed just to obtain an adequate tissue sample for diagnosis and management. Different biopsy techniques, including FNAB, core biopsy, and excisional biopsy, are utilized depending on the need of the patient [14]. Many papers have been written on biopsy procedures, tissue processing techniques, and benefits of special studies. The reader is referred to these references for detailed information. One imperative requisite for the surgeon is to contact the pathologist prior to surgery and inquire about specific processing requirements and the capabilities of the laboratory.

Tissue Removal/Ablation

In all quadrants of the orbit, once the sufficient exposure of well-delineated masses (and cysts) is accomplished the lesion is stabilized with forceps, cryoprobe, and/or sutures to be removed. This allows the surgeon to apply gentle traction while dissecting the surrounding tissue attachments to the lesion (Fig. 11.5).

The lesions of the anterior orbit are surgically approached directly over the lesion. About 80% of the mid and posterior orbital pathologies can be easily accessed surgically with time-honored techniques of lateral and conjunctival medial (caruncular) orbitotomies (Table 11.1 and Videos 11.1 and 11.2). Only the rare tumors in unusual locations in the orbit require special surgical methods including combined craniotomies which are not covered in this chapter.

Although the classical lateral orbitotomy approach with retraction or removal of the zygomatic arch is useful in many cases, benign orbital tumors of the intraconal space may be removed effectively through medial transconjunctival and superomedial lid crease incisions even with local anesthesia. According to some surgeons, this approach has a number of advantages over the lateral orbitotomy, including ease of dissection, incision-to nerve distance, and angle of approach to the optic nerve [1, 15, 16].

Unlike well-encapsulated tumors, infiltrating lesions cannot be removed totally but can only be removed in a piecemeal fashion for diagnostic or debulking purposes. Partial removals can be accomplished by isolating areas of the tumor and excising sections that are not infiltrating vital structures.

Well encapsulated lesions can often be removed completely. Most small and medium size cysts are best dissected with an intact capsule, although it may be advisable in very large cysts to deflate the cystic structure for removal. In certain space-occupying lesions of the orbit, such as pleomorphic adenoma of the lacrimal gland, hemangiopericytoma, and echinoccocal cysts, it would be compulsory to remove the lesion within its capsule to avoid seeding into the surgical field.

Innovative surgical techniques for the management of orbital mass lesions have been expanding in the literature. Such methods include direct embolization techniques via the superior ophthalmic vein for cavernous sinus-dural fistulas, image-guided orbital surgery, endoscopic orbitotomy, and percutaneous sclerotherapy [17–22]. These techniques can be extremely useful in specific situations, and however may require specific material and technical capacities that can be institution dependent.

Complications of Orbit Surgery

Intraoperative Complications

The most serious complication during surgery is the unintentional laceration of a vital structure such as a peripheral nerve, muscle, blood vessel, the optic nerve, or the globe. Although this kind of injury is rare, the damage should be repaired before the procedure is continued. Scleral lacerations are exceedingly rare and should be treated as an open globe repair. Optic nerve damage may not appear immediately and can be related to vascular occlusion or vasospasm. Vascular lacerations are difficult if not impossible to restore with an end-to-end anastomosis because of the small size of the orbital blood vessels and the difficulty in locating the severed ends. If a major peripheral nerve is cut accidentally, it is ideal to anastomose the nerve under high magnification (preferably

with the microscope) with 9-0 nylon suture from perineurium to perineurium after the cut ends of the nerve have been aligned. If anastomosis is not possible, the nerve edges should be approximated to facilitate healing. Tissue glue is another option if available. If an extraocular muscle is cut or damaged inadvertently, it should be approximated and sutured with a 6-0 Vicryl suture.

Lacerations to the nasolacrimal drainage system may also lead to postoperative problems. Here as well every attempt should be made to repair the laceration, and canalicular silicone stent should be placed in a position to maintain the patency of the LDS. If the damage is limited at the canaliculus level, both ends of the cut canaliculus should be aligned and repaired with fine sutures under the operating microscope. If the damage is serious, at the lacrimal sac or nasolacrimal duct level, and judged to be irreparable, a DCR may be the choice of treatment at the end of the orbital exploration or at a later date.

If dural laceration is suspected during surgery, it should be identified to rule out CSF leak. Although small lacerations can be repaired with direct suturing, the visualization is usually not good enough to allow this procedure. The best way to repair the dural rents is to apply free grafts from temporalis fascia or muscle, which can be applied with or without tissue adhesives. For small leaks, orbital fat may be sufficient to plug the leak. If the CSF leak cannot be controlled, neurosurgical consultation should be sought intraoperatively. A lumbar puncture may be of some help to reduce the CSF pressure and thereby allow the surgeon to control the leak better [23].

Intraoperative hemorrhage due to vascular laceration or generalized oozing is the most challenging part of orbital surgery, as it interferes with direct visualization. Therefore, intraoperative bleeding during orbit surgery should be addressed methodically until hemostasis is regained. The first objective is the identification of the bleeding source. Alternating suction and pressure by hand may accomplish this. If any obvious bleeding from blood vessels is detected, these can be cauterized or tied off. If no direct source can be seen, generalized pressure with epinephrine-soaked gauze or thrombin-soaked Gelfoam can be applied with gentle pressure.

Bleeding from the bone may be controlled with unipolar cautery. If this is not successful, bone wax may be applied. Excess bone wax should be carefully removed as it can lead to postoperative foreign body reaction [24].

Postoperative Complications

Emergent Postoperative Complications

One of the most serious complications in orbital surgery is a unilateral or (rarely bilateral) orbital hemorrhage leading to compartment syndrome and visual loss. The orbit is a small, non-expansile space, and an expanding hematoma can create a compartment syndrome, which is a potentially vision-threatening condition. The use of orbital drains is somewhat controversial, and their effect in preventing orbital compartment syndrome is not well established (Fig. 11.6).

Generous application of ice and elevation of the head of the bed during the first 24–48 h of the postoperative period may reduce the likelihood of orbital bleeding and can assist with swelling. However, postoperative hemorrhage may occur even in patients treated in this way, who do not have risk factors such as hypertension or hypocoagulability.

Physician's orders should be clearly written to alert the nursing staff to recognize symptoms of acute postoperative hemorrhage, including loss of vision, pain, and rapidly increasing proptosis. Small postoperative hematomas that produce some proptosis and chemosis but no pain or

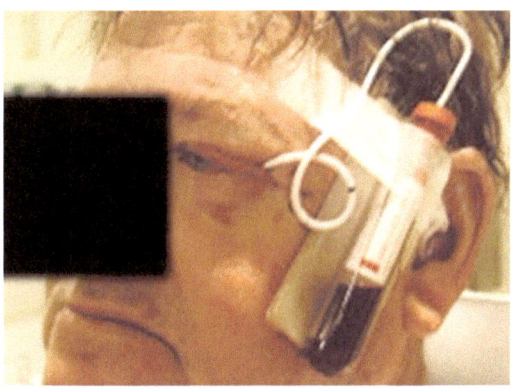

Fig. 11.6 Hemovac™ drain in position one day after surgery. (From Karcioglu [29], with permission)

afferent pupillary defect can be observed under conservative treatment. If a large postoperative hematoma is suspected, the eye should be examined immediately by checking the visual acuity, intraocular pressure, and pupillary light reflex. If the patient complains of visual loss in the presence of rapidly developing painful proptosis, one should check the intraocular pressure, which correlates with orbital pressure in the acute setting [25]. Even when the imaging studies do not reveal obvious nerve compression but the clinical symptoms suggest an acute increase in intraorbital pressure, the patient should be managed urgently.

Acute increase in orbital pressure is an emergency. In case of suspicion of a postoperative bleed in a patient with a drain in place, adjustment and/or irrigation of the drain should be tried before surgical intervention. If the high pressure persists, it should be relieved surgically. Opening the surgical wound may be effective as an egress point for the hemorrhage. However, the simplest and the most effective way of relieving the orbital pressure is by performing a lateral canthotomy and cantholysis [26]. This should be performed without delay based on clinical findings [27].

Catholysis splits the lateral canthal tendon in parallel and allows for access to the superior and inferior crus of the tendon, it does not relieve pressure in itself. In cantholysis procedure, the orbital volume expansion is best accomplished with the lysis of the inferior crus of the lateral canthal tendon. This should include generous portions of the inferior retinaculum, essentially 90° of the orbital rim. If the pressure is not relieved, the superior crus can be cut in the same fashion. When the canthotomy is done, the lids may not cover the cornea which should be protected with ointment, collagen shield, bandage contact lens, or light patching. If the increased orbital pressure cannot be relieved, the patient should be taken back to the operating room so that the wound can be opened to evacuate the blood. If active bleeding is observed, hemostasis should be accomplished and new drains should be placed before re-closure. The addition of mannitol and acetazolamide can be considered to lower the intraocular pressure as well.

Non-emergent Postoperative Complications

Excessive traction or blind dissection of the orbital tissues may damage the nerves, causing postoperative sensory and motor complications. In one study, the greatest incidence of complications was recorded in lateral orbitotomies (35%). Complications of lateral orbitotomy included extraocular motility problems, particularly abduction deficit (17.5%), and loss of pupillary reflex (10%). The majority of complications were associated with the lateral surgical approach to excise an intraconal mass and tumor type did not appear to be a factor. Ptosis may also be a problem following lateral and superior orbitotomy, typically resolving in weeks to months. However, damage to the superior division of the III CN and injury in the orbital apex can also produce long-term ptosis [28]. Anterior orbitotomy, not surprisingly, had much lower incidence of complications in only 3% of surgeries reported.

Dissection in the lateral orbit may injure the ciliary ganglion, particularly after removal of intraconal lesions, and the patient may develop dilated, nonreactive pupil postoperatively. This may take up to 6 months to resolve, or can be permanent. In superior medial orbitotomy, if the trochlea is injured, the patient may develop acquired Brown's syndrome postoperatively. This usually resolves spontaneously. In superior lateral orbitotomy, the lacrimal gland or its connecting ductules may be damaged, potentially resulting in dry eye. This is usually a permanent problem and should be managed with artificial tears, ointments, and punctal plugs.

Another long-term complication in any surgical procedure is scar formation, which in general can be minimized with strict attention to precise surgical technique. The surgical approach for orbital tumor biopsies is usually well planned and accomplished with relatively small skin incisions. Therefore, scars are seen less often after orbital tumor surgery than following treatment for other orbital problems, such as trauma and inflammation.

Acknowledgments We are grateful to Dr. Daniel Rootman, Assistant Professor, Orbital and Ophthalmic Plastic Surgery, Doheny Eye Institute, University of California, Los Angeles, for his contribution as the expert reviewer for this section. The author also appreciates the lifelong surgical counsel he has received from Dr. Bita Esmaeli of Houston, Texas, and Dr. J Chris Fleming of Memphis, Tennessee. He also warmly remembers Dr. Barrett G. Haik of New Orleans, Louisiana, a world leader in ocular and orbital oncology, as a great mentor and a valued friend. Dr. Barrett G. Haik died on July 22, 2016.

Videos 11.1 and 11.2 have been included with contribution from Santosh G Honavar MD, FACS Ocular Oncology Service, Centre for Sight, Banjara Hills, Hyderabad, India and Raksha Rao MS, FICO Department of Orbit and Ophthalmic Oncology, Narayana Nethralaya, Bangalore, India.

References

1. Goldberg RA, Rootman DB, Nassiri N, Shadpour JM. Orbital tumors excision without bony marginotomy under local and general anesthesia. J Ophthalmol. 2014;2014:1–5. https://doi.org/10.1155/2014/424852.
2. Bilyk JR, Sutula FC. Anesthesia for ophthalmic plastic surgery. In: Stewart WB, editor. Surgery of the eyelid, orbit and lacrimal system, vol. 1. San Francisco: American Academy of Ophthalmology; 1993. p. 26–55.
3. Morris R, McKay W, Mushlin P. Comparison of pain associated with intradermal and subcutaneous infiltration with various local anesthetic solutions. Anesth Analg. 1987;66(11):1180–2.
4. Gupta A, Tomlins PJ, Ng A TW, Reuser TT. Alleviating pain in oculoplastic procedures by reducing the rate of injection of local anaesthetic. Open Ophthalmol J. 2015;9:156–8.
5. Ascaso FJ, Peligero J, Longás J, Grzybowski A. Regional anesthesia of the eye, orbit, and periocular skin. Clin Dermatol. 2015;33(2):227–33.
6. Kumar CM, Dowd TC. Complications of ophthalmic regional blocks: their treatment and prevention. Ophthalmologica. 2006;220(2):73–82.
7. Borges AF. Relaxed skin tension lines (RSTL) versus other skin lines. Plast Reconstr Surg. 1984;73(1):144–50.
8. Appling WD, Patrinely JR, Salzer TA. Transconjunctival approach vs subciliary skin-muscle flap approach for orbital fracture repair. Arch Otolaryngol Head Neck Surg. 1993;119(9):1000–7.
9. Schor HI, Baylis HI, Goldberg RA, Perry JD. Transcaruncular approach to the medial orbit and orbital apex. Ophthalmology. 2000;107(8):1459–63.
10. Moe KS. The precaruncular approach to the medial orbit. Arch Facial Plast Surg. 2003;5(6):483–7.

11. Kim JW, Yates BS, Goldberg RA. Total lateral orbitotomy. Orbit. 2009;28(6):320–7.
12. Goldberg RA, Shorr N, Arnold AC, Garcia GH. Deep transorbital approach to the apex and cavernous sinus. Ophthal Plast Reconstr Surg. 1998;14(5):336–41.
13. Rootman J, Stewart B, Goldberg RA. Orbital surgery: a conceptual approach. Philadelphia: Lippincott-Raven; 1995.
14. Bourne TD, Karcioglu ZA. Orbital biopsy. In: Karcioglu ZA, editor. Orbital tumors: diagnosis and treatment. New York: Springer; 2015. p. 121–43.
15. Kıratlı H, Bulur B, Bilgiç S. Transconjunctival approach for retrobulbar intraconal orbital cavernous hemangiomas. Orbital surgeon's perspective. Surg Neurol. 2005;64:71–4.
16. Pelton RW, Patel BCK. Superomedial lid crease approach to the medial intraconal space: a new technique for access to the optic nerve and central space. Ophthal Plast Reconst Surg. 2001;17:241–53.
17. Goldberg RA, Goldey SH, Duckwiler G, Vinuela F. Management of cavernous sinus-dural fistulas. Indications and techniques for primary embolization via the superior ophthalmic vein. Arch Ophthalmol. 1996;114(6):707–14.
18. Karcioglu ZA, Mascott CR. Computer-assisted image-guided orbit surgery. Eur J Ophthalmol. 2006;16:446–52.
19. Berger M, Char DH. Interactive image guidance for surgical localization of orbital apical tumors. Orbit. 2002;21:199–203.
20. Murchison AP, Rosen MR, Evans JJ, Bilyk JR. Endoscopic approach to the orbital apex and periorbital skull base. Laryngoscope. 2011;121:463–7.
21. Hill RH, Shiels WE, Foster JA, et al. Percutaneous drainage and ablation as first line therapy for macrocystic and microcystic orbital lymphatic malformations. Ophthal Plast Reconstr Surg. 2012;28(2):119–25.
22. Naik MN, et al. Foam sclerotherapy for periorbital dermoid cysts. Ophthal Plast Reconstr Surg. 2014;30(3):267–70.
23. Tse DT, Panje WR, Anderson RL. Cyanoacrylate adhesive used to stop CSF leaks during orbital surgery. Arch Ophthalmol. 1984;102(9):1337–9.
24. Karcioglu ZA, Nasr AM. Diagnosis and management of orbital inflammation and infections secondary to foreign bodies: a clinical review. Orbit. 1998;17(4):247–69.
25. Nassr MA, Morris CL, Netland PA, Karcioglu ZA. Intraocular pressure change in orbital disease. Surv Ophthalmol. 2009;54(5):519–44.
26. Goodall K, Brahma B, Bates A, Leatherbarrow B. Lateral canthotomy and inferior cantholysis: an effective method of urgent orbital decompression for sight threatening acute retrobulbar haemorrhage. Injury. 1999;30:485–90.
27. Oester AE Jr, Sahu P, Fowler B, Fleming JC. Radiographic predictors of visual outcome in orbital compartment syndrome. Ophthal Plast Reconstr Surg. 2012;28(1):7–10.
28. Purgason PA, Hornblass A. Complications of surgery for orbital tumors. Ophthal Plast Reconstr Surg. 1992;8(2):88–93.
29. Karcioglu ZA. Orbital tumors: clinical diagnosis and treatment. 2nd ed. New York: Springer; 2015.

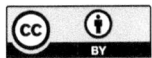

Santosh G. Honavar and Raksha Rao

Enucleation and exenteration for the management of intraocular and orbital malignancies, respectively, was the standard treatment of care before the advent of radiotherapy and chemotherapy. Over the past few decades, enhanced knowledge on the biology of the tumors, advances in the histopathologic and cytological techniques, use of various diagnostic modalities for an early and a more precise diagnosis, implementation of protocol-based management, and use of multimodal treatment including chemotherapy, radiotherapy, immunotherapy, and conservative surgeries, have greatly contributed to the reduction in the need for enucleation and exenteration. This paradigm shift toward less radical treatment has brought about a refinement in the absolute indications for enucleation and exenteration.

Electronic supplementary material The online version of this chapter (https://doi.org/10.1007/978-3-030-18757-6_12) contains supplementary material, which is available to authorized users.

S. G. Honavar (✉)
Ocular Oncology Service and National Retinoblastoma Foundation, Centre for Sight, Hyderabad, India

R. Rao
Department of Orbit and Ophthalmic Oncology, Narayana Nethralaya, Bangalore, India

Overview and Indications of Enucleation

Enucleation is defined as the removal of the eyeball while preserving the rest of the orbital tissues, including the extraocular muscles. Following enucleation, the aim is to achieve a good cosmesis by placing a prosthesis which matches the contralateral eye. A well-planned surgical technique with adequate volume replacement provides gratifying static and dynamic cosmesis. The characteristics of an ideal anophthalmic socket include a centrally placed well-covered implant of adequate volume, a socket lined with healthy conjunctiva, deep fornices to help retain the prosthesis, normal eyelid position with symmetric lid crease, and good implant motility which is transmitted to the overlying prosthesis.

In oncology practice, enucleation is routinely performed for the management of malignant intraocular tumors with an aim for complete tumor control [1–12]. To achieve this end, it sometimes entails the removal of an additional and adequate length of the optic nerve, excision of any adherent conjunctiva and tenon's fascia to the underlying tumor, or sacrificing a part of the orbital tissue, and this is termed as extended enucleation. Over the past few decades, advances in chemotherapy and radiotherapy have led to eye-salvaging treatment options for intraocular tumors, and the indications for enucleation have thus become specific [9, 10, 13–15].

© The Author(s) 2019
S. S. Chaugule et al. (eds.), *Surgical Ophthalmic Oncology*,
https://doi.org/10.1007/978-3-030-18757-6_12

Enucleation continues to play a major role in the management of retinoblastoma and uveal melanoma (Table 12.1). In retinoblastoma, indications for primary enucleation include advanced unilateral retinoblastoma without salvageable vision (group E of international classification of retinoblastoma [ICRB]), unilateral retinoblastoma with diffuse anterior chamber involvement, unilateral retinoblastoma with total vitreous hemorrhage, unilateral retinoblastoma with accompanying neovascular glaucoma, and retinoblastoma with a phthisical eye [1–3]. Secondary enucleation is performed for recurrent retinal tumor not controlled with current treatment modalities, vitreous seeds or subretinal seeds with suboptimal response to chemotherapy and/or radiotherapy, eyes with opaque media (total hyphema or dense vitreous hemorrhage) after an initial failed response to chemotherapy and/or radiotherapy, and as a part of the treatment protocol in orbital retinoblastoma [2–4].

Enucleation for ciliochoroidal melanoma as a primary treatment is indicated in very large tumors (>18 mm in diameter and >10 mm in thickness) which are not amenable to plaque radiotherapy (Table 12.1) [5, 6]. Choroidal melanomas with optic nerve invasion are also an indication for enucleation [7]. Enucleation may be necessary in recurrent posterior melanoma, which has not responded favorably to radiation treatment [5, 6]. Extraocular extension of melanoma also warrants enucleation, although there has been a recent trend to manage such cases by plaque brachytherapy where the size of the extraocular extension is less than 3 mm [8, 9]. Ciliochoroidal melanomas presenting with dense vitreous hemorrhage, or as a painful blind eye due to extensive necrosis or secondary glaucoma, are other indications for enucleation [5, 6].

Enucleation in iris melanoma is generally reserved for tumors which have progressed to a size where surgery or radiotherapy is not feasible (Table 12.1) [10, 11]. These include eyes where

Table 12.1 Indications for enucleation

Tumor	Primary	Secondary
Retinoblastoma	Advanced unilateral retinoblastoma without salvageable vision Diffuse anterior chamber involvement Total vitreous hemorrhage Total hyphema Unilateral retinoblastoma with accompanying neovascular glaucoma Retinoblastoma with a phthisical eye	Recurrent retinal tumor, vitreous seeds or subretinal seeds with suboptimal response to chemotherapy and/or radiotherapy Eyes with opaque media (total hyphema or dense vitreous hemorrhage) after an initial failed response to chemotherapy and/or radiotherapy As a part of the treatment protocol in orbital retinoblastoma
Ciliochoroidal melanoma	Very large tumors (>18 mm in diameter and >10 mm in thickness) Optic nerve invasion Extraocular extension of melanoma more than 3 mm in size Dense vitreous hemorrhage Painful blind eye secondary to extensive necrosis or secondary glaucoma	Recurrent posterior melanoma, which has not responded favorably to radiation
Iris melanoma	Tumor involving all iris quadrants Eyes with uncontrolled secondary glaucoma with angle seeding Eye with large extrascleral extension	Recurrent iris melanoma, which has not responded favorably to radiation
Others	Large medulloepithelioma Intraocular extension of conjunctival squamous cell carcinoma Blind painful eyes harboring large benign or malignant intraocular tumors	Recurrent tumors, which has not responded favorably to other conservative treatment

the tumor involves all iris quadrants, eyes with uncontrolled secondary glaucoma with angle seeding, or in the presence of extrascleral extension [10, 11]. In a long-term analysis of 144 patients with iris melanoma treated by plaque radiotherapy, Shields et al. noted that glaucoma was present at the initial visit in 40% of cases, and by Kaplan-Meier estimate at 7 years, enucleation was necessary in 12% [11].

Enucleation is sometimes necessary in other conditions including medulloepithelioma, intraocular extension of conjunctival squamous cell carcinoma, and blind painful eyes harboring large benign or malignant intraocular tumors (Table 12.1) [7, 12]. In a two-institutional study of 41 eyes with medulloepithelioma, 26 eyes (63%) required enucleation, and it was mainly indicated in larger tumors ($n = 21$), and in smaller tumors that failed to respond to conservative treatment ($n = 5$) [12].

Overview and Indications of Exenteration

Orbital exenteration is the surgical removal of the orbital contents, including the eyeball. Exenteration is performed as a life-saving measure for primary or secondary orbital malignancies where conservative treatment has failed or is not feasible. Exenteration maybe sub-total, total, extended, or radical exenteration depending on the amount of orbital contents excised. Subtotal exenteration entails removal of only the anterior orbital tissue. In total exenteration, the orbital contents are removed in their entirety. In extended exenteration, removal of orbital bones is also performed. In radical exenteration, adjacent structures like the paranasal sinuses are also sacrificed.

Exenteration is generally considered to be a radical procedure that should be performed only when there is a valid indication (Table 12.2) [16–20]. It is indicated in advanced primary orbital malignancies, eyelid tumors with orbital extension, conjunctival tumors with orbital extension, and intraocular tumors with orbital extension. Rarely, it may even be indicated in advanced benign tumors like neurofibromatosis or arteriovenous malformation with orbital deformity [19].

Table 12.2 Indications for exenteration

Advanced primary or recurrent orbital malignancies
Advanced primary or recurrent eyelid tumors with orbital extension
Advanced primary or recurrent conjunctival tumors with orbital extension
Advanced primary or recurrent intraocular tumors with orbital extension
Advanced benign tumors like neurofibromatosis with orbital deformity

Preoperative Evaluation

Preoperative evaluation of a patient with an ocular tumor includes documentation of symptoms, vision, pressure, slit lamp findings, and fundus findings. Additionally, transillumination test is performed for a suspected ciliary body tumor. The extent and nature of the tumor is assessed with the help of fundus images, ultrasound, fluorescein angiography (FA), and ocular coherence tomography (OCT). Examination of a child with a suspected intraocular tumor is always done under anesthesia, with complete evaluation including external photographs, RetCam images, and ultrasound performed in the same sitting. A large fundus diagram of the tumor replicating its extent in the eye with the measurements listed is used at the time of surgery.

For orbital tumors, careful inspection and palpation is necessary including evaluation of ocular motility, globe and lid position. Examination of the regional lymph nodes and other possible relevant details must be done. Radiological images of the orbit to study the tumor extent are obtained which must be available at the time of surgery. Malignancies with the potential for systemic spread must undergo a complete metastatic workup. In tumors which require adjunctive treatment with chemotherapy, radiotherapy or immunotherapy, a collaborative team consisting of medical and radiation oncology is essential. An incisional biopsy for the histopathologic diagnosis of the malignancy is recommended before proceeding with exenteration.

Technique of Enucleation (Video 12.1)

It is pertinent that fundus examination be done by the operating surgeon at the time of surgery to identify and mark the correct eye. Enucleation can be performed under general anesthesia or local anesthesia with intravenous sedation. Even for cases done under general anesthesia, it is advised that retrobulbar injection of 2% lignocaine in combination with 1:100,000 epinephrine, mixed with 75% bupivacaine (1:1), be administered (8–10 mL).

After the patient is prepared and draped, a wire speculum is placed to exclude the eyelashes from the field. A lateral canthotomy is performed when additional space is required, as in an eye with retinoblastoma where the globe maybe enlarged [2, 21]. A 360° peritomy is performed using a blunt tipped Westcott scissors, cutting as close to the limbus as possible to preserve the conjunctiva (Fig. 12.1a). The underlying posterior tenon's fascia is undermined in all four quadrants between the recti muscles in a spreading action using a blunt tipped tenotomy scissors. The medial rectus muscle is hooked using a muscle hook and freed from the surrounding intermuscular septa by blunt dissection. The muscle is then identified, hooked and double-tagged, first with 6-0 silk suture 2 mm from the insertion and then with 6-0 vicryl suture 4 mm from the insertion (Fig. 12.1b, c) [2, 21]. 6-0 silk sutures serve as traction sutures while 6-0 vicryl sutures would later be used to suture the muscles through the implant or the conjunctiva (described later). The muscle is then transected between the two sutures. This is followed by similar tagging and transection of inferior rectus, lateral rectus, and superior rectus. Superior oblique and inferior

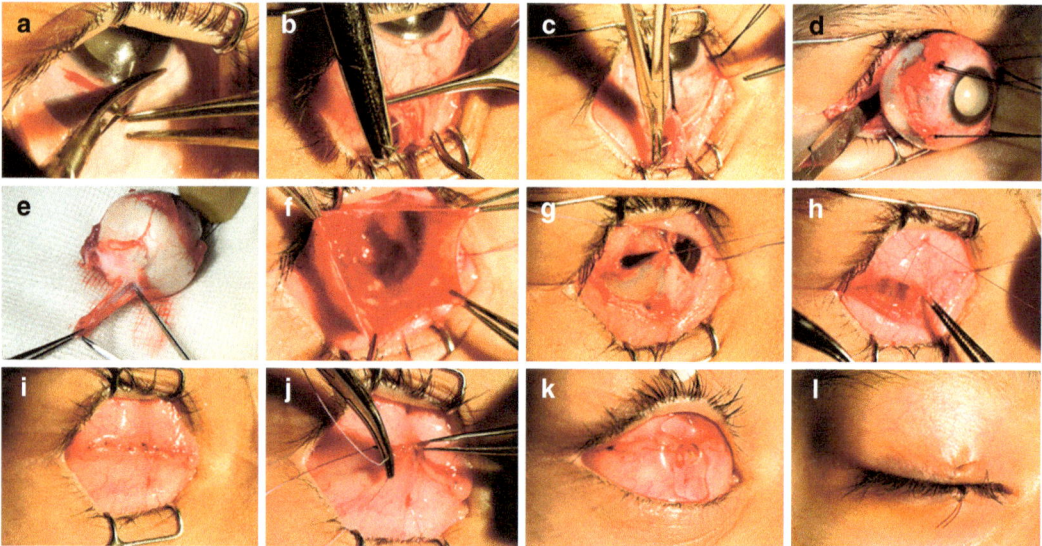

Fig. 12.1 Technique of enucleation in a 5-year-old male with right eye advanced retinoblastoma. (**a**) A 360° peritomy is performed using a blunt-tipped Westcott scissors, cutting as close to the limbus as possible. After undermining the posterior tenon's fascia, each rectus is double tagged, (**b**) first with 6-0 silk suture 2 mm from the insertion and then with (**c**) 6-0 vicryl suture 4 mm from the insertion. After transecting the muscles, (**d**) the eyeball is prolapsed between the blades of the speculum, and the optic nerve divided just a little anterior to the superior orbital fissure. (**e**) The transected optic nerve length is measured in all cases of retinoblastoma before the eyeball is submitted for histopathology. (**f**) Hemostasis is achieved and (**g**) the orbital implant placed within the posterior tenon's fascia, closing it with interrupted 6-0 vicryl suture. (**h**) Each rectus is sutured to the conjunctiva in its respective fornix by passing the tagged 6-0 vicryl suture through the conjunctiva. (**i**) Anterior tenon's closure is done with interrupted 6-0 vicryl suture and (**j**) conjunctival closure with a continuous key-suturing pattern. (**k**) An appropriate-sized conformer is placed in the socket and (**l**) a temporary median tarsorrhaphy performed with 6-0 vicryl suture

oblique muscles are transected and allowed to retract posteriorly. Each of the sutures is clamped with a bulldog clip.

A conjunctival relaxing incision is made for easy manipulation in large globes [21]. The eyeball is then prolapsed between the blades of the speculum (Fig. 12.1d). With a forward traction on the eyeball using the four silk sutures, a gently curved blunt-tipped tenotomy scissors is passed along the lateral wall and the optic nerve is strummed along its length. With one bold cut, the optic nerve is transected at the desired length. In retinoblastoma, the transection is performed just a little anterior to the superior orbital fissure, to gain a good length of the nerve (15–20 mm) and at the same time avoiding injury to the superior orbital fissure contents [2]. Adequate hemostasis is achieved using firm pressure for 5–10 min. The enucleated globe is inspected thoroughly for any scleral thinning, perforation, extraocular tumor extension, and dilated vessels. The transected optic nerve length is measured (Fig. 12.1e), and the eyeball is then sent for histopathologic examination in 10% formalin.

An implant of adequate size and the surgeon's preferred material is placed posterior to posterior tenon's fascia (intraconal fat space). Posterior tenon's fascia is closed with interrupted 6-0 vicryl sutures (Fig. 12.1f, g). The recti are then attached to the implant using the 6-0 vicryl sutures by passing the needles through posterior tenons including the implant wrapping material as anteriorly as possible. Alternately, the muscles can be sutured to the conjunctiva in their respective fornices by passing the needle through the conjunctiva (Fig. 12.1h). These are the myoconjunctival sutures and the technique is known as the myoconjunctival technique [21]. The advantage of this technique is that it allows the use of a non-integrable orbital implant (silicone or PMMA sphere) which offers a safe and cost-effective alternative, with prosthesis motility comparable to biointegrable implants while minimizing the complications of implant extrusion and migration [21].

Following this, anterior tenon's is closed with interrupted 6-0 vicryl sutures (Fig. 12.1i). Conjunctival closure is done in a continuous key-suturing pattern with 6-0 vicryl suture (Fig. 12.1j). An appropriate sized conformer is placed in the socket (Fig. 12.1k) and a temporary median tarsorrhaphy performed with 6-0 vicryl suture (Fig. 12.1l). The suture tarsorrhaphy is removed after 1 week, and a customized prosthesis can then be placed in the socket after 6 weeks [21].

Choice of Implant

Currently available implants can be categorized as:

1. Non-integrable: Implants that do not integrate with either the prosthesis or the orbital tissues. Examples for this include PMMA spheres, silicone spheres, and titanium spheres.
2. Semi-integrable: Implants that integrate with either the prosthesis or the orbital tissues. Allen's implant is an example for a semi-integrable implant.
3. Fully integrable: Implants that integrate with both the prosthesis and the orbital tissues. Cutler's implant is an example for a fully integrable implant.
4. Biointegrable: Implants that induce fibrovascularization within their substance and thus get integrated, for example, hydroxyapatite spheres.
5. Biogenic: Implants that are of biological origin, for example, dermis fat graft.

Non-integrated spherical implants by the conventional technique have a higher chance of migration, and also of poor implant and prosthesis motility. But when used in conjunction with the myoconjunctival technique, as described above, excellent static and dynamic cosmesis can be obtained [21]. Allen's implant and Cutler's implants are complicated by a high incidence of infection and extrusion [22]. Traditionally, dermis fat grafts are used in long-standing anophthalmic sockets with volume loss and surface loss [22].

Hydroxyapatite implants represent a new generation of integrated spheres that allow fibrovascular growth, which theoretically reduces the chances of migration, infection, and extrusion

[23–25]. Also, these biointegrated implants with pegging achieve satisfactory excellent motility [23–25]. Porous polyethylene offers a good alternative to hydroxyapatite implants, as they cause less irritation to the conjunctiva owing to their smoother surface [22]. Porous implants, although in wide use, are known to cause certain complications. These include conjunctival irritation, discharge, pyogenic granuloma formation, implant exposure, scarring, implant infection, and persistent discomfort [22–25]. These implants are also not suitable in immunocompromised individuals, diabetics, or in those who have had or require periorbital radiation therapy [22]. The choice of implant used is left to the surgeon's discretion.

Technique of Exenteration (Video 12.2)

Exenteration can be performed by either an eyelid-sacrificing or eyelid-sparing technique. With the eyelid-sacrificing method, the orbital cavity has to be lined by temporalis muscle, forehead flaps or grafts. Some surgeons advocate spontaneous granulation, and this offers comparable cosmetic results. However, healing by granulation takes longer and requires intensive postoperative care.

To circumvent this problem, an eyelid-sparing technique maybe used when possible. This method, popularized by Coston and Small, is a modification of the total exenteration technique which spares parts of both the eyelids, with transverse blepharorrhaphy to cover the orbit, thus ensuring better cosmesis and early rehabilitation [17]. In addition, sparing of the orbicularis muscle provides an excellent vascular supply to the skin flap, enabling early wound healing [17, 20].

Assistance from an otorhinolayrngologist or a neurosurgeon may be necessary in patients with extensive maxillary sinus involvement or roof erosion by the orbital tumor. The correct eye is identified and marked. Exenteration is always performed under general anesthesia. After the patient has been prepped and draped, the incision marking is placed 2 mm behind the lash line, joining them at the medial and lateral commissures (Fig. 12.2a) [17]. Three double-armed trac-

tion sutures with 4-0 silk are placed through the upper and lower tarsi to provide traction on the orbital contents. The incision is then made with a radiofrequency probe along the skin marking (Fig. 12.2b). Dissection is carried in the preseptal plane which decreases the likelihood of perforating the orbital septum, which is especially important in tumors present in the anterior orbit (Fig. 12.2c) [17]. Also, it leaves the orbicularis muscle intact, which provides a source for vascular supply to the skin flap.

Dissection is done till the orbital rim is reached, and the periosteum just outside the arcus marginalis is incised all around (Fig. 12.2d). Periosteal elevators are used to dissect the periosteum off the bony orbit, beginning at the incised margin along the orbital rim and continuing all the way back to the orbital apex (Fig. 12.2e). Most of the periosteum is loosely adherent to the underlying bone, with tight adhesions seen at certain anatomic locations, including the bony sutures and orbital fissures, as also in areas where the tumor has spread to the periosteum. At these points, gentle dissection is done to prevent any rip in the periosteum. Along the superior rim, dissection is gently carried around the supraorbital notch. The supraorbital and supratrochlear neurovascular bundle are identified and cauterized. Subperiosteal dissection is then carried from anterior to posterior lacrimal crest and beyond. Dissection is performed carefully along the medial wall, so as to not fracture the thin lamina papyracea. After negotiating the frontozygomatic suture with gentle dissection, zygomaticofacial and zygomaticotemporal neurovascular bundles are identified and cauterized. Dissection should be performed carefully along the orbital floor, so as to not fracture the thin bone and create a communication with the maxillary sinus. The sac is approached by dissecting medial to it and dividing the common canaliculus and orbicularis attachments. It is dissected from the lacrimal sac fossa and divided from the nasolacrimal duct with cautery. The exposed nasolacrimal duct is obliterated by cautery to reduce the risk of postoperative fistula formation (Fig. 12.2f).

Further deeper along the medial wall, anterior and posterior ethmoidal vessels are identified and

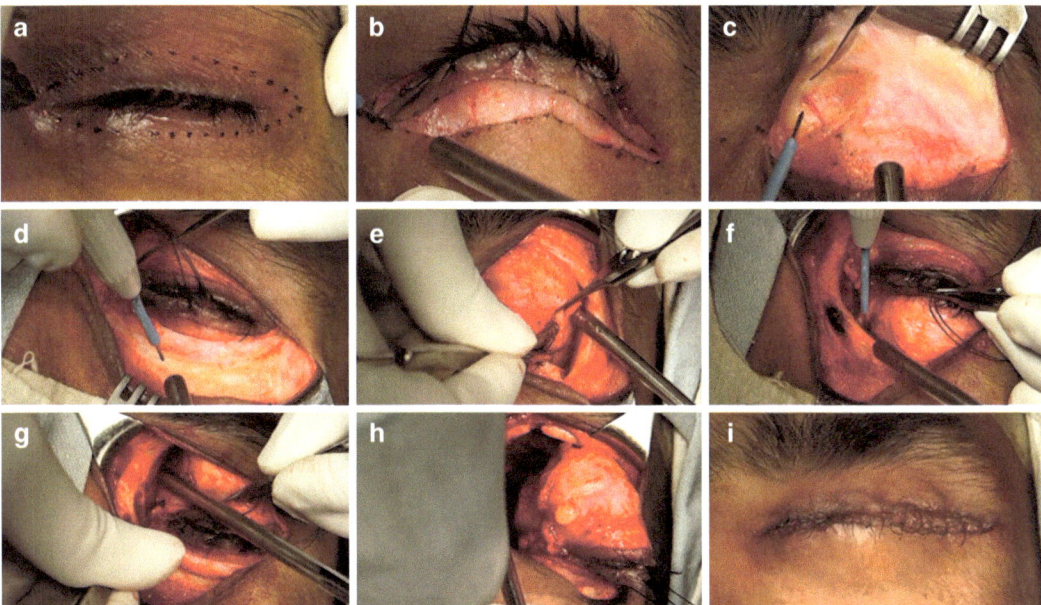

Fig. 12.2 Eyelid-sparing orbital exenteration technique in a 49-year-old male with the left orbital extension of conjunctival squamous cell carcinoma. (**a**) An incision marking is placed 2 mm behind the lash line in both the upper and lower eyelids, joining them at the medial and lateral commissures. (**b**) The incision is made with a radiofrequency probe along the skin marking. (**c**) Dissection is carried in the preseptal plane till the orbital rim is reached. (**d**) The periosteum just outside the arcus marginalis is incised all around. (**e**) A periosteal elevator is used to dissect the periosteum off the bony orbit, begin-ning at the incised margin along the orbital rim and con-tinuing all the way back to the orbital apex. (**f**) After dividing the nasolacrimal duct, the exposed duct is oblit-erated by cautery. (**g**) Along the deeper medial wall, ante-rior and posterior ethmoidal vessels are identified and cauterized. (**h**) The orbital tissue is held in forward trac-tion while dividing the posterior structures. (**i**) After ade-quate hemostasis, the eyelid flaps are reapproximated in two layers, with the orbicularis closure using 4-0 vicryl and skin closure using 6-0 silk suture

cauterized (Fig. 12.2g). In the inferotemporal orbit, the inferior orbital fissure is encountered and penetrating vessels divided with cautery. Next, the infraorbital nerve is identified and cau-terized. Ensure that the periosteum has been dis-sected to the apex, by passing a lid speculum all around in the orbit. A pair of curved enucleation scissors is then introduced into the posterior orbit. The optic nerve, superior orbital fissure contents, and posterior orbital tissues are divided (Fig. 12.2h). Hemostasis can be obtained with ice-cold wet gauze, pressure, and/or cautery. If necessary, additional hemostasis is achieved with surgicel or bone wax. The socket is carefully inspected for any residual tumor. The adequacy of resection may be judged with the aid of frozen-section control. The resection of additional orbital apical tissue may be done as deemed nec-essary. The eyelid flaps are reapproximated in two layers, with orbicularis closed using 4-0 vic-ryl, and the skin using 6-0 silk suture (Fig. 12.2i) [17]. Aspiration of the orbital cavity is done at the end of the procedure using a 10 cc syringe which yields some amount of blood and serum, and pro-vides a concave lid flap. The wound is then patched using an antibiotic ointment.

Following surgery, aspiration of the socket for any blood or serum is done every day using a 10 cc syringe till a dry aspiration is obtained. The socket usually heals quickly over the course of 3–6 weeks and is ready for a prosthesis at the end of 6–8 weeks. Eyelid-sparing orbital exen-teration enables early wound healing and cos-metic rehabilitation thus minimizing patient morbidity.

For lid-sacrificing exenteration, the incision marking is placed along the orbital rim. Dissection is then carried till the periosteum.

The periosteum just outside the arcus marginalis is incised, and the rest of the steps are similar as above. After excision of the orbital contents, the orbital cavity is left open to granulate in which case epithelialization generally occurs over 3–4 months, or reconstruction using split skin lining or skin flaps is done.

Following enucleation and orbital exenteration, the challenge lies in providing a good cosmesis. Once complete healing of the wound has occurred, a customized ocular prosthesis in an enucleated socket can be placed in 6 weeks. A good surgical technique is essential to provide a concave, smooth, and stable skin cover, over which an orbital prosthesis can be placed [17, 20].

In conclusion, enucleation and exenteration in ocular oncology are mainly performed in advanced malignant tumors. These procedures can be life-saving and are used as a part of multimodal treatment in achieving complete local remission. The cosmetic disfigurement caused by these radical procedures must be rehabilitated by a well-matched prosthesis.

References

1. Shields CL, Shields JA. Retinoblastoma management: advances in enucleation, intravenous chemoreduction, and intra-arterial chemotherapy. Curr Opin Ophthalmol. 2010;21(3):203–12.
2. Honavar SG, Singh AD. Management of advanced retinoblastoma. Ophthalmol Clin N Am. 2005;18:65–73.
3. Murthy R, Honavar SG, Naik MN, Reddy VA. Retinoblastoma. In: Dutta LC, editor. Modern ophthalmology. New Delhi: Jaypee Brothers; 2004. p. 849–59.
4. Honavar SG. Orbital retinoblastoma. In: Singh AD, Murphee LA, Damato BE, editors. Clinical ophthalmic oncology-retinoblastoma. 2nd ed. New York: Springer; 2015.
5. Shields CL, Shields JA. Ocular melanoma: relatively rare but requiring respect. Clin Dermatol. 2009;27(1):122–33.
6. Shields J, Shields C. Posterior uveal melanoma: clinical features. In: Shields J, Shields C, editors. Atlas of intraocular tumors. 3rd ed. Philadelphia: Lippincott, Wolters Kluwer; 2016. p. 45–59.
7. Lingam G. Options for management of intra ocular tumors. Indian J Ophthalmol. 2015;63(3):204–10.
8. Rini FJ, Jakobiec FA, Hornblass A, Beckerman BL, Anderson RL. The treatment of advanced choroidal melanoma with massive orbital extension. Am J Ophthalmol. 1987;104:634–40.
9. Gündüz K, Shields CL, Shields JA, Cater J, Brady L. Plaque radiotherapy for management of ciliary body and choroidal melanoma with extraocular extension. Am J Ophthalmol. 2000 Jul;130(1):97–102.
10. Popovic M, Ahmed II, DiGiovanni J, Shields CL. Radiotherapeutic and surgical management of iris melanoma: a review. Surv Ophthalmol. 2017;62:302–11. pii:S0039-6257(16)30152-7.
11. Shields CL, Shah SU, Bianciotto CG, et al. Iris melanoma management with iodine-125 plaque radiotherapy in 144 patients: impact of melanoma-related glaucoma on outcomes. Ophthalmology. 2013;120:55e61.
12. Kaliki S, Shields CL, Eagle RC Jr, et al. Ciliary body medulloepithelioma: analysis of 41 cases. Ophthalmology. 2013;120(12):2552–9.
13. Shields JA, Shields CL, Sivalingam V. Decreasing frequency of enucleation in patients with retinoblastoma. Am J Ophthalmol. 1989;108:185–8. 32.
14. Ferris FL 3rd, Chew EY. A new era for the treatment of retinoblastoma. Arch Ophthalmol. 1996;114:1412.
15. Epstein JA, Shields CL, Shields JA. Trends in the management of retinoblastoma: evaluation of 1,196 consecutive eyes during 1974 to 2001. J Pediatr Ophthalmol Strabismus. 2003;40:196–203.
16. Kennedy RE. Indications and surgical techniques for orbital exenteration. Ophthalmology. 1979;86(5):967–73.
17. Coston TO, Small RG. Orbital exenteration—simplified. Trans Am Ophthalmol Soc. 1981;79:136–52.
18. Rathbun JE, Beard C, Quickert MH. Evaluation of 48 cases of orbital exenteration. Am J Ophthalmol. 1971;30;72(1):191–9.
19. Levin PS, Dutton JJ. A 20-year series of orbital exenteration. Am J Ophthalmol. 1991;112(5):496–501.
20. Shields JA, Shields CL, Demirci H, Honavar SG, Singh AD. Experience with eyelid-sparing orbital exenteration: the 2000 Tullos O. Coston lecture. Ophthal Plast Reconstr Surg. 2001;17(5):355–61.
21. Shome D, Honavar SG, Raizada K, Raizada D. Implant and prosthesis movement after enucleation: a randomized controlled trial. Ophthalmology. 2010;117(8):1638–44.
22. Leatherbarrow B. Enucleation and evisceration. In: Leatherbarrow B, editors. Oculoplastic surgery. 2nd ed. Informa Healthcare; London, 2011. p. 479–98.
23. Kim YD, Goldberg RA, Shorr N, Steinsapir KD. Management of exposed hydroxyapatite orbital implants. Ophthalmology. 1994;101:1709–15.
24. Shields JA, Shields CL, De Potter P. Hydroxyapatite orbital implant after enucleation—experience with 200 cases. Mayo Clin Proc. 1993;68:1191–5.
25. Kaltreider SA, Newman SA. Prevention and management of complications associated with the hydroxyapatite implant. Ophthal Plast Reconstr Surg. 1996;12:18–31.

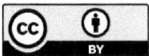

Kasturi Bhattacharjee, Manab Jyoti Barman
and Sripurna Ghosh

Loss of an eye is an immense psychological setback for any patient. Providing an appropriate implant with a well fitted mobile prosthesis can go a long way to alleviate this pain. Orbital implants are medical prosthetics used to replace the lost orbital volume as well as maintain it and allow some amount of realistic movement of a prosthetic eye following enucleation (or evisceration). In 1884 implants were first described by Mules, and ever since then different implant materials, designs and shapes have been tried [1]. An orbital implant may be autologous or alloplastic, integrated, or semi- or non-integrated [2]. The shapes of the implants are usually spherical and range from 12 to 24 mm in diameter. The wrapping materials act as buffer to shield the conjunctiva as well as act as a conducive niche for the attachment of the extraocular muscles.

Wrapping materials may be either organic (autologous and heterologous) or alloplastic. Advantages and disadvantages of wrapping an implant and choice of wrapping material are still matter of debate among the surgeons [3]. While human donor sclera is commonly used as a readily available cost-effective

wrapping material, it entails some potential risk of disease transmission. Specially processed and marketed allografts like human donor pericardium, fascia lata, sclera, bovine pericardium, and acellular dermis have been implemented as safe alternatives with variable success rate. These materials increase the cost of surgery. Autologous materials like temporalis fascia, rectus abdominus sheath, fascia lata, etc. have also been tried as wrapping materials. However use of these autologus tissues needs a second donor operative site resulting in prolonged operation time and increased morbidity. Synthetic wrapping materials (e.g., undyed polyglactin 910 mesh) are gaining popularity due to eliminated risk of disease transmission, no need of second surgical site, simple technique, and relatively inexpensive nature.

Enucleation especially in retinoblastoma patients undergoing adjuvant radio or chemotherapy has a higher risk of long-term complication [4]. Enucleation at a young age enhances the perils of volume deficiency both in terms of bone and soft tissue [5, 6]. Hence, careful selection of implant material and meticulous surgical technique is a necessity for these patients.

Various types of implants like gold, silver, glass, silicone, cartilage, bone, fat, cork, titanium mesh, acrylics, rubber, catgut, peat, agar, silicon, hydroxyapatite, and polyethylene have been described. At present most popular integrated implants are the hydroxyapatite and polyethylene and the non-integrated being the acrylic and silicon.

K. Bhattacharjee (✉) · S. Ghosh
Department of Orbit, Ophthalmic Plastic
and Reconstructive Surgery, Sri Sankaradeva
Nethralaya, Guwahati, India

M. J. Barman
Ocular Oncology Services, Sri Sankaradeva
Nethralaya, Guwahati, India

© The Author(s) 2019
S. S. Chaugule et al. (eds.), *Surgical Ophthalmic Oncology*,
https://doi.org/10.1007/978-3-030-18757-6_13

Hydroxyapatite Implant

Natural coralline hydroxyapatite material is used as the hydroxyapatite (HA) ocular implant. It contains approximately 500 μm diameter pores structurally that simulate the haversian system of human bone. The microstructure of this implant allows fibrovascular ingrowth of host tissues in the anophthalmic socket [7]. Once the implant is well vascularized and integrated, it can be drilled and fitted with a motility peg implant. This motility peg is then coupled to the ocular prosthesis to enhance prosthesis motility and cosmesis.

The hydroxyapatite implant is usually wrapped in donor sclera or fascia. The socket is measured using sterile trial spheres. Usually an 18–22 mm implant is appropriate. Wrapping the implant adds approximately 1–1.5 mm to the overall diameter.

The scleral shell is cut to the appropriate size and shape to enclose the implant securely with the corneal window placed posteriorly. Multiple interrupted 6-0 Vicryl sutures are used for securely closing the sclera; 2–4 mm rectangular windows are cut through the sclera within 8–10 mm from the anterior most apex of the implant. Multiple holes are then drilled manually into the implant using a 20-gauge needle to promote further fibrovascular ingrowth at the site of each window and at the site of the posterior corneal window [8]. The four recti muscles are sutured and fixed to the anterior lip of the corresponding scleral windows. Anterior Tenon's fascia is sutured with multiple interrupted 6-0 Vicryl sutures. The conjunctiva can be closed with continuous 6-0 plain suture. Some authors report a relatively high exposure rate with hydroxyapatite compared with alloplastic sphere implants emphasizing the need for a meticulous closure in layers as well as placement of the implant posterior to the posterior tenon deep in the socket [9–12].

Polyethylene (Medpor®) Implant

Polyethylene is a high-density straight-chain hydrocarbon material, formed by polymerization of ethylene molecules. It is nontoxic, nonaller-genic, and biocompatible. Medpor (Porex Surgical Inc., Georgia, USA) is a lightweight, polyporous form (150–400 μm) of polyethylene. This material enables fibrovascular proliferation of orbital tissue allowing biointegration of the implant with the host's body, thus reduces the risk of migration, exposure and extrusion. Unlike hydroxyapatite, it is much resilient, allowing muscles to be sutured directly to it without wrapping. Many studies have reported favorable surgical outcomes after Medpor orbital implantation [13–15].

A range of implant diameters of 14–22 mm are available. A set of resterilizable sizer is available for measuring the appropriate implant diameter.

The classic Medpor has a rough surface with some tendency to cause erosion of overlying Tenon's capsule and conjunctiva. To compensate for this, other types of Medpor have been designed. Medpor-SST is a further refinement with a smooth, porous anterior surface, which helps minimize late-implant exposure, and the preplaced suture tunnels allow for easy anchoring of the rectus muscles. Medpor-MCOI is cone-shaped, to provide extra volume in the orbit with a similar diameter implant. They have proved to be more effective in patients with phthisis bulbi or microphthalmos.

Bio-ceramic Implant

Bioceramic orbital implant is made of the porous, nonbrittle biomaterial alumina (Al_2O_3). It has uniform interconnected pores of approximately 500 μm in size. Unlike hydroxyapatite, it is manufactured with no disruption to marine ecosystems.

Advantages of bio-ceramic implants include:

- Easy to manufacture, structurally strong, and free of contaminants.
- Porous, strong, and resilient composition
- Rapid fibrovascular ingrowth
- No risk of disease transmission
- Lightweight and easy manuverability during surgery
- Easy suturing of extra ocular muscles to implant
- Effortlessly hand-drilled

- Noninflammatory, nonallergenic
- Improved motility of the artificial eye
- After implantation, a biofilm develops over the implant that acts as a barrier and helps in prevention of rejection.

Self-Inflating Tissue Expanders

Self-inflating tissue expanders are hydrogel implants which follow principle of osmotic gradient leading to volume enhancement. After implantation, absorbs body fluid and grow consistently to a predefined volume. The swelling capacity of the implant is between 7- and 12-fold, depending on the product type. These implants are indicated in the treatment of clinical anophthalmia, post enucleation socket syndrome, and congenital microphthalmia. Their advantages are as follows:

- Procedure is safe, quick, and minimally invasive
- High biocompatibility
- Lesser postoperative complications
- Optimized swelling
- Various shapes available for various indications

Being a relatively new technique, long-term safety of the material as an orbital implant has yet to be established, but early results are promising.

References

1. Mules PH. Evisceration of the globe, with artificial vitreous. Trans Ophthalmol Soc UK. 1885;5:200.
2. Baino F, Perero S, Ferraris S, Miola M, Balagna C, Verné E, et al. Biomaterials for orbital implants and ocular prostheses: overview and future prospects. Acta Biomater. 2014;10(3):1064–87.
3. Long JA, Tann TM 3rd, Bearden WH 3rd, Callahan MA. Enucleation: is wrapping the implant necessary for optimal motility? Ophthal Plast Reconstr Surg. 2003;19(3):194–7.
4. Shildkrot Y, Kirzhner M, Haik BG, Qaddoumi I, Rodriguez-Galindo C, Wilson MW. The effect of cancer therapies on pediatric anophthalmic sockets. Ophthalmology. 2011;118(12):2480–6.
5. Hintschich C. Bony orbital development after early enucleation in humans. Br J Ophthalmol. 2001;85(2):205–8.
6. Chojniak MM, Chojniak R, Testa ML, Min TT, Guimarães MD, Barbosa E, et al. Abnormal orbital growth in children submitted to enucleation for retinoblastoma treatment. Pediatr Hematol Oncol. 2012;34(3):102–5.
7. Perry AC. Integrated orbital implants. Adv Ophthalmic Plast Reconstr Surg. 1990;8:75–81.
8. Ferrone PJ, Dutton JJ. Rate of vascularization of coralline hydroxyapatite ocular implants. Ophthalmology. 1992;99:375–9.
9. Buettner H, Bartley GB. Tissue breakdown and exposure associated with orbital hydroxyapatite implants. Am J Ophthalmol. 1992;113:669–73.
10. Goldberg RA, Holds JB, Ebrahimpour J. Exposed hydroxyapatite orbital implants, reports of six cases. Ophthalmology. 1992;99:831–6.
11. Nunery WR, Heinz GW, Bonnin JM, et al. Exposure rate of hydroxyapatite spheres in the anophthalmic socket: histopathologic correlation and comparison with silicone sphere implants. Ophthalmic Plast Reconstr Surg. 1993;9:96–104.
12. Nunery WR, Cepela MA, Heinz GW, et al. Extrusion rate of silicone spherical anophthalmic socket implants. Ophthalmic Plast Reconstr Surg. 1993;9:90–5.
13. Baek SH. Clinical effect of porous polyethylene (Medpor®) orbital implant. J Korean Ophthalmol Soc. 2000;41:1858–63.
14. Blaydon SM, Shepler TR, Neuhaus RW, et al. The porous polyethylene (Medpor®) spherical orbital implant: a retrospective study of 136 cases. Ophthal Plast Reconstr Surg. 2003;19:364–71.
15. Kim DH, Koh YM, Na KS. Comparison of clinical results between hydroxyapatite and Medpor® orbital implant. J Korean Ophthalmol Soc. 2002;43:349–56.

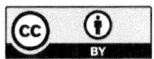

Ophthalmic Radiotherapy: Plaques and Implants

Paul T. Finger, Mark J. Rivard, Sonal S. Chaugule,
P. Mahesh Shanmugam, Svetlana Saakyan,
Hatem Krema, Mandeep S. Sagoo,
and Wolfgang A. G. Sauerwein

Radiation therapy is an indispensable tool used by eye cancer specialists around the world [1, 2]. However, ophthalmic radiation therapy can be expensive and typically requires collaboration between an ophthalmic oncologist, radiation oncologist, and a medical physicist. This chapter provides an overview of a basic ophthalmic radiation therapy program as well as indications for irradiation of common ocular malignancies.

Ionizing radiation has been used to destroy cancers of the eyelids, conjunctiva, iris, retina, choroid, optic nerve, and orbit [3–5]. The most common applications are brachytherapy (implanted and surface applicators), external beam radiation therapy (EBRT), and rarely interstitial orbital brachytherapy techniques. Most of these approaches have a surgical component.

Electronic supplementary material The online version of this chapter (https://doi.org/10.1007/978-3-030-18757-6_14) contains supplementary material, which is available to authorized users.

P. T. Finger (✉)
The Eye Cancer Foundation, Inc., The New York Eye Cancer Center, New York University School of Medicine, New York, NY, USA
e-mail: pfinger@eyecancer.com

M. J. Rivard
Department of Radiation Oncology, Brown University School of Medicine, Providence, RI, USA
e-mail: mark.j.rivard@gmail.com

S. S. Chaugule
Ophthalmic Plastic Surgery, Orbit and Ocular Oncology, PBMA's H V Desai Eye Hospital, Pune, India
e-mail: schaugule@eyecancercure.com

P. M. Shanmugam
Vitreoretinal and Oncology Service, Sankara Eye Hospital, Bangalore, India
e-mail: shanmugam1998@yahoo.com

S. Saakyan
Department of Ocular Oncology, Moscow Helmholtz Research Institute of Eye Diseases, Moscow, Russia
e-mail: svsaakyan@yandex.ru

H. Krema
Department of Ophthalmology and Vision Sciences, Princess Margaret Hospital, Toronto, ON, Canada
e-mail: Hatem.krema@unh.ca

M. S. Sagoo
Ocular Oncology Service, Moorfields Eye Hospital and Retinoblastoma Service, Royal London Hospital , UCL Institute of Ophthalmology, London, UK
e-mail: Mandeep.sagoo@moorfields.nhs.uk

W. A. G. Sauerwein
Department of Radiation Oncology, Strahlenklinik, University Hospital Essen, Essen, Germany
e-mail: w.sauerwein@uni-due.de

Programmatic Overview

Herein, we describe technical aspects required to start a radiation therapy program. These include specific imaging protocols for treatment planning of the various lesion types, specifically tumor-imaging or simpler nonimaging methods, quality assurance for the radiation sources encompassing the implanted brachytherapy device, and sterilization methods and radiation surveys of the operating theater and patient before/after implantation and explantation. Once the agreed-upon workflow is established and formalized in writing, it must be approved by the appropriate local radiation control agencies. All participants in each process should have reached a consensus as how to proceed. Any new staff should be trained, and there should also be annual retraining for all participants. It is helpful to have test conditions to evaluate staff comfort and proficiency with the multitude of tasks comprising ocular brachytherapy. An open environment will aid the long-term objective of having a safe and successful ocular brachytherapy program.

Costs

To be successful, all programs should perform a financial analysis before starting any procedures and then reviewed at least annually to ensure that prior assumptions were accurate and to capture looked-over items. In doing this financial analysis, a proposed workflow should be defined and include the following components: initial patient consultation, image acquisition, treatment planning, source ordering, quality assurance measures, treatment device sterilization, device implantation, radiation surveys, patient discharge (if applicable), device explant, post-explant wound care, device cleaning, and source disposal (if applicable). Estimates for each component cannot be given herein as every center will have unique circumstances that should be carefully assessed in the financial analysis. However, it is known that brachytherapy is both a cost-effective and clinically successful means of treating numerous ocular diseases. With consistent high-quality care and reproducible treatments for a given prescription, there should be a simple means for billing code entry by the staff performing the procedures or their designates.

In general, a brachytherapy program is typically less expensive to start than EBRT. Brachytherapy requires the purchase of implantable materials. For example, ruthenium-106 (^{106}Ru) applicators are solid brachytherapy sources, which are relatively inexpensive because they can be reused for multiple temporary implants over their longer half-life (372 days). In contrast, low-energy eye plaques [e.g., palladium-103(^{103}Pd), iodine-125 (^{125}I)] are relatively more expensive because radioactive seeds must be purchased, inserted in plaque shells, and calculated to the prescribed dose. ^{125}I and ^{103}Pd seeds exhibit half-lives of 59.4 and 17 days, respectively [2]. Therefore, they can be reused but only after reassessment of their current strength. It is important to note that seeded plaques are more versatile compared to solid sources. Seeded plaques are capable of treating larger tumors, can be customized to load the seeds eccentrically to try to spare normal tissues from radiation exposure, seeds can be mixed to modulate intraocular radiation distribution and require smaller margins (2–3 mm) [1, 6–8]. Thus, low-energy seeds can be affixed into custom-designed plaques to treat tumors of the iris, ciliary body, optic disc and conjunctiva more pre-cisely than a solid source plaque. Though most western centers use one plaque for each patient, high volume centers have decreased the cost per patient by reusing low-energy seeds and seed carriers.

In contrast, EBRT (e.g., photon, electron, proton) carries the highest startup cost [9]. In addition to the large capital cost of the linear or particle radiation accelerator, EBRT typically requires large, expensive facilities and radiation-shielded rooms. Although brachytherapy and proton EBRT provide comparable tumor control rates, brachytherapy produces the most conformal radiation dose distributions (within the eye) with less long-term radiation toxicity, particularly to anterior ocular and adnexal structures [6, 10–12].

Personnel

The Team: Medical Physicist, Radiation Oncologist, and Ophthalmic Oncologist

Radiation therapy personnel are required. The medical physicist (MP) and radiation oncologist (RO) are typically responsible for collaborating on radiation source selection, dose calculation (dose rate, implant duration, and target volume) [1, 2]. The MP usually constructs radioactive sources prior to implantation and/or administering EBRT. However, it is the ophthalmic oncologist (OO) who selects the patients and monitors for radiation side-effects. Therefore, the OO should become familiar with both MP and RO aspects of therapy [1]. For the purpose of this chapter, the OO's primary role is to make or confirm the diagnosis, biopsy tumors (when necessary), and surgically insert radioactive devices. In some countries, the OO can obtain licensing for the selection and prescription of radioactive plaques. Similarly, the RO may assume the role of MP.

Indications for Surgery

Available Evidence-Based Guidelines

Uveal Melanoma

Commonly treated with eye and vision-sparing surgical "plaque" irradiation [13]. In 2014, consensus guidelines were published by an international multicenter Ophthalmic Oncology Task Force (OOTF) that included 47 radiation oncologists, medical physicists, and ophthalmic oncologists from 10 countries. From this work, there was level 1 consensus that all centers:

1. Adopt the use of the American Joint Committee on Cancer (AJCC) or Union for International Cancer Control (UICC) staging systems to facilitate communication.
2. Brachytherapy procedures are performed at specialized medical centers with expertise.
3. These centers were defined as having a subspecialty-trained ophthalmic surgeon, a radiation oncologist, and a medical physicist who are all familiar with the AAPM TG-129 report [2].

Uveal Melanoma Case Selection

1. A clinical diagnosis of uveal melanoma is adequate (biopsy is not needed).
2. Small melanomas can be treated at the eye cancer specialist's discretion.
3. AJCC-UICC T1, T2, T3, and T4a-d uveal melanoma patients can be treated after counseling about likely vision, eye retention, and local control outcomes.
4. Patients with peripapillary, sub-, and perifoveal melanoma and those with exudative retinal detachments should be counseled about poorer resultant vision and local control outcomes.
5. Tumors with T4e extraocular extension, diameters that exceed the limits of brachytherapy, blind painful eyes, or no light perception vision are not suitable.

ABS = American Brachytherapy Society; AJCC = American Joint Committee on Cancer, UICC = Union International for Cancer Control; ^{106}Ru and ^{90}Sr plaques are less accommodating for nodular extra-scleral extension. (Reprinted by permission of *Brachytherapy* [1].)

Retinoblastoma Case Selection

The most common reasons to use plaque radiation for retinoblastoma is for eye and vision salvage after systemic, regional, or intraocular chemotherapy [1, 14]. An example: residual or relapsed RB that failed local control with chemoreduction and large enough not to be controlled by focal laser and/or cryotherapy. Prospects for sight-threatening complications should be discussed with the family as part of the consent process, through retinoblastoma typically requires a lower tumor apex dose than uveal melanoma. Further, the ABS groups achieved Level 2 consensus that the most common indication for plaque treatment of retinoblastoma is when the tumor is anterior to the equator in unilaterally affected children [1]. Exceptions include when there is evidence of anterior chamber tumor. The ABS-OOTF recommended that children at risk for extraocular RB undergo systemic staging [1]. Episcleral brachytherapy can be used to treat unilateral unifocal tumor or as an adjunct to treat chemoresistant tumors, post-chemotherapy residue showing signs of recurrence, and too large to treat with laser or cryotherapy. However, note chemotherapy treated eyes appear more likely to develop intraocular radiation vasculopathy. Lastly, specialized orbital applicators have been devised to irradiate orbital RB recurrence [1].

Orbital Brachytherapy Case Selection

There are three general indications for orbital brachytherapy implants: extrascleral extension of uveal melanoma, orbital invasion of adnexal tumors and recurrent retinoblastoma [15, 16]. Extrascleral extension of intraocular cancers presents unique challenges. Small amounts of uveal melanoma extrascleral extension are often treated with local plaque therapy with or without subsequent scleral patch grafting. However, in cases where the eye has been removed and residual tumor (microscopic disease) is suspected, postoperative radiation therapy has been employed to sterilize any remaining orbital cancer. EBRT ($\approx$40–50 Gy) with 6 MV photons has been prescribed [4]. However, such treatment typically results in entry dose-associated eye lash and brow loss, dry socket, a sunken orbit, or orbital bone dysgenesis (in children) [4]. There exist alternative high-dose-rate interstitial brachytherapy methods to temporarily implant the radiation within the orbit. These techniques increase the dose within the targeted orbit while decreasing the dose to the eye lids and brow [15]. More cosmetically acceptable, this technique has been reported to yield equivalent local control and improved cosmesis [4, 15, 16].

Intraocular Tumors

Uveal Melanoma

Uveal melanoma is the most primary common ocular tumor treated with implant radiation therapy in the developed world [17]. Methods of radiation plaque construction and dosimetry were reviewed by the American Association of Physicists in Medicine (AAPM) Task Group 129 in 2012 [2]. Similarly, open-access consensus clinical treatment guidelines were published in 2013 by the American Brachytherapy Society (ABS) [1].

Both of these guidelines offered the most widely accepted, evidence-based consensus from teams of eye cancer specialists. Invaluable for a new center, this information includes methods of dosimetry, quality assurance, and case selection [1, 2]. Though both apply to uveal melanoma, aspects also are relevant for selected intraocular retinoblastomas, as well as other intraocular tumors.

Vascular Tumors of the Retina and Choroid

Peripapillary or large retinal angiomas can be treated with brachytherapy. Circumscribed or diffuse choroidal hemangiomas smaller than the largest available episcleral brachytherapy implant can also be treated. However, when compared to brachytherapy, low-dose (16–24 Gy), photon-based external beam radiation therapy of choroidal hemangiomas will typically offer relative-sparing vision-critical intraocular structures [4, 18, 19, 31].

Uveal Metastasis

While most choroidal metastases are treated with nonsurgical EBRT, indications for plaque radiation therapy include radiation resistant tumors (e.g., renal cell, adenoid cystic carcinoma), when prior ocular radiation does not permit treatment of subsequent metastasis and when a patient refuses EBRT [4].

Ocular Adnexal Tumors

Conjunctival Tumors (Melanoma, Squamous Carcinoma)

Conjunctival tumors (melanoma, squamous carcinoma) can be treated with radiation. Melanomas are more commonly treated with these methods in that squamous carcinomas are more amenable to surgery with adjuvant cryotherapy and more recently topical chemotherapy [20]. Specialized plaques have been used to treat the ocular surface malignancies in select centers using a variety of radionuclides. Though the use of [106]Ru and ^{125}I plaques has been reported, by far the least expensive (but not widely available) method is strontium-90 (^{90}Sr) brachytherapy due to its 28.9-year half-life.

Orbital Tumors (Melanoma, Retinoblastoma)

Orbital Tumors (melanoma, retinoblastoma) can also receive curative and/or adjuvant ophthalmic brachytherapy [4]. Albeit rare, most commonly reported are treatments of residual tumors after enucleation of the eye. In addition, orbital adenoid cystic and basal cell carcinomas have been treated with orbital radiation implants. By far the most common use of orbital radiation therapy (EBRT) is for lymphoma (not covered in this chapter).

Presurgical Preparations

Ocular Imaging

Intraocular tumor imaging is used to determine whether or not the patient is eligible for brachytherapy treatment and then to dictate how the treatment should proceed [1]. Tumor dimensions are determined by clinical examination, photographic imaging, and ultrasonographic measurements. Typically performed with ultrasound (US) in A-scan or B-scan modes eye cancer specialists determine the largest basal dimension and furthest apical height of intraocular tumors. Other preimplant imaging modalities include optical coherence tomography and fundus autofluorescence imaging which offer more information about tumor extent (within tissues).

Small iris tumors are best localized and measured by slit lamp and gonioscopic photography as well as high-frequency ultrasound imaging. The clinically measured size and extent should be mapped in the chart. In addition, the tumour can be measured with calipers. Immidiately prior to surgery, the tumour borders should be drawn on the cornea and sclera with a marking pen. Transillumination may be used to help define the posterior extent of anterior segment tumours that allow production of an episcleral shadow. The surgeon should place the transilluminator in the quadrant opposite that of the tumor (or through the pupil if better) to produce a tumor shadow to be marked with a marking pen. Transillumination is often difficult in individuals with pigmented fundi and with tumors obscured by the ciliary body band.

In such situations and posteriorly placed tumors, the anterior and lateral margins of the tumor may be localized on to the scleral surface using indirect ophthalmoscopy with scleral depression. Such localization techniques are equivalent to those used for scleral buckling surgery [1].

Treatment Planning

Tumor measurements and distances to critical intraocular structure drive the resultant radiation treatment plan. Depending on the center, treatment planning can range from a simple calculation of the time to deliver the prescribed radiation dosage to a desired depth, to the sophisticated fusion of multiple radiographic imaging modalities used to measure the lesion, its location and distances to critical intraocular structures. Such computer-based radiographic imaging can be helpful for calculation of 3D dose distributions and the biologic effective dose.

As time marches forward, there have been significant advances in ocular brachytherapy treatment planning. The COMS approach derived dose to points based on characterizing ^{125}I brachytherapy seeds as point sources on a template diagram in a liquid water environment without concern for high-Z materials such as the treatment device or bony anatomy [21]. More recently, image-guided (CT/MRI) brachytherapy treatment planning has permitted more accurate approximations of volumetric dose information throughout the lesion and adjacent healthy structures. At this time, there exists no widely accepted radiographic image guided method or application for intraocular tumors [1].

To our knowledge, there is only one treatment planning system (TPS) created for eye plaque brachytherapy [22]. Many centers employ generic brachytherapy systems altered to perform for ocular use. Commissioning of any treatment planning system will include checks on the linearity of dose with prescription, tests of exponential decay based on the radionuclide half-life, spot checks of the reference dose distribution for a given source or brachytherapy treatment device with that replicated by the TPS, checks of volumetric calculations for accurate structure assessments, checks of dose-volume calculations for depiction of accurate 3D volumetric information, and many other basic features as prevalent in brachytherapy TPSs. Further, modern systems may include the ability to depict source collimation or dose differences between tissue and water [23].

Device Preparation

Most centers purchase solid or assemble seeded treatment devices. Therefore, each center must have a protocol to validate their treatment devices to match what is expected and characterized within the brachytherapy TPS. Commissioning the device will include comparisons of the manufacturer-reported dimensions and compositions to hands-on measurements and also those used in the TPS.

COMS-type plaques and other multicomponent treatment devices consist of a combination of several components that must be compatible. Sometimes the components (such as the glue necessary to hold the device together) are not explicitly approved by local governmental or regulatory agencies for medical purposes such as sterilization and implantation. To be proactive for regulatory audits, the center will need to document the suitability of all components and their intended use in their ocular brachytherapy program.

Some brachytherapy devices such as $^{106}Ru/^{106}Rh$ episcleral plaque have a built-in radiation source and are intended to be used on multiple patients. Other devices may have a nonradioactive plaque into which low-energy photon-emitting brachytherapy seeds (i.e., ^{103}Pd, ^{125}I, or ^{131}Cs) are loaded. These seeds may be reused depending on the source half-life, rate of patient accrual, and variety of prescriptions. In both cases, care must be taken to inspect (preceding first use and subsequent reuse) to ensure radioactive capsule integrity. Evaluation (mathematical or physical) of source strength is generally made prior to each use. Measurements of source strength require a re-entrant well-type air ionization chamber and seed holder with calibration for a given source model that is traceable to a primary standards calibration laboratory. In the United States of America, this is achieved through calibrating the chamber and seed holder at one of three Accredited Dosimetry Calibration Laboratories, which are traceable to the National Institute of Standards and Technology (NIST) [24]. Centers located elsewhere should follow local regulations. While not technically challenging, sterilization of the ocular brachytherapy device requires diverse attributes and coordination across multiple disciplines (Video 14.1).

Multicomponent devices will have differing or unspecified sterilization procedures with a limited number of permissible sterilization cycles (pertinent for devices to be used on multiple patients). Given the sensitive nature of some components such as glue or a seed holder, care must be taken to establish a sterilization program that accommodates limitations of all components yet provides timely and effective sterilization [1, 2].

Whichever approaches are taken, it is recommended that a patient database be established from the inception of an ocular brachytherapy program to capture information on various patient specific aspects of the procedure. This database can include imaging datasets and treatment planning information in addition to simple fields like implant/explant dates and times; names of participating staff; lesion height and basal dimensions; prescription dose, extent, and radionuclide; and dose-volume information for adjacent healthy structures. These data may be stored within the electronic health record system for later query.

Therapy Techniques

Orbital Brachytherapy for Residual Orbital Melanoma

We recommend that this procedure be performed 4–6 weeks after enucleation or other subtotal excisional surgery to allow wound healing [15]. When used for orbital extrascleral melanoma extension, the temporary prosthesis or conformer is removed and the patient placed under general anesthesia. The eyelids and conjunctival surfaces are prepared with povidone-iodine antiseptic (Table 14.1). The orbit is inspected for the condition of the conjunctival wound and the position of the orbital implant. A marking pen is used to define evenly spaced (1 cm) sites for catheter placement. The sites should be located just within the bony rim of the orbital bone by palpation. Care is taken to avoid critical structures (e.g., lacrimal drainage system, superior and inferior orbital nerves, and anterior ethmoid artery). Using the marks as a guide, transcutaneous #11 blade incisions should be performed (sequentially) as to create 3-mm wide orbitotomy sites. The aforementioned brachytherapy catheters were marked with ink to indicate when they are <4.5cm deep into the orbit. A brachytherapy button is placed onto the catheter to aid cutaneous fixation.

Then, a bimanual catheter implantation technique is used to guide the trochar toward the orbital apex. While the catheter enters the orbit, the surgeon uses on finger to palpate the catheter tip as it traverses through the orbital soft tissues. Once in place, with the catheter tip at the orbital apex, a cutaneous 4-0 suture is placed though the brachytherapy button to anchor it in place. Then, the catheters trocar is withdrawn. This series of steps is repeated with each catheter until there are 8–10 evenly spaced catheters in place. Then medical grade glue is placed to affix the trocars to the brachytherapy buttons and allowed to dry (Video 14.2).

Prior to being discharged to the recovery room, the catheters are trimmed to 5 cm in length and covered with a protective gauze dressing. Upon recovery from anesthesia, the orbit is imaged by computed tomography for treatment planning by the medical physicist.

Orbital Brachytherapy for Extrascleral Uveal Melanoma

High-dose-rate (HDR) brachytherapy is performed in a shielded room using a remote after

Table 14.1 Ophthalmic radiosurgery equipment and devices

Surgical equipment/materials
Anesthesia
Sterilization fluid for the plaque or Autoclave for solid plaques
Indirect ophthalmoscope
20 diopter lens
Scleral depressor
Ocular muscle suture material
Conjunctival suture material
Transilluminator and cable
Sterile Q-tips
Schepens Retractors
Scissors, forceps, speculum
Orbital brachytherapy materials
Anesthesia
#11 blade and Adsen forceps
8–10 brachytherapy catheters with trochars
8–10 brachytherapy buttons
4-0 silk sutures
Surgical marking pen
Medical grade epoxy or cyanoacrylate
Surgical dressing
Radiation isolation room
Computed axial tomography scans
HDR Iridium-192 system/treatment planning software/applicator(s)/shielded room
Select commercial vendors
Gold plaque shells http://www.trachseldentalstudio.com
Bebig ruthenium plaques http://www.bebig.com/home/products/ophthalmic_brachytherapy/ru_106_eye_applicators
Tantalum clips http://www.novoprecision.com/products/tantalum-markers
Preloaded plaques https://www.isoaid.com/prod_pages/eye-plaque
Survey meters https://www.environmental-expert.com/companies/keyword-geiger-counter-27616
Radioactive seeds
Best Medical http://www.teambest.com
BEBIG http://www.bebig.com/home/products/seed_brachytherapy
IsoAid https://www.isoaid.com
Theragenics https://www.theragenics.com
BXTAccelyon https://www.bxt-accelyon.com
Resotech http://www.resotech.ru

loader that houses an ^{192}Ir source. Under mild sedation and with pain medication, the orbital catheters are attached to the mechanical remote after-loader which sends the source down the catheters into the orbit for the prescribed dwell time, and are then retracted. Nine to ten treatment fractions are typically delivered (BID) over 5 consecutive days. At the end of treatment, 3–5 cm³ of lidocaine is placed into the orbit 15 min prior to extraction of the catheters. Once removed, the 3 mm cutaneous wounds are treated with topical antibiotic ointment and the ocular prosthesis is replaced.

Orbital Brachy-Boost Technique

In an effort to treat microscopic residual radiation-resistant tumor (e.g., adenoid cystic carcinoma, hemangiopericytoma, invasive carcinomas) HDR radiation can be applied to the tumor bed [4]. While the surgery is similar to the aforementioned technique (for treatment of melanomatous orbit extension), a lower brachytherapy dose is employed in addition to a subsequent overlay of EBRT. The result intensifies treatment of the tumor bed with relative sparing of the rest of the orbit. This eye and vision sparing HDR orbital brachytherapy technique is typically employed as an alternative to orbital exenteration.

Anesthesia for Radioactive Plaque Surgery

General anesthesia is preferred. This is because introduction of 3–5 cm³ of orbital fluid can limit the surgeons view and increase the difficulty of plaque placement. However, these procedures can be performed with local assisted surgery if needed, particularly for iris, ciliary body and anterior uveal tumors.

In that episcleral brachytherapy can be performed under peribulbar or retrobulbar anesthesia, we recommend using a mixture of 2% xylocaine and 0.5% bupivacaine. Caution to be taken to avoid inadvertent globe perforation which can increase the risk of orbital tumor dissemination. Vitreoretinal management of complications of globe perforation is both complicated and controversial.

Surgical Steps for Radioactive Plaque Surgery

The chart should be reviewed immediately prior to implantation surgery. Eye lid skin and periorbital area is sterilized with 10% povidone iodine solution with application of 5% povidone iodine eye drops in the conjunctival cul de sac. Then the patient should be draped with only the operative eye exposed for surgery. Then a secondary examination (ophthalmoscopy or ultrasound imaging) should be performed to confirm the presence of the tumor and condition of the eye. An eyelid speculum is placed. Then a limbal conjunctival periotomy is followed by opening of the intermuscular septa (Tenon's fascia) in all four quadrants. This is performed using a curved tenotomy scissors which is placed with closed blades in the episcleral space between the muscles. The scissors are opened in the orbit and withdrawn with open blades thereby lysing the intermuscular septa.

Anterior Plaques

Melanomas of the anterior uvea, ciliary body, and iris are commonly treated with plaque radiation [1, 17] (Video 14.3). Such treatment offers a method to cure the patient without intraocular surgery and often preserves the iris and its function. However, epicorneal plaque position can be painful and cause corneal erosions. This is why centers place a thin layer of donor tissue (e.g., amniotic membrane) as a buffer between the plaque and the cornea [25, 26]. In addition, insertion is complicated by "backward" plaque placement where the plaque eyelets are rotated onto the sclera as to avoid eyelet corneal suturing (see youtube.com/watch?v=B8IxecQCGOQ).

Circumpapillary Plaques

While the intraocular optic disc diameter is typically 1.8 mm, behind the eye the optic nerve is encased within the optic nerve sheath (ONS). The retrobulbar optic nerve sheath diameter is typically 5–6 mm, which means that a plaque placed against the ONS can only reach to 1.5 mm from the optic disc [3, 27–29]. The ONS presents a significant obstruction to normal radioactive plaque placement, defined by the ABS as covering the tumor plus a 2–3 mm margin. In order for a plaque to overcome the ONS diameter, 8-mm wide (variable depth) slots have been cut from COMS-type plaques. In that the seeds are the radioactive sources, the space within the slot can be filled with radiation. However, this requires more complex medical physics planning that guides placement of seeds within the plaque [27]. Due to their sharp penumbra and the 8-mm slot distance, complete tumor coverage or "normal plaque placement" cannot be achieved with solid ^{106}Ru plaques.

Radioactive Plaque Placement

Most uveal melanomas are located in the posterior choroid. Herein we include a movie showing plaque insertion for a posterior choroidal melanoma (Video 14.4). However, melanomas can occur beneath a variety of extraocular muscles as well as near the optic nerve. Any muscles that might interfere with plaque placement or displace the plaque during treatment should be temporarily relocated to a location that will not disturb the plaque. This typically requires standard disinsertion on locking sutures. They will be returned to their original insertions at the time of plaque removal. Permanent diplopia is uncommon [30].

Transillumination of the eye (transocular or transpupillary) will allow the surgeon to view the tumors shadow. The edges of the shadow are marked as well as the 2–3 mm surrounding free margin with tissue dye on the sclera. Scleral depression, diathermy marking, and/or focal light transillumination may be required for patients with darkly pigmented choroid.

A dummy plaque is placed on the sclera overlying the tumor and is anchored to the sclera using sutures passed through the eyelet of the plaque. Temporary knots are used to secure the dummy plaque. Intraoperative ultrasound (with the probe wrapped in a sterile sleeve) should be performed to ensure accurate localization of the plaque. Once ensured, the dummy plaque is removed and the radioactive plaque is secured in place using the aforementioned sutures.

In some centers, the radioactive plaque is used instead of a dummy plaque, thus avoiding one step. This change increases irradiation of the surgeon, eliminates possible differences in dummy-active plaque suture-related placement, allows for ultrasonographic verification of the actual radioactive device and decreases surgical time. After plaque placement, the conjunctiva is closed with absorbable sutures. Peribulbar infusion and topical antibiotic and steroid are placed. The eye is covered with a soft pad and a lead shield. Removal of the plaque can also be performed under local or general anesthesia. When the plaque has been placed to treat conjunctival lesions, it can be removed under topical anesthesia.

The Russian Experience with Strontium-90

Case Selection

Conjunctival melanoma, squamous carcinoma, and lymphomas may be treated. Brachytherapy of biopsy proven tumors with the exception of uveal melanoma. Tumor thickness should not exceed 3–4 mm. Maximum diameter is practically irrelevant, because the irradiation can be performed in several fields. Margins extend 3–4 mm beyond the visible tumor (on every side). In cases of thicker conjunctival tumors, surgical removal is performed prior to brachytherapy.

Contraindications:

1. Full lid-thickness infiltration.
2. Intraocular and orbital extension.

Methods:

1. Brachytherapy performed in a reclining chair.
2. Local anesthesia.
3. Head fixation.
4. Strontium-90 plaque (Resotech) is applied to the targeted zone, using a rod (plaque holder) fixed to a headlamp retainer.
5. Single dose applied over 10–30 min.

Dose (cumulative dose at depth):

1. For melanoma, 200 Gy; carcinoma, 120–150 Gy; lymphoma, 90–110 Gy.
2. Single dose in a depth, 10–15 Gy.

Strontium-90 for uveal melanoma:

1. Tumor thickness up to 3.5 mm.
2. Dose to the apex 200–230 Gy.

Strontium-90 for retinoblastoma:

1. Tumor thickness up to 3.5 mm.
2. Dose to the apex, 120–150 Gy.

Postsurgical Procedures

The patient is treated with topical steroid antibiotic eye drops on a tapering schedule for 4 weeks and is examined periodically depending on the type of tumor and plaque treatment.

Radiation Surveys and Regulations

After each case (insertion and removal), the patient's eye and operating room are assessed to ensure that emitted radiation falls within the prescribed and acceptable range. Precautions and safety measures are detailed to the patient and attenders. Please consult your governmental regulatory authority governing the use of radiation. Each locality typically prescribes the practices related to patient handling after brachytherapy. For instance, in India patients are hospitalized for the duration of treatment. In

New York City, using ^{125}I and ^{103}Pd, they are sent home or to a hotel until plaque removal.

Governing regulatory agencies for most centers require radiation surveys to ensure a radiologically safe environment for the staff, patient, and general public. You should consult your government regulatory agency to determine require radiation safety procedure. The practice of radiation surveys should follow the radiation source(s) towards documenting the environment before and after their introduction.

Specifically, this may include receipt of the sources from the manufacturer with wipe tests and radiation survey of the shipping package; wipe tests and radiation survey of the brachytherapy source(s) upon opening the shipping package; radiation survey of the assembled brachytherapy treatment device preceding sterilization; radiation survey of the operating theater and the patient preceding implant; radiation survey of the operating theater, patient, and sterilization container following implant; radiation survey of the operating theater, patient, and sterilization container preceding explant; and radiation survey of the operating theater, patient, and sterilization container following explant. Expected and maximum permissible exposure rates should be included in a standardized form. Survey instrumentation should be calibrated for the radiation quality and expected exposure rates.

Summary

The authors of this chapter recognize the significant challenges that face any center starting a new ophthalmic radiation therapy program. However, those who are willing to organize this effort will likely see generations of patients benefitting from sight and life-saving treatment.

This chapter was created to serve as a starting point for ophthalmologists, radiation oncologists, and medical physicists around the world. Herein, we pledge to share our knowledge in support to your efforts.

References

1. American Brachytherapy Society – Ophthalmic Oncology Task Force. The American Brachytherapy Society consensus guidelines for plaque brachytherapy of uveal melanoma and retinoblastoma. Brachytherapy. 2014;13(1):1–14.
2. Chiu-Tsao ST, Astrahan MA, Finger PT, et al. Dosimetry of ^{125}I and ^{103}Pd COMS eye plaques for intraocular tumors: report of task group 129 by the AAPM and ABS. Med Phys. 2012;39(10):6161–84.
3. Finger PT. Radiation therapy for choroidal melanoma. Surv Ophthalmol. 1997;42(3):215–32.
4. Finger PT. Radiation therapy for orbital tumors: concepts, current use, and ophthalmic radiation side effects. Surv Ophthalmol. 2009;54(5):545–68.
5. Saakyan SV, Amiryan AG, Valskiy VV, Mironova IS. Plaque radiotherapy for anterior uveal melanomas. Vestn Oftalmol. 2015;131(2):5–12.
6. Rivard MJ, Melhus CS, Sioshansi S, Morr J. The impact of prescription depth, dose rate, plaque size, and source loading on the central axis using ^{103}Pd, ^{125}I, and ^{131}Cs. Brachytherapy. 2008;7(4):327–35.
7. Fluhs D, Anastassiou G, Wening J, Sauerwein W, Bornfeld N. The design and the dosimetry of binuclide radioactive ophthalmic applicators. Med Phys. 2004;31(6):1481–8.
8. Gagne NL, Rivard MJ. Quantifying the dosimetric influences of radiation coverage and brachytherapy implant placement uncertainty on eye plaque size selection. Brachytherapy. 2013;12(5):508–20.
9. None. Proton therapy appears to be less cost-effective. Cancer Discov. 2013;3(2):OF2.
10. Krema H, Heydarian M, Beiki-Ardakani A, et al. A comparison between ^{125}Iodine brachytherapy and stereotactic radiotherapy in the management of juxtapapillary choroidal melanoma. Br J Ophthalmol. 2013;97(3):327–32.
11. Yousef YA, Finger PT. Lack of radiation maculopathy after palladium-103 plaque radiotherapy for iris melanoma. Int J Radiat Oncol Biol Phys. 2012;83(4):1107–12.
12. Wilson MW, Hungerford JL. Comparison of episcleral plaque and proton beam radiation therapy for the treatment of choroidal melanoma. Ophthalmology. 1999;106(8):1579–87.
13. Kivela T, Simpson ER, Grossniklaus HE, Jager MJ, Singh AD, Caminal JM, Pavlick, et al. Uveal melanoma. In: Amin M, Edge SB, Greene FL, et al., editors. The American Joint Committee on cancer staging manual. 8th ed. New York: Springer; 2017. p. 805–18.
14. Mallipatna AC, Gallie BL, Chevez-Barrios P, Lumbroso-Le Rouic L, Chantada GL, Doz F, Brisse HJ, et al. Retinoblastoma. In: Amin MB, Edge S, Greene F, Byrd DR, Brookland RK, Washington MK, et al., editors. The AJCC cancer staging manual. 8th ed. New York: Springer; 2017. p. 819–31.
15. Finger PT, Tena LB, Semenova E, Aridgides P, Choi WH. Extrascleral extension of choroidal melanoma: post-enucleation high-dose-rate interstitial brachytherapy of the orbit. Brachytherapy. 2014;13(3):275–80.
16. Stannard C, Maree G, Munro R, Lecuona K, Sauerwein W. Iodine-125 orbital brachytherapy with a prosthetic implant in situ. Strahlenther Onkol. 2011;187(5):322–7.
17. Finger PT. Intraocular melanoma. In: DeVita JVT, Lawrence TS, Rosenberg SA, editors. Cancer: principles and practice of oncology, vol. 1. 10th ed. Philadelphia: Wolter Kluwer, Lippincott, Williams and Wilkins; 2014. p. 1770–9.
18. Madreperla SA. Choroidal hemangioma treated with photodynamic therapy using verteporfin. Arch Ophthalmol. 2001;119(11):1606–10.
19. Aizman A, Finger PT, Shabto U, Szechter A, Berson A. Palladium 103 (^{103}Pd) plaque radiation therapy for circumscribed choroidal hemangioma with retinal detachment. Arch Ophthalmol. 2004;122(11):1652–6.
20. Pe'er J. Ocular surface squamous neoplasia: evidence for topical chemotherapy. Int Ophthalmol Clin. 2015;55(1):9–21.
21. Collaborative Ocular Melanoma Study Group. Ch 12: radiation therapy. In: Service NTI, editor. COMS manual of procedures PB95-179693. Springfield: National Technical Information Service; 1995.
22. Astrahan MA. Improved treatment planning for COMS eye plaques. Int J Radiat Oncol Biol Phys. 2005;61(4):1227–42.
23. Rivard MJ, Chiu-Tsao S-T, Finger PT, et al. Comparison of dose calculation methods for brachytherapy of intraocular tumors. Med Phys. 2011;38(1):306–16.
24. DeWerd LA, Huq MS, Das IJ, et al. Procedures for establishing and maintaining consistent air-kerma strength standards for low-energy, photon-emitting brachytherapy sources: recommendations of the Calibration Laboratory Accreditation Subcommittee of the American Association of Physicists in Medicine. Med Phys. 2004;31(3):675–81.
25. Finger PT. Finger's amniotic membrane buffer technique: protecting the cornea during radiation plaque therapy. Arch Ophthalmol. 2008;126(4):531–4.
26. Semenova E, Finger PT. Amniotic membrane corneal buffering during plaque radiation therapy for anterior uveal melanoma. Ophthalmic Surg Lasers Imaging Retina. 2013;44(5):477–82.
27. Finger PT, Chin KJ, Tena LB. A five-year study of slotted eye plaque radiation therapy for choroidal melanoma: near, touching, or surrounding the optic nerve. Ophthalmology. 2012;119(2):415–22.
28. Sagoo MS, Shields CL, Emrich J, Mashayekhi A, Komarnicky L, Shields JA. Plaque radiotherapy for juxtapapillary choroidal melanoma: treatment complications and visual outcomes in 650 consecutive cases. JAMA Ophthalmol. 2014;132(6):697–702.
29. Sagoo MS, Shields CL, Mashayekhi A, et al. Plaque radiotherapy for choroidal melanoma encircling the optic disc (circumpapillary choroidal melanoma). Arch Ophthalmol. 2007;125(9):1202–9.
30. Nagendran ST, Finger PT, Campolattaro BN. Extraocular muscle repositioning and diplo-

pia: associated with ophthalmic plaque radiation therapy for choroidal melanoma. Ophthalmology. 2014;121(11):2268–74.

31. PaulT Finger, Radiation therapy for exudative choroidal hemangioma. Indian Journal of Ophthalmology 2019;67(5):579.

Suggested Reading

http://www.ijo.in/article.asp?issn=0301-4738;year=2019;volume=67;issue=5;spage=579;epage=581;aulast=Finger

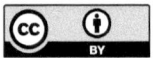

Ocular Pathology

15

Hardeep Singh Mudhar

The partnership between an ophthalmologist and an ophthalmic pathologist is critical to ensure that the final histopathology report is accurate and intelligible and contains as much relevant information to ensure safe patient management. At all stages of this process, clear verbal and written communication is key; every link in the chain must be robust to ensure the patient comes to no harm. To quote Professor Christopher Fletcher, Director of Surgical Pathology at Harvard Medical School, 'the reality is that the histology report is the principal determinant of diagnosis, likely clinical course and therapy in any patient found to have a mass....' [1].

Ocular pathology specimens travel through three phases: pre-analytical (pre-surgery communication, surgery, request form, specimen handling prior to fixation, fixation and transportation), analytical (processing of specimen, stains, ancillary investigations and histological interpretation by pathologist) and post-analytical (histopathology report, post-report discussion at multidisciplinary meeting, supplementary reporting).

This chapter will cover the following topics:

- Pre-analytical phase
  - Pre-surgical planning.
  - The ophthalmic pathology request form.
  - Handling specimens in theatre before fixing.
  - Fixation.
  - Transportation of specimens to the histopathology laboratory.
- Post-analytical phase
  - Basic histopathology terminology and understanding the histopathology report.
  - The use of ancillary investigations in ophthalmic pathology.
  - Ocular tumour prognostic factors.

As this chapter is meant to be a practical guide for clinicians, it will not cover the analytical aspects of how the specimen is grossed/cut up, its processing or staining in the ocular pathology laboratory. Many texts are available that cover these steps in detail and interested readers should consult these.

Pre-analytical Phase

Discussion of Cases Prior to Surgery

Some cases (complex margins), specimens requiring frozen sections or those requiring special requirements (e.g. certain fixatives), are best discussed in advance with the ocular pathology laboratory. This will ensure the pathology

H. S. Mudhar (✉)
National Specialist Ophthalmic Pathology Service (NSOPS), Department of Histopathology,
Royal Hallamshire Hospital, Sheffield, UK
e-mail: hardeep.mudhar@sth.nhs.uk

© The Author(s) 2019
S. S. Chaugule et al. (eds.), *Surgical Ophthalmic Oncology*,
https://doi.org/10.1007/978-3-030-18757-6_15

laboratory can meet the needs of the surgical procedure and ensure adequate handling without compromising the specimen.

How to Complete the Ophthalmic Pathology Request Form [2]

A pathology request form is a referral letter and a primary source of communication between the ophthalmologist and pathologist. It is also a medico-legal document. For all specimens submitted to the laboratory, a fully completed request form should accompany each case. Request forms are designed to provide:

- Unique identification of the patient.
- A destination for the report and any charging information.
- The laboratory with the clinician contact details if discussion of the case is required.
- Date and time of specimen collection/removal and investigations required (e.g. histology/cytology).
- Type of specimen and anatomical site of origin. This is especially important for multiple map biopsies taken from the conjunctiva to establish the extent of ocular surface squamous, sebaceous and melanocytic malignancies. It is critical that the request form include a diagram indicating the precise origin of each biopsy.
- Clinical information so that the pathologist may handle the specimen appropriately and interpret microscopic findings in the proper context.
- An awareness of any health and safety issues with a given specimen.
- Complete information must be supplied on the request form. Each specimen container, no matter how small, should also be labelled with the appropriate patient identification data (minimum of three identifiers, e.g. first and last name, date of birth/age and gender and preferably patient's hospital no).
- The information must be consistent with the request form, to prevent errors in specimen and patient identification.

See Fig. 15.1a–e showing examples of well-filled out and suboptimally filled out pathology request forms.

Specimen Handling in Operation Theatre Prior to Fixation

Multiple Specimens from a Surgical Procedure

As a general principle, specimens from different locations should be placed in separate fixation pots. If multiple pieces of tissue from different sites are placed in the same fixation pot and one of the pieces of tissue turns out to be malignant, it is impossible to ascertain where the tissue has been sampled from.

Orientation of Specimens

Orientation of specimens is required, to ensure the pathologist can report the margins of excision accurately. This is best done by placing sutures at particular margins and then specifying the sutured margin on the pathology request form in writing or as a diagram (Fig. 15.2a).

Conjunctival Mapping Biopsies

Conjunctival biopsies comprise thin strips of epithelium and stroma and are prone to curling if placed straight into fixative. They should be attached to sponge or card before placing into the fixative, so that they arrive in the ocular pathology laboratory in a flattened state. The latter facilitates orientation during embedding

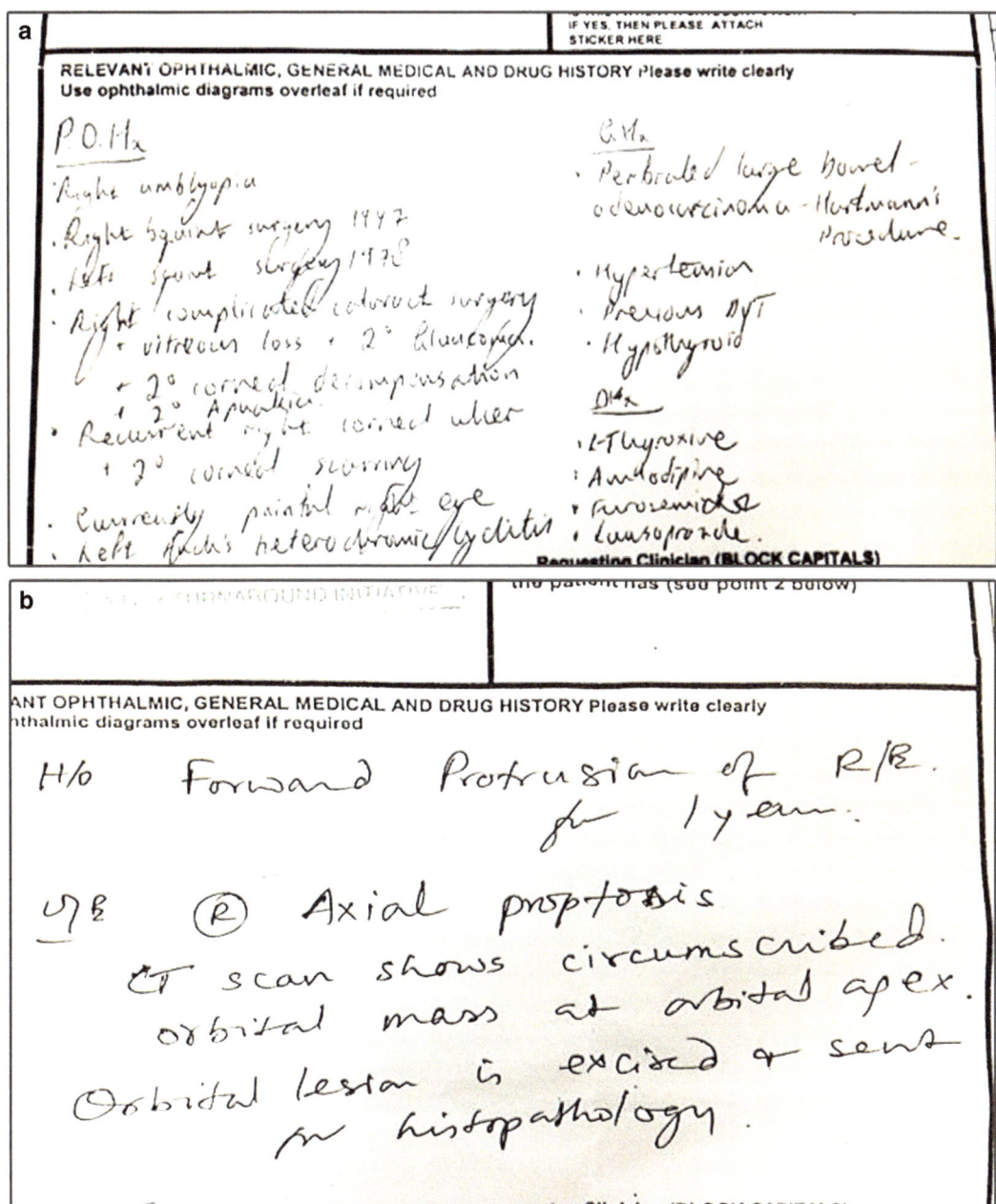

Fig. 15.1 (**a–c**) These are examples of well-filled out pathology request forms that detail all the relevant information. (**c**) The surgeon has drawn a very useful diagram, to indicate the orientation of the specimen. (**d, e**) Suboptimally filled out pathology request forms that merely state the procedure carried out with no indication of the disease process, no differential diagnosis and no further history

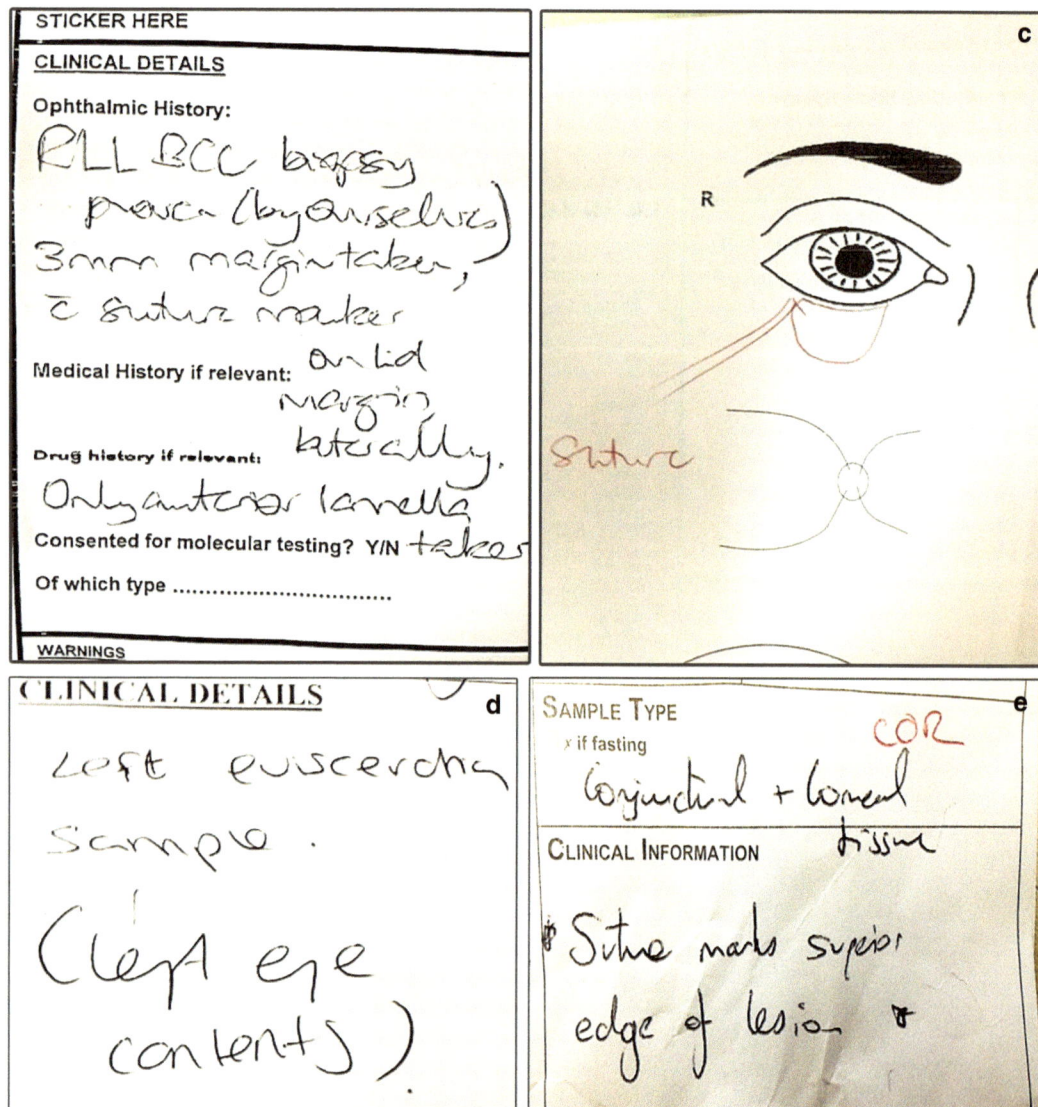

Fig. 15.1 (continued)

and greatly facilitates the histological assessment for the presence or absence of invasion by tumour. If multiple mapping biopsies are performed, the pathology request form must state the precise location of the biopsies. Figure 15.2b shows a very helpful diagram drawn by the surgeon that shows the extent of this patient's conjunctival lesion (shaded areas) and the precise location of the mapping biopsies.

Sampling Fresh Tissue Prior to Fixation

Some tumours require to be sampled fresh for special genetic/ molecular investigations (diagnostic and prognostic testing) or for research.

- In the case of an enucleation, sample the optic nerve first and place in a separate pot of formalin. This is to prevent fresh tumour

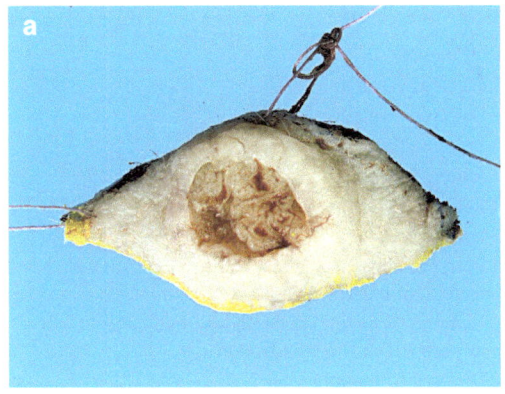

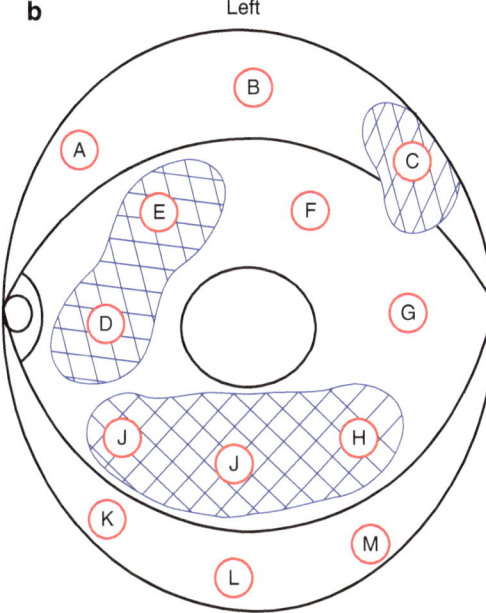

Fig. 15.2 (**a**) shows an eyelid skin ellipse excision orientated by the surgeon using two sets of sutures. (**b**) A conjunctival mapping biopsy diagram sketched by the surgeon in theatre. The hash shading denotes the distribution of the lesion and the letters denote the locations of the biopsies that correspond to the formalin pots into which the biopsies have been placed/fixed

contaminating the optic nerve resection margin.
- The globe is transilluminated and using a scalpel, a sclera-choroidal flap is created beneath the tumour, leaving the scleral-choroidal flap hinged along one side. Fresh tumour is harvested with scissors and forceps.
- Fresh tumour is placed in an appropriate medium and vessel.

- Some use a corneal trephine to cut a window into the sclera and choroid.
- After harvesting fresh tumour, the specimen is fixed.
- An alternative strategy is to submit the intact specimen unfixed to the ocular pathology laboratory, where the above steps can be carried out.

Fixation of Ocular Pathology Specimens

Routine Surgical Specimens

Standard 10% phosphate-buffered formalin in a leak-proof container is the fixation of choice (Table 15.1) [3–5]. This will allow routine haematoxylin and eosin staining (H&E), other special tinctorial stains and immunohistochemistry. In addition, numerous molecular studies for diagnosis and prognosis can be performed on formalin-fixed tissue (Fig. 15.3a).

- If certain molecular biological diagnostic techniques or research is to be done on unfixed tumour samples, the clinician or assistant must remove fresh tumour from the specimen prior to fixing in formalin.
- The formalin should ideally be 10x the volume of the specimen to allow timely penetration of the tissues at room temperature. To ensure this, an adequate sized plastic container is required. Most well-stocked pathology labs have a variety of sizes of plastic container to facilitate this. Many containers come prefilled with formalin (Fig. 15.3a).
- Specimens should be placed into the container that has been pre-filled with formalin. If formalin is poured into a dry container that has the specimen in it, there is a chance that the specimen will be ejected by the formalin and will end up on the bench or floor.
- Specimen containers must then be sealed tightly with the lids to avoid spillage of hazardous formalin.
- Smaller containers are then usually placed in a plastic bag which also accommodates a side compartment for the request form. Follow

Table 15.1 Various surgical specimen types and fixations used

Type of specimen	Type of fixative
Eyelid tumour incisional biopsy	10% buffered formalin
Eyelid tumour excision	10% buffered formalin
Conjunctival tumour biopsy	10% buffered formalin
Conjunctival tumour excision	10% buffered formalin
Intraocular solid tissue biopsy (not FNA)	10% buffered formalin
Localised resection of intraocular tumour	10% buffered formalin
Tumour enucleation	10% buffered formalin—remember to sample any fresh tumour prior to fixation if indicated
Tumour exenteration	10% buffered formalin—remember to sample any fresh tumour prior to fixation if indicated
Orbital tumour biopsy	10% buffered formalin
Orbital tumour excision	10% buffered formalin—remember to sample any fresh tumour prior to fixation if indicated
Lacrimal drainage system/sac biopsy or excision	10% buffered formalin
Aqueous tap for cytology	Equal volume of CytoLyt or similar methanol-based fixative
Aqueous tap for flow cytometry	RPMI
Vitreous tap or pars plana vitrectomy specimen for cytology	Equal volume of CytoLyt or similar methanol-based fixative
Vitreous tap or pars plana vitrectomy specimen for flow cytometry	RPMI
FNA intraocular of solid tumour (e.g. retinal, subretinal uveal tumour and orbital)	CytoLyt or similar methanol-based fixative

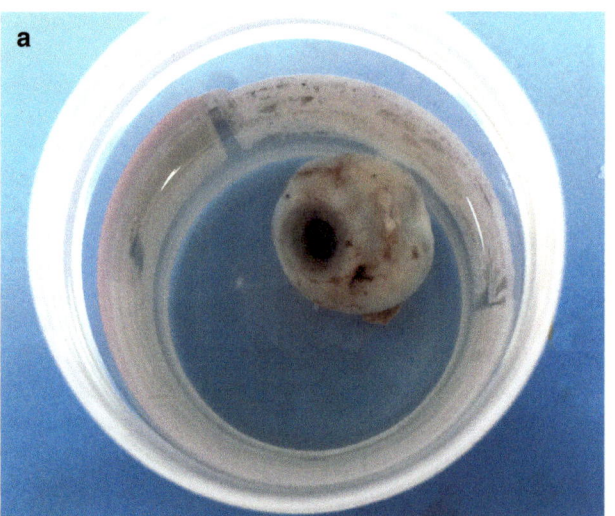

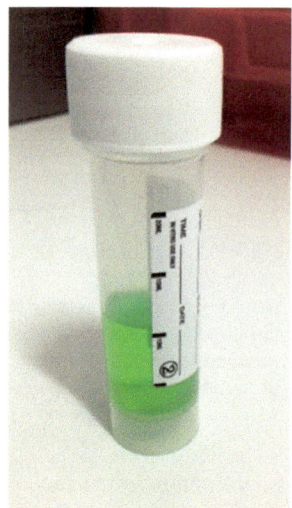

Fig. 15.3 (**a**) shows a globe specimen (containing a uveal melanoma) in a standard plastic pot, containing 10% buffered formalin for fixing the specimen. (**b**) This is a universal tune that contains green, methanol-based cytofixative for intraocular tumour aspiration cytology. The colour of the fluid varies according to the manufacturer. (**c**) The arrows point to black specs of an aspirated melanotic tumour, fixed in cytofixative in a universal tube. (**d**) This is a vitrectomy cassette containing vitreous washings from a patient with suspected intraocular lymphoma, fixed in green cytofixative of a volume equal to the volume of the vitreous washings. (**e**) This shows an impression cytology plastic ring, fixing in 10% buffered formalin. (**f**) A small plastic tube containing buffered glutaraldehyde for the fixation of specimens for transmission electron microscopy

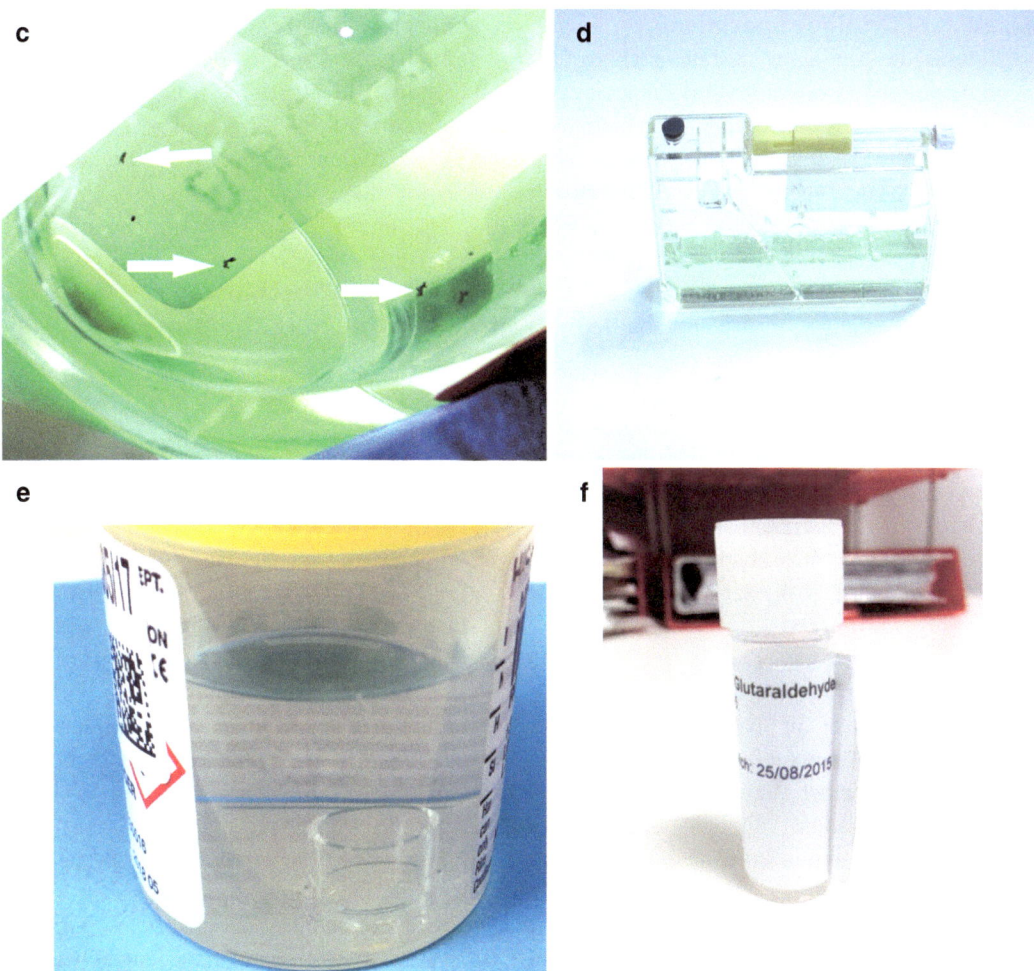

Fig. 15.3 (continued)

your institutional standard operation protocols for additional packaging.

- The appropriate institutional health and safety protocols must be followed when handling formalin.

Which Specimens Should Not Be Fixed?

- Tissue destined for frozen sections (to assess margins of excision for eyelid, adnexal and orbital tumours).
- Tissue for research or tissue banking.
- Some tumours requiring prognostic information (e.g. sarcomas, paediatric small round blue cells tumours, retinoblastoma) may require special studies on fresh tissue.
- Biopsies destined for flow cytometry (e.g. vitreous and fine-needle aspiration specimens for assessment of lymphoma). In this situation, many practitioners send the cell sample in Roswell Park Medical Institution medium (RPMI) to enhance the survival of the cells.
- Some labs still do Oil Red O staining for suspected cases of sebaceous carcinoma. However, this is being superseded by haematoxylin and eosin-stained (H&E) sections and immunohistochemistry.

Fixation of Cytology Specimens

- Fine-needle aspiration specimens (FNA) are preferably fixed in CytoLyt or Shandon cytofixative (or equivalents) which are methanol-based mild fixatives (Table 15.1). They preserve the cyto-morphology well and permit good-quality DNA to be extracted for molecular diagnostic tests. CytoLyt preserved specimens can be used to make thin-prep slides as well. FNA samples are usually squirted into pre-filled universal tubes that contain the fixative. The syringe used in the collection of the sample may be submitted with the fluid inside. Needles must be removed and the syringe capped. If the specimen is to be fixed, an equal volume of cytology fixative may be drawn up into the same syringe, capped and then agitated gently to mix the sample with the fixative (Fig. 15.3b, c).
- Vitrectomy specimens: It is preferable to receive a pars plana vitrectomy specimen in a vitreous cassette or bag. If samples are required for microbiology, virology, PCR, etc., please remove these from the cassette/bag before fixation, although, ideally, these should have been sent from the initial core vitreous tap. Vitrectomy samples need to be preserved/fixed in an equal or excess volume of RPMI or cytology fixative. It is important to seal the bag or cassette to prevent leaks in transit (Fig. 15.3d).
- Impression cytology plastic rings can be dropped into a small pot of formalin for fixation (Fig. 15.3e).

Fixation of Specimens Requiring Transmission Electron Microscopy

- Buffered 2.5–3% glutaraldehyde is used to fix fresh specimens for transmission electron microscopy. This would be done for cases that are intended for research or in which the original interpretation of an initial tumour biopsy was equivocal and clarification is sought from ultrastructure. It is best to place only part of the fresh tissue into buffered glutaraldehyde, as whilst it is an excellent fixative for ultrastructure, it adversely affects antigen retrieval for immunohistochemistry and extraction of DNA for molecular studies (Fig. 15.3f).

Transporting Specimens to the Pathology Laboratory

High Risk/Danger of Infection Specimens

- It is the ophthalmologist's responsibility to indicate on the request form and the specimen pot if the patient is known or suspected to be a 'High Risk/Danger of Infection' category (e.g. HIV, TB, hepatitis B, hepatitis C), to facilitate appropriate handling in the laboratory.
- It is the ophthalmologist's responsibility to ensure that all specimens are submitted to the laboratory in suitable and approved containers.
- Approved specimen containers have leakproof lids and the appropriate hazard warning signs for the fixative, e.g. formalin.
- Specimen containers should be closed securely and placed inside a sealed specimen bag.
- Specimens received leaking or damaged are a danger to all those who come into contact with them, including theatre staff, porters and laboratory staff and can also compromise the diagnosis.

Mailed or Couriered Specimens

- Specimens mailed or couriered should be packaged in approved containers in accordance with the requirements of the delivery service. To confirm receipt of specimen(s) in the department, it is good practice that a 'confirmation of receipt fax-back' form, providing the senders' confidential fax number, is enclosed with the specimen(s).

Post-analytical Phase

Understanding the Ophthalmic Histopathology Report

The ophthalmic histopathology report contains a lot of specialised pathology terminology that can seem rather bewildering. To understand histopathologic terminology related to tumours, it is best to return to basics. Table 15.2 outlines the tissue of origin and their related tumours that are commonly encountered [6] (Fig. 15.4a–j).

Knowledge of this basic table does go a long way to understanding the various tumours encountered in ocular oncology practice and their behaviour and prognosis. It also allows for a conversation with your local pathologist, who is often equally keen to learn specialised ophthalmology terminology to enhance the quality and clarity of the professional interaction.

Examples of Histopathology Reports with Explanations of Specialised Terminology

Set out below are examples of ophthalmic histopathology reports that may be encountered in a busy ocular oncology practice with specialised terms defined and figures provided for clarity [6].

Eyelid Tumour Histopathology Report Example

This full thickness wedge excision contains an *invasive neoplasm*. It is arising from the Meibomian gland and is composed of *pleomorphic* cells, with *vacuolated* cytoplasm, indenting the nuclei. Numerous mitotic figures are present. The individual tumour cells exhibit *hyperchromatic chromatin* and nucleoli are prominent. Foci of *intraepithelial pagetoid* spread are seen over the invasive tumour, involving the tarsal conjunctival epithelium and the epidermis of the skin. The invasive tumour shows focal *comedo*-like *necrosis* and shows *vascular and perineural invasion*.

Immunohistochemistry shows that the invasive tumour is positive for adipophilin, EMA and shows nuclear androgen receptor positivity.

The features are those of an invasive sebaceous *carcinoma*, derived from the meibomian gland. The excision of the invasive component is complete (nearest margin is 3 mm). However, the pagetoid spread contaminates the tarsal conjunctival margin and is therefore incompletely excised.

Sebaceous neoplasms can be associated with the Muir-Torre syndrome. Is there a history of internal malignancies in this patient or is there a family history of malignancies?

Table 15.2 Tissues of origin and related tumours

Tissue of origin	Benign	In situ	Invasive malignancy
Squamous Epithelium	Squamous cell papilloma	In situ squamous carcinoma	Invasive squamous cell carcinoma
Sebaceous gland epithelium	Sebaceous adenoma	In situ sebaceous carcinoma	Invasive sebaceous carcinoma
Melanocytes	Nevus	In situ melanoma	Invasive malignant melanoma
Blood cells	Reactive lymphoid hyperplasia		Lymphoma or leukaemia
Soft tissue	Lipoma		Liposarcoma
	Haemangioma		Angiosarcoma
	Rhabdomyoma		Rhabdomyosarcoma

a

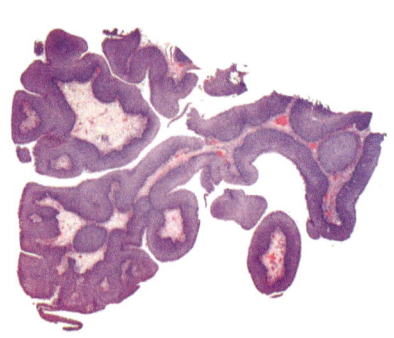

b

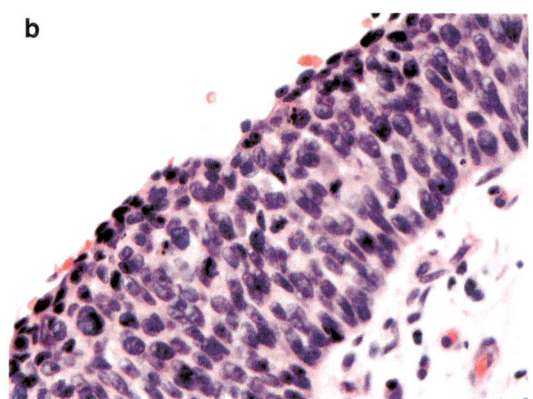

Fig. 15.4 (**a**) Haematoxylin & eosin (H&E)-stained histology image of a typical viral squamous papilloma of the conjunctiva. Note the typical cauliflower-like appearance caused by the fibrovascular cores covered in thickened epithelium. (**b**) H&E-stained section showing conjunctival in situ squamous carcinoma. The epithelium is thicker than usual and packed full of atypical nuclei, with no maturation at all. (**c**) H&E section showing conjunctival invasive squamous cell carcinoma with keratin formation. The latter is the orange material in the centre of the irregular invasive islands of tumour. (**d**) H&E of a cystic conjunctival nevus. The asterisk is the cystic space and the arrow points to the bland, monotonous nevus cells. (**e**) H&E of conjunctival in situ melanoma. The arrow points to the melanoma cells confined to the epithelium. (**f**) H&E of invasive conjunctival melanoma. The asterisk indicates an invasive nodule of melanoma in the substantia propria. (**g**) H&E of reactive lymphoid hyperplasia. The thicker arrow shows the paler germinal centre lymphocytes of the well-organised nodular lymphoid tissue. The thinner arrow indicates the darker staining mantle lymphocytes, surrounding the germinal centre lymphocytes. (**h**) H&E of a conjunctival extranodal marginal zone lymphoma. Note the sheet-like population of monotonous lymphoid cells. (**i**) H&E of an alveolar variant rhabdomyosarcoma of the orbit. (**j**) H&E of a higher power of Fig. 15i showing small round blue cells with occasional larger pink (eosinophilic cells) present. (**k**) H&E of a squamous cell carcinoma of the conjunctiva that illustrates nuclear size, shape and colour variation-called pleomorphism and is a feature of malignant cells. (**l**) H&E of the same tumour in plate K showing a typical tumour mitotic figure (arrow). (**m**) H&E showing cytoplasmic vacuolation (clear spaces) of sebaceous tumour cells (arrow). (**n**) H&E of a sebaceous carcinoma with the arrow pointing to a hyperchromatic nucleus (darker in shade compared to other nuclei in image). (**o**) H&E of a sebaceous carcinoma showing intraepithelial 'Pagetoid' spread (arrows). (**p**) H&E of a retinoblastoma. The asterisk indicates pink irregular necrotic tumour. (**q**) H&E of an adenoid cystic carcinoma of the orbit showing tumour around a nerve (arrow). This is perineural invasion. (**r**) Melanoma cells (stained red) are within the lumen of a lymphatic channel (stained brown). This is intra-lymphatic spread of tumour. (**s**) H&E of conjunctival squamous dysplasia (mid- to right aspect of image). The latter epithelium is thicker compared to the epithelium on the left which is much thinner. (**t**) H&E of a spindle-rich uveal melanoma. (**u**) H&E of an epithelioid rich uveal melanoma. The cells are much rounder and larger compared to the spindle cells in plate T. This is because they possess larger nuclei and more cytoplasm. (**v**) This is a Periodic Acid Schiff's (PAS) stain of a uveal melanoma showing rounded clones of tumour cells surrounded by pink/purple basement membrane boundaries, so-called loops. (**w**) This is a fluorescence in situ hybridisation (FISH) image showing different chromogenic-labelled DNA probes (green, red, blue, yellow) hybridising with various gene loci. (**x**) This is an orbital lymphoma stained with a B-cell marker antibody called CD20, by the technique of immunohistochemistry. The positive cells stain brown (different coloured chromogens can be employed such as red, brown, blue, etc.). Note how it is the cell membranes that stain, imparting a chicken-wire appearance. (**y**) This is an orbital lymphoma stained with Ki67 antibody by immunohistochemistry. The antibody stains the nuclei brown. The proliferation fraction of the tumour can be estimated by counting the number of stained nuclei out of 100 cells. (**za**) This trace shows a typical polyclonal population of B-cells when assessed for B-cell IgH rearrangement by PCR. Note the spread of varying sized peaks in a Gaussian dumbbell curve configuration. The histology showed a reactive lymphocytic population in the vitreous with a final diagnosis of chronic vitritis. (**zb**) This trace shows a typical monoclonal population of B-cells when assessed for B-cell IgH rearrangement by PCR. The final diagnosis was vitreo-retinal high-grade B-cell lymphoma

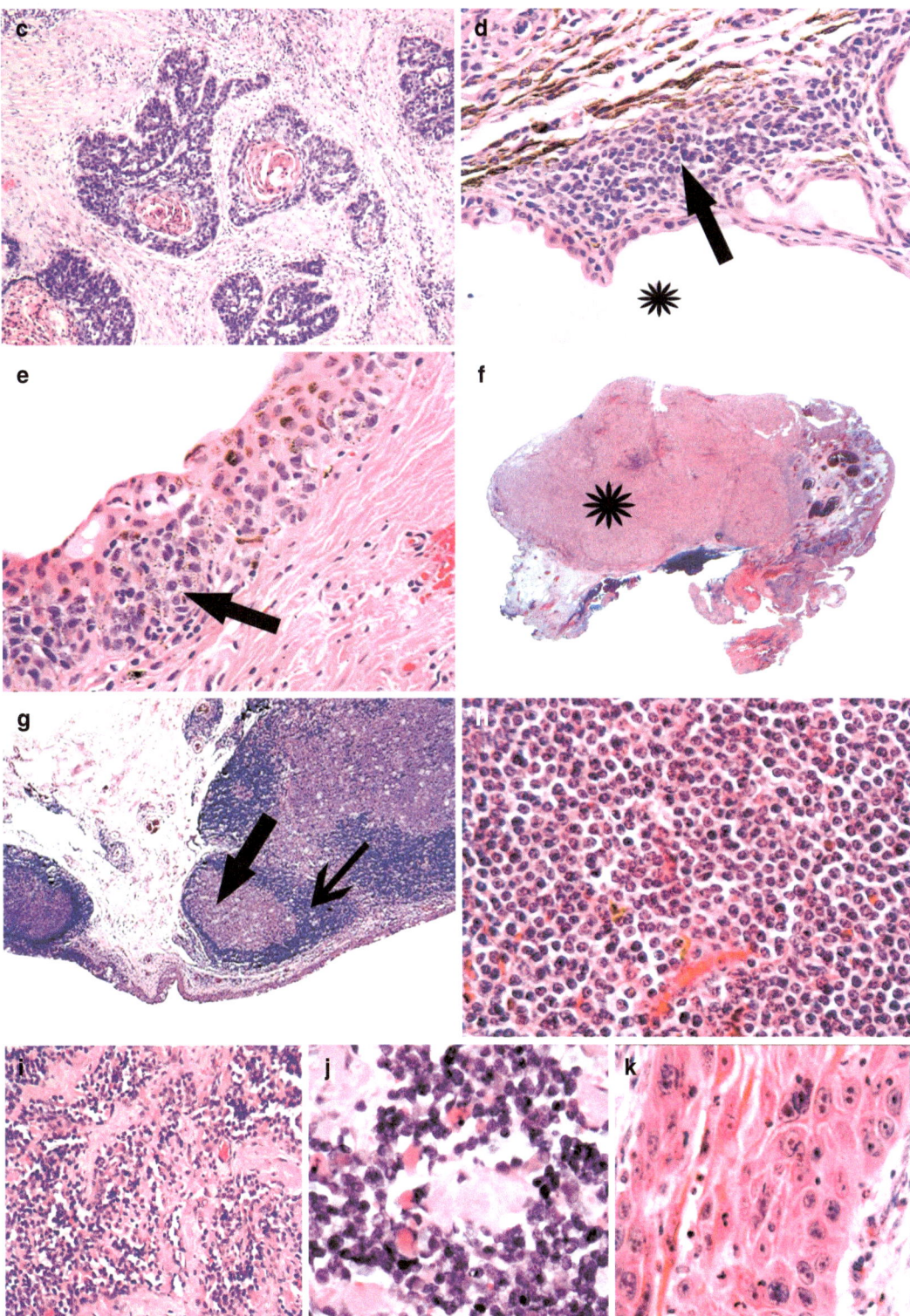

Fig. 15.4 (continued)

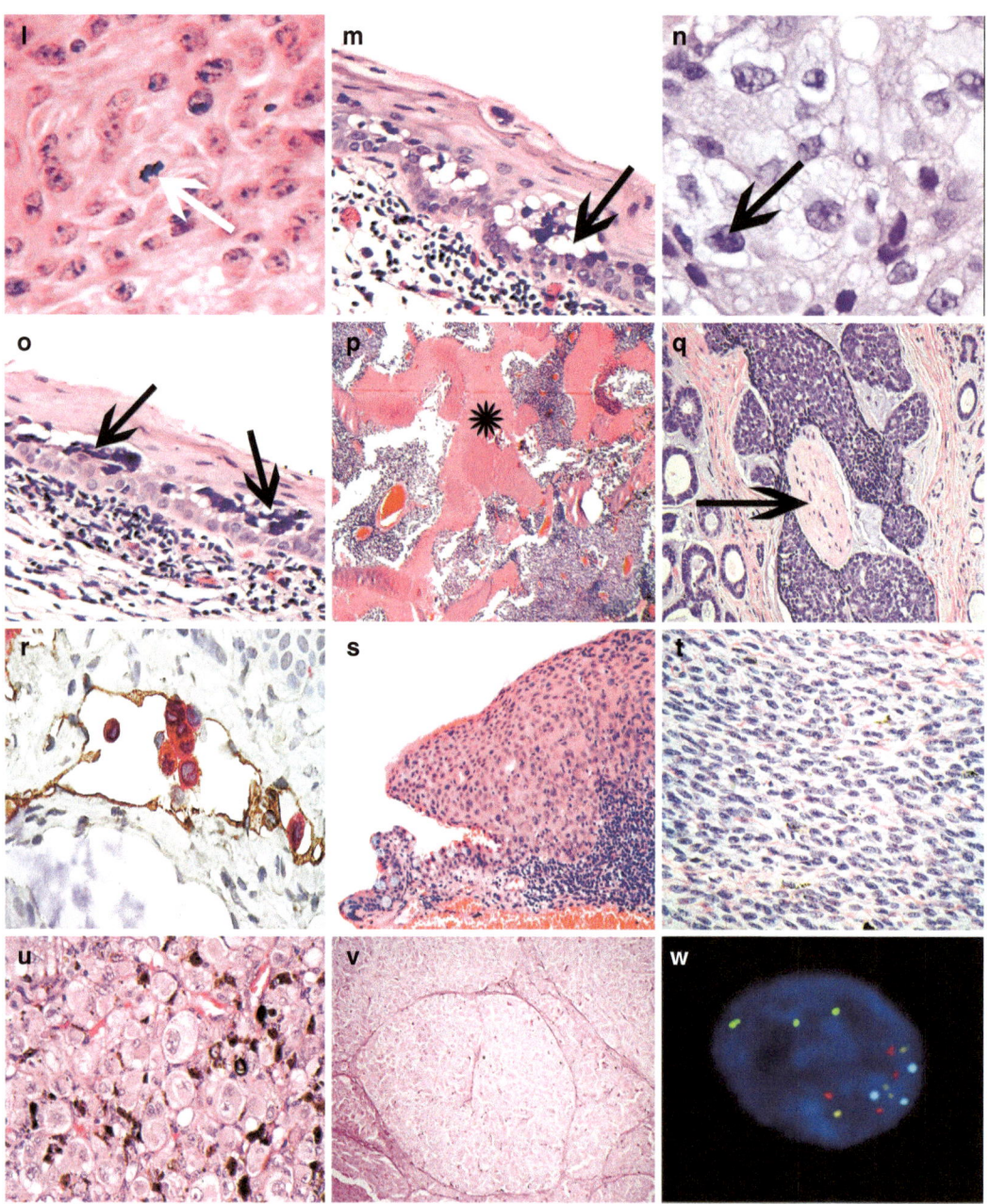

Fig. 15.4 (continued)

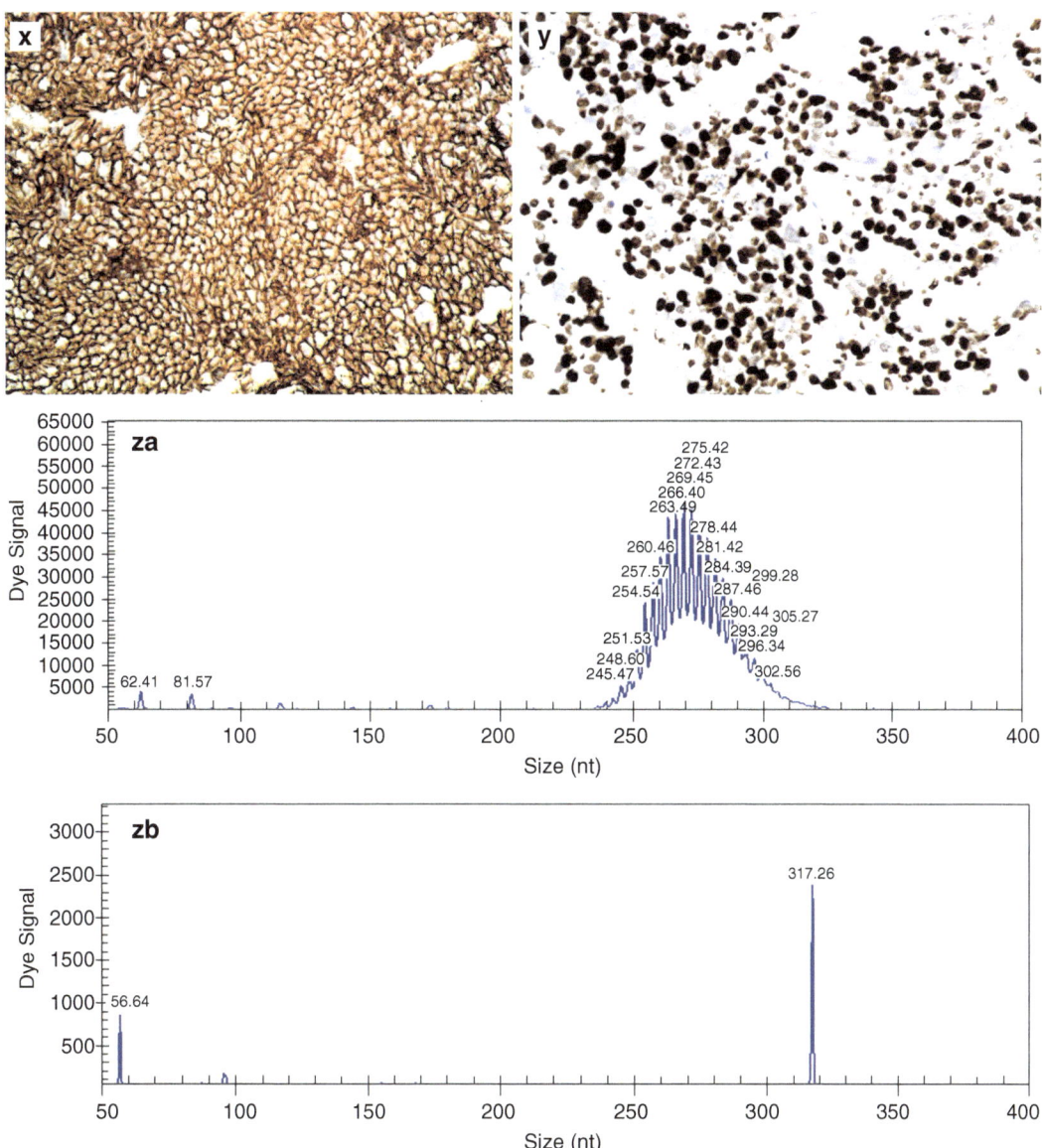

Fig. 15.4 (continued)

Terminology Explained

Invasive Malignant tumours invade through basement membranes into the surrounding tissue and can metastasise by invading into blood vessels and lymphatics.

Neoplasm Literally means 'new growth' (derived from Greek).

Pleomorphic Variation is size and shape of the nucleus and cytoplasm of the individual tumour cells. This is a feature of malignant cells that have lost their normal constraining signals (Fig. 15.4k).

Mitotic Figures Prophase, metaphase, anaphase, telophase and cytokinesis are the five phases of mitosis (refer to any intermediate biology textbook).

Mitotic figures are seen in normal and repairing tissues. An example of a normal tissue containing mitotic figures is the proliferative phase of endometrial glands and stroma. When injured tissue is regenerating, it is common to see many mitotic figures, e.g. regenerating epithelium in skin after trauma. Benign and malignant tumours contain mitotic figures. Malignant tumours tend to have more mitotic figures than benign tumours. Of the malignant tumours, poorly differentiated tumours tend to have higher mitotic figure counts compared to better differentiated tumours. In malignant tumours, the mitotic figures can have an abnormal morphology that is not seen in benign, normal or regenerating tissues. These include tripolar or multipolar forms (Fig. 15.4l).

Vacuolated A bubbly appearance to the cytoplasm due to the presence of various substances. In this case, it is lipid as the diagnosis is sebaceous carcinoma. It could be mucin (mucin forming carcinomas) or glycogen (e.g. renal cell carcinoma). The products made by tumour cells can be very helpful for classification (Fig. 15.4m).

Hyperchromatic Chromatin Simply means dark staining DNA in the nucleus. This is a feature of malignant cells (Fig. 15.4n).

Intraepithelial Within the confines of the epithelium.

Pagetoid Horizontal and vertical spread of malignant tumour cells as individuals or groups within epithelium. Named after Sir James Paget, an English surgeon and pathologist who described Paget's disease that shows this pattern of spread. Tumours that show this pattern of spread include malignant melanoma and sebaceous carcinoma (Fig. 15.4o).

Comedo Literally means like a 'zit'. Malignant tumour cells forming sheets are hypoxic in the middle and undergo necrosis. The appearance is that of a necrotic centre surrounded by a viable rim of malignant tumour cells. If the tissue is squeezed gently during handling, the necrotic tumour centre oozes out of the cut surface like zits being squeezed.

Necrosis Cell death with loss of cell contents to the exterior. Malignant tumours that outstrip their blood supply often become necrotic (Fig. 15.4p).

Vascular and Perineural Invasion Malignant tumours can invade into vessels and metastasise to distant locations. They also follow the paths of least resistance and spread along natural tissue scaffolds such as nerves (Fig. 15.4q, r).

Immunohistochemistry A common ancillary technique employed in histopathology to detect signature proteins using antibodies in various disease processes. In malignant tumours, it can help to type the tumour (e.g. carcinoma, lymphoma, melanoma, sarcoma) and can also reveal vital prognostic and therapeutic information.

Carcinoma A malignant epithelial neoplasm.

Further Comments

The last comment in the report relates to the surgical margins. In this case, the contamination of the conjunctival margin may necessitate mapping biopsies to ascertain the extent of the pagetoid spread that would inform subsequent therapy choices.

Conjunctival Tumour Histopathology Report Example

The bulbar conjunctiva contains a focus of in situ squamous carcinoma, arising in a background of various degrees of *dysplasia*. No invasion is identified in the planes examined. The surgical margins are clear. The background stromal tissue shows solar elastosis.

Terminology Explained

Dysplasia Derived from Greek meaning 'disordered growth'. Dysplasia is a term that is applied to epithelium. Histologically, the individual epithelial cells show pleomorphism (defined above), can have hyperchromatic nuclei and have a disorganised distribution within the epithelium. Mitotic figures may be seen. Pathologists can grade epithelial dysplasia according to how much of the epithelial thickness is occupied by the dysplastic cells. For example, common classifications of epithelial dysplasia are mild, moderate and severe or low-grade and high-grade. When the full thickness of the epithelium is consumed by dysplastic cells and the basement membrane has not been breached, it is called carcinoma in situ and is said to be pre-invasive. Invasion is not present. Therapeutic intervention at this stage of the disease is potentially curative (Fig. 15.4s).

Intraocular Tumour Histopathology Report Example

This enucleation contains a malignant melanoma of uveal type. It is located in the ciliary body and choroid and has a diffuse component. It is composed of *spindle and epithelioid cells* and has up to 15 mitotic figures *per 10 hpf. Closed loops and networks matrix patterns are seen.* Focal tumour necrosis is present. The tumour does not breach Bruch's membrane. There is no scleral invasion. The vortex veins are tumour-free. *FISH* analysis on the tumour has shown monosomy 3 and a gain of iso-chromosome 8q in 90% of the cells.

Summary: A *pathological stage pT3b* uveal melanoma of the ciliary body and choroid. The presence of monosomy 3 and iso-chromosome 8q indicates a poor prognosis.

Terminology Explained
Spindle and Epithelioid Cells This refers to the shape of the cells found in uveal melanoma, referred to as the Callender classification. This is of prognostic significance; more epithelioid cells carry a worse prognosis [7] (Fig. 15.4t, u).

Per 10hpf This is a mitotic count performed in 10 'high-power fields' (each with an area of 0.152 mm^2 and usually corresponding to a ×40 lens on a high-quality light microscope).

Closed Loops and Networks' Matrix Patterns This refers to the presence of specific basement membrane patterns stained with a periodic acid-Schiff (PAS) stain, present around expanding nests of melanoma cells. These matrix patterns are related to a poorer prognosis in uveal melanoma [8] (Fig. 15.4v).

FISH: *Fluorescence In Situ Hybridisation* FISH has been used in this case to gain genetic data on the status of chromosomes 3 and 8 in this uveal melanoma. Uveal melanoma genetics data is a powerful predictor of prognosis [9–13] (Fig. 15.4w).

Pathological Stage pT3b This refers to the TNM pathological classification of the stage of the uveal melanoma [14].

Further Comments
Ophthalmic pathologists will use the TNM[14] or AJCC [15] cancer staging manuals to include all of the relevant tumour prognostic information required for prognosis and treatment planning for uveal melanoma.

Also note how the report has combined histopathological and genetic data. This is increasingly common and is called integrated reporting, in the context of individualised oncology practice.

Orbital Tumour Histopathology Report Example

This orbital fat biopsy contains numerous *reactive lymphoid aggregates*. On this background, there is a larger expansile nodule composed of small lymphocytes, with a *monocytoid appearance*, associated with cells exhibiting lymphoplasmacytic *differentiation*. These monocytoid cells are positive for *B-cell markers* using immunohistochemistry (CD20 and CD79a positive) and are negative for CD5, CD10, Cd23 and Cyclin D1. *The Ki67 fraction* is 5%. *PCR for IgH rearrangement* shows clonal peaks in FR1, FR2 and FR3 confirming an unequivocal *clonal population of B lymphocytes*.

The appearances are those of an indolent B-cell lymphoma, sub-classification: extranodal marginal zone lymphoma of MALT type

(MALToma-WHO classification). This patient requires referral to your haemato-oncology service for further management.

Terminology Explained

Reactive Lymphoid Aggregates These are non-lymphomatous collections of lymphocytes comprising a germinal centre of larger lymphocytes undergoing apoptosis surrounded by a mantle of smaller lymphocytes. They indicate chronic antigenic stimulation and contain polyclonal groups of B lymphocytes.

Monocytoid Appearance It is common for a pathologist to describe the appearance of certain tumour cells with peculiar adjectives. Monocytoid means a lymphocyte nucleus within a clear cytoplasm, resembling a fried egg.

B-cell Markers This refers usually to immunohistochemistry markers for staining B-cells. Common markers include CD20 and CD79a. It is vitally important that any lymphoma should be differentiated into B or T cell type for diagnostic, prognostic and treatment purposes (Fig. 15.4x).

The Ki67 Fraction This refers to the % of cells that express Ki67. This protein is expressed in cells in all non-G0 phases of the cell cycle. It gives an indication of how fast tumour cells are proliferating. A higher Ki67 fraction tends to predict aggressive tumour behaviour (Fig. 15.4y).

PCR for IgH Rearrangement PCR, polymerase chain reaction. IgH-heavy chain of the immunoglobulin molecule. This is a common molecular diagnostic test performed in cases of suspected lymphoma.

Clonal Population of B Lymphocytes This means a population of B-cells all expressing the same heavy chain of immunoglobulin. Monoclonality usually means lymphoma but not always. Reactive lymphoid populations can contain monoclonal lymphocyte populations. The pathologist will always interpret the results of ancillary diagnostic/supportive molecular tests in the context of the clinical and histopathological findings (Fig. 15.4za, zb).

Further Comments

Lymphoma diagnosis often requires histopathological, immunohistochemical and molecular diagnostic tests to secure a firm diagnosis. An ophthalmic pathologist will often discuss the case with a specialist lymphoma pathologist and the case reviewed at the local multidisciplinary team meeting to plan further investigations (e.g. staging) and treatment. Again, note how the report contains integrated items of histopathological and molecular data and a suggestion for referral to an appropriate clinical team.

Common Ancillary Investigations Used in Ophthalmic Histopathology

Ancillary investigations are used to assist in making a diagnosis and to give prognostic information. The results of ancillary tests must always be interpreted alongside the light microscopic histological features in order to avoid an over or under diagnosis.

Immunohistochemistry

This is the application of antibodies to antigens in formalin-fixed, paraffin-embedded sections, visualised with various coloured chromogens. The antibodies are directed toward certain proteins that are expressed by specific cell types. Tumour cells express specific proteins allowing the tumour type to be established, which otherwise may be difficult on light microscopic examination alone.

Diagnostic Application

Example 1 Figure 15.5a shows a biopsy of the conjunctiva. The morphology shows atypical cells occupying the full thickness of the epithelium. The morphological differential diagnosis includes in situ melanoma, in situ squamous carcinoma and in situ sebaceous carcinoma. These are tumours with varying behaviour, prognosis and treatments so the diagnosis must be refined. Application of a small panel of antibodies allows discrimination. In this case, the tumour is positive for Melan A antibody

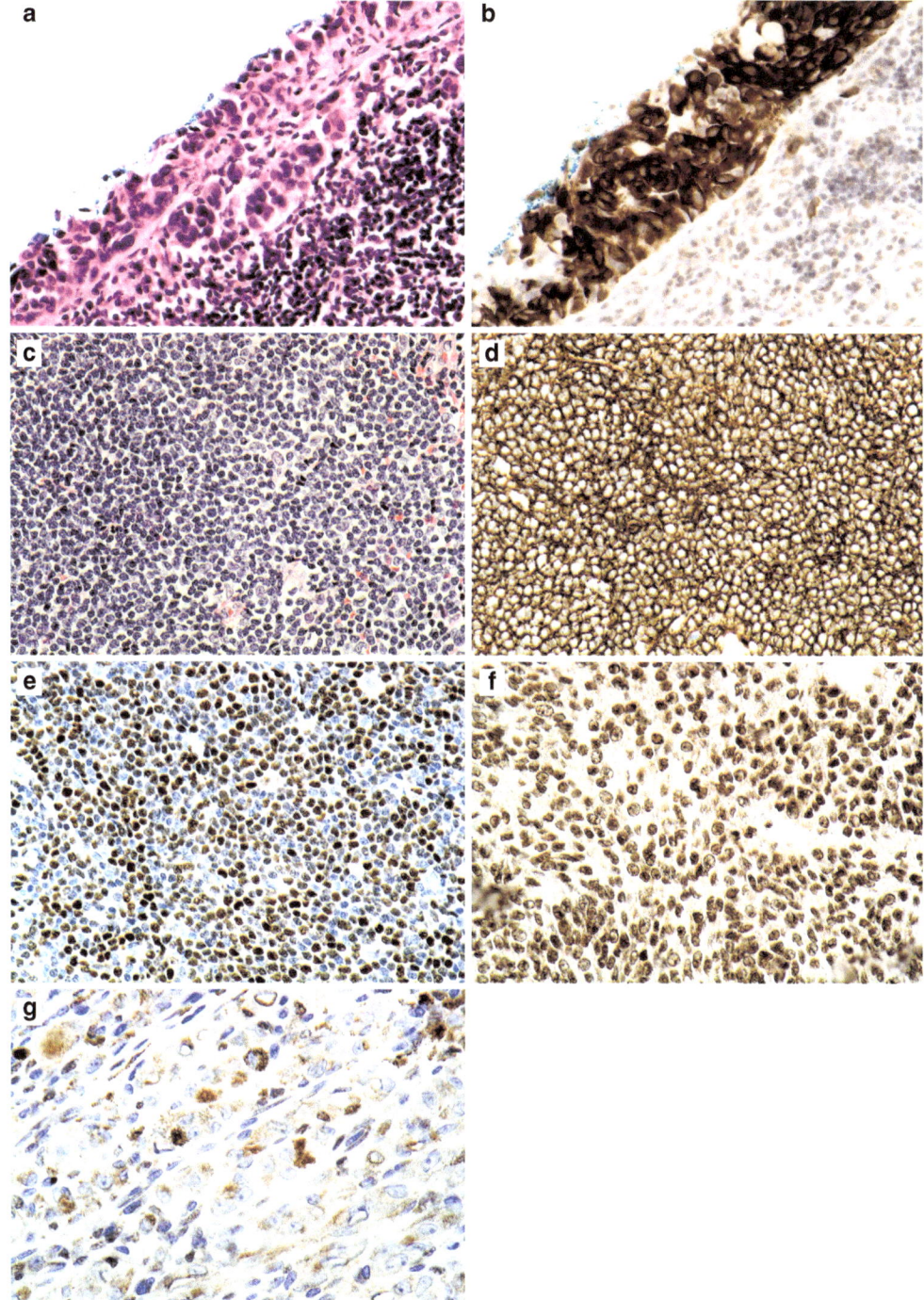

Fig. 15.5 (**a**) H&E of a conjunctival biopsy showing amelanotic atypical cells occupying the full thickness of the epithelium. (**b**) Melan A immunohistochemistry shows positivity in the atypical intraepithelial cells (brown signal), indicating in situ melanoma. (**c**) H&E showing a diffuse sheet of round lymphoid cells. (**d**) The lymphoid cells in Fig. (**c**) are positive for CD20. (**e**) The lymphoid cells in panel **c** are positive for nuclear Cyclin D1, indicating a diagnosis of Mantle cell lymphoma. (**f**) BAP 1 immunohistochemistry on a uveal melanoma showing nuclear positivity. (**g**) BAP 1 immunohistochemistry on another uveal melanoma showing a lack of nuclear staining. (**e**, courtesy of Dr. Karen Sisley, Senior Lecturer, Department of Oncology, Sheffield University, Sheffield, UK)

(Fig. 15.5b) and negative for cytokeratin and androgen receptor. Melan A is a protein specific to melanoma cells. Cytokeratins are expressed by epithelial malignancies (in situ squamous and sebaceous carcinoma), and androgen receptor is expressed strongly by in situ sebaceous carcinoma. The final diagnosis is in situ melanoma.

Example 2 This orbital biopsy shows a lymphocytic infiltrate that histologically is a lymphoma (Fig. 15.5c). However, every lymphoma must be precisely sub-typed as each lymphoma has a specific morphology, immunohistochemical phenotype, molecular signature, prognosis and treatment (WHO classification). Application of a panel of lymphoid markers shows that this lymphoma is of B-cell phenotype (positive for CD20, Fig. 15.5d) and furthermore is positive for Cyclin D1 (Fig. 15.5e) which indicates the precise diagnosis of mantle cell lymphoma [16].

Prognostic Application

Figure 15.5f shows a uveal melanoma that shows nuclear positivity for BAP1. Figure 15.5g shows nuclear BAP-1 absence in another uveal melanoma, an indication that the tumour is of probable monosomy 3 genotype, associated with a poor prognosis [17].

Polymerase Chain Reaction (PCR)

Diagnostic Application

Sometimes, it is difficult to ascertain on light microscopy whether a lymphoid infiltrate is reactive or neoplastic. Formalin-fixed, paraffin-embedded extracted DNA can be tested for lymphocyte clonality, to establish whether a population of lymphoid cells are polyclonal (reactive-not lymphoma) or monoclonal (likely lymphoma) (Fig. 15.6a).

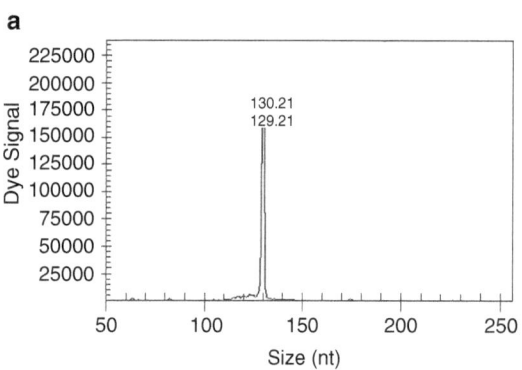

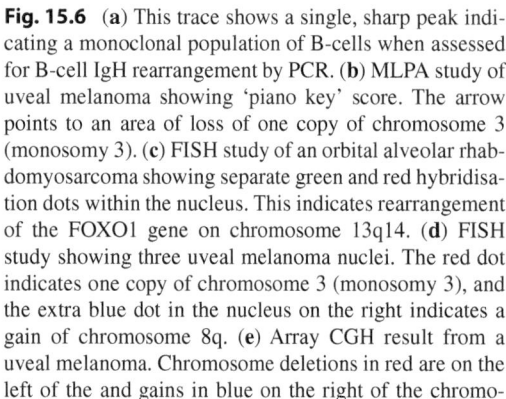

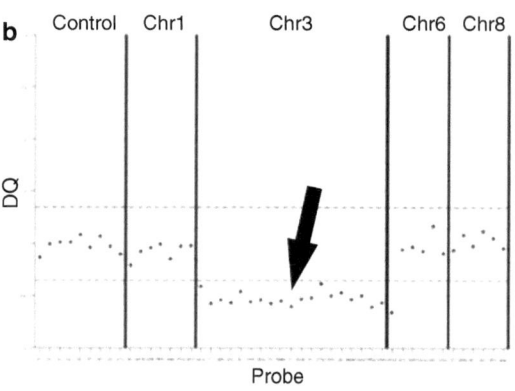

Fig. 15.6 (a) This trace shows a single, sharp peak indicating a monoclonal population of B-cells when assessed for B-cell IgH rearrangement by PCR. (b) MLPA study of uveal melanoma showing 'piano key' score. The arrow points to an area of loss of one copy of chromosome 3 (monosomy 3). (c) FISH study of an orbital alveolar rhabdomyosarcoma showing separate green and red hybridisation dots within the nucleus. This indicates rearrangement of the FOXO1 gene on chromosome 13q14. (d) FISH study showing three uveal melanoma nuclei. The red dot indicates one copy of chromosome 3 (monosomy 3), and the extra blue dot in the nucleus on the right indicates a gain of chromosome 8q. (e) Array CGH result from a uveal melanoma. Chromosome deletions in red are on the left of the and gains in blue on the right of the chromo-

somes. This study shows a loss of chromosome 3 (left arrow) and a loss of 8p and gain of 8q (right arrow). Other changes include deletion of chromosome 1 and gains of chromosome 20 and 21. (f) SNP array data from a uveal melanoma showing loss of one copy of chromosome 3 (left arrow) and loss of 8p and gain of 8q (right arrow). (Courtesy of: **b**, Professor Sarah E Coupland-Professor of Ophthalmic Pathology, Liverpool University, Liverpool UK; **c**, Dr Duncan Baker, Cytogeneticist, Sheffield Children's Hospital, Sheffield UK; **d**, Dr Karen Sisley, Senior Lecturer, Department of Oncology, Sheffield University, Sheffield UK; **f**, Dr Natasha van Poppelen and Dr Rob Verdijk, Department of Pathology, Erasmus Medical Centre, Rotterdam, Netherlands)

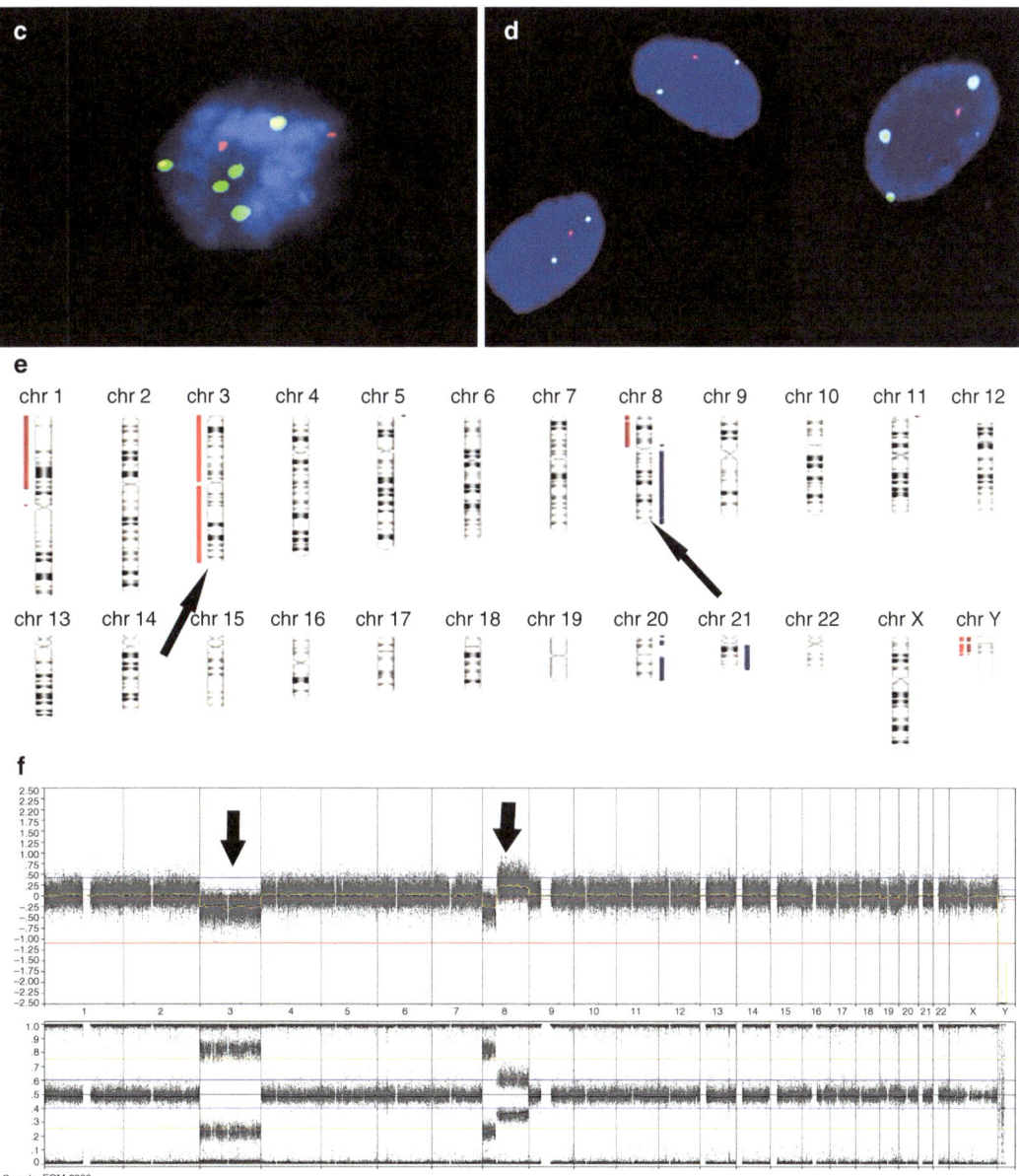

Fig. 15.6 (continued)

Prognostic Application

The states of chromosomes 1, 3, 6 and 8 allow uveal melanoma to be stratified into good and bad prognostic categories. A technique called MLPA (multi-ligation-dependent probe amplification), which is a variation of PCR, can be used to test for these chromosomal changes [18] (Fig. 15.6b).

Flow Cytometry

Diagnostic Application

This technique is used in some centres to ascertain whether a neoplastic population of B or T cells are present in vitreous or aqueous biopsies, in limited material. It is a powerful technique for the diagnosis of lymphoma [19]. Multiple antibodies directed to various lymphoid cell proteins, including kappa and lambda light chains, are applied as a cocktail to an unfixed suspension of lymphoid cells.

Fluorescence In Situ Hybridisation (FISH)

This technique uses fluorescent-tagged DNA or RNA probes to detect the presence or absence of a specific chromosome or the identification of two genes involved in a translocation. It can be used on cytology and paraffin-embedded tissue.

Diagnostic Application

Many sarcomas have distinctive, diagnostic recurrent genetic translocations. The example in Fig. 15.6c shows a FISH analysis of an orbital alveolar rhabdomyosarcoma with the diagnostic 1:13 translocation, which is also important as a prognostic marker in this tumour [20].

Prognostic Application

Uveal melanoma can have its chromosome 3 and 8 status tested by FISH [10, 12, 13] (Fig. 15.6d).

Chromosomal Microarray Analysis (aCGH and SNP)

Techniques such as array comparative genomic hybridisation (aCGH)[21] and single nucleotide polymorphism (SNP) chromosomal arrays [22] are powerful tools to detect genome-wide copy number changes in chromosomes. Furthermore, SNP arrays can detect copy-neutral changes and loss of heterozygosity. These techniques can be applied to fresh and paraffin-embedded tumour tissue successfully.

Diagnostic Applications

Can be used to help differentiate benign nevus from melanoma of the skin.

Prognostic Application

Can be used in uveal melanoma prognostic chromosomal analysis (Fig. 15.6e, f).

Tumour Prognostic Factors

Histopathology reports contain critical bits of information that will reflect the biological behaviour of the tumour; hence, its prognosis will trigger specific clinical management. What follows are brief descriptions of prognostic factors for some ocular tumours impacting on clinical management.

Every prognostic factor for every ocular tumour cannot be reproduced here. The relevant chapters in the TNM classification of Malignant Tumours (8th edition -UICC) [14] and the *AJCC Cancer Staging Manual* (8th edition) [15] have comprehensive lists of prognostic factors for all major ophthalmic tumours. Additionally, the tumour-reporting guidelines/datasets from the College of American Pathologists [23, 24] and the Royal College of Pathologists UK [25, 26] are a very comprehensive guide to macroscopic and microscopic prognostic factors for ocular tumours. Tumour prognostic factors from a pathological perspective can be macroscopic, microscopic and molecular/genetic.

Examples of Tumour Prognostic Factors Encountered in Ophthalmic Histopathology Reports

Eyelid Basal Cell Carcinoma [14, 15, 27]

The growth pattern of basal cell carcinoma will be mentioned in a report. Infiltrating and/or sclerosing/morphoea and/or micronodular growth patterns are high-risk growth patterns. These growth patterns correlate with a significantly increased risk for local recurrence and very occasionally metastasis, hence high risk. The clearance of the tumour in 'mm' from specific margins will be mentioned in the report. Contaminated margins will trigger further treatment to ensure clearance.

Conjunctival Melanoma [14, 15]

For conjunctival melanoma, the site and depth of invasion determine the 'pT' staging of these tumours. Tumours of the palpebral, forniceal and caruncular conjunctiva are higher risk compared to bulbar conjunctival tumours. The higher risk relates to recurrence and metastatic rates. The deeper the invasive component, the higher the pT stage.

Retinoblastoma [14, 15, 23, 24]

The presence of 'high-risk' histopathological factors on a histopathology report of a retinoblastoma enucleation includes 'massive choroidal invasion', 'extra-scleral tumour extension', 'optic nerve invasion' and 'anterior chamber extension'. These features will lead to post-enucleation chemotherapy.

Uveal Melanoma [14, 15, 25, 26]

Iris melanomas have a much better prognosis that ciliary body and choroidal located tumours. Ciliary body and choroidal uveal melanomas with monosomy 3 and iso-chromosome 8q gain will have a poor prognosis, compared to tumours with balanced genetics.

Orbital Alveolar Rhabdomyosarcoma

Histology reports will make the distinction between the different subtypes of orbital rhabdomyosarcoma as they have different prognoses. An alveolar growth pattern which shows a 1:13 or 2:13 translocation [28] has is more aggressive and of higher risk for recurrence and metastasis compared to the embryonal variant.

References

1. Fletcher CDM. Diagnostic histopathology of tumors. 4th ed. Philadelphia: *Elsevier Saunders*; 2013.
2. Maudgil A, Salvi SM, Tan JH, Mudhar HS. Improving the interaction between the ophthalmology and histopathology departments. Eye (Lond). 2011;25(8):998–1004.
3. Suvarna KS, Layton C, Bancroft JD. Bancroft's theory and practice of histological techniques. 7th ed. Oxford: Churchill Livingstone; 2013.
4. Ford AL, Mudhar HS, Farr R, Parsons MA. The ophthalmic pathology cut-up part 1: the enucleation and exenterations specimen. Curr Diagn Pathol. 2005;11:284–90.
5. Ford AL, Mudhar HS, Farr R, Parsons MA. The ophthalmic pathology cut-up part 2: the enucleation and exenterations specimen. Curr Diagn Pathol. 2005;11:340–8.
6. Kumar V, Abbas AK. Fausto N Aster Robbins and Cotran pathological basis of disease. 8th ed. Philadelphia: Elsevier/Saunders; 2015.
7. McLean IW, Foster WD, Zimmerman LE, Gamel JW. Modifications of Callender's classification of uveal melanoma at the armed forces Institute of Pathology. Am J Ophthalmol. 1983;96:502–9.
8. Folberg R, Rummelt V, Parys-Van Ginderdeuren R, Hwang T, Woolson RF, Pe'er J, et al. The prognostic value of tumor blood vessel morphology in primary uveal melanoma. Ophthalmology. 1993;100:1389–98.
9. Prescher G, Bornfield N, Becher R. Non-random chromosomal abnormalities in primary uveal melanoma. J Natl Cancer Inst. 1990;82:1765–9.
10. Sisley K, Rennie IG, Parsons MA, Jacques R, Hammond DW, Bell SM, et al. Abnormalities of chromosomes 3 and 8 in posterior uveal melanoma correlate with prognosis. Genes Chromosomes Cancer. 1997;19:22–8.
11. Onken MD, Worley LA, Char DH, Augsburger JJ, Correa ZM, Nudleman E, et al. Collaborative ocular oncology group report number 1: prospective validation of a multi-gene prognostic assay in uveal melanoma. Ophthalmology. 2012;119:1596–603.
12. Coupland SE, Lake SL, Zeschniqk M, Damato BE. Molecular pathology of uveal melanoma. Eye (Lond). 2013;27:230–42.
13. Vaarwater J, van den Bosch T, Mensink HW, van Kempen C, Verdijk RM, Naus NC, et al. Multiplex ligation-dependent probe amplification equals fluorescence in-situ hybridization for the identification of patients at risk for metastatic disease in uveal melanoma. Melanoma Res. 2012;22:30–7.
14. Brierley J, Gospodarowicz MK, Wittekind C. TNM classification of malignant tumors. 8th ed. Oxford UK: Wiley; 2017.
15. Amin MB. AJCC Cancer staging manual. 8th ed. Cham: Springer; 2017.
16. Swerdlow SH, Campo E, Harris NL, Jaffe ES, Pileri SA, Stein H, Thiele J. World Health Organization of tumors-tumors of the haematopoietic and lymphoid tissues. 4th ed. Lyon: IARC press; 2017.
17. Shah AA, Bourne TD, Murali R. BAP1 protein loss by immunohistochemistry: a potentially useful tool for prognostic prediction in patients with uveal melanoma. Pathology. 2013;45(7):651–6.
18. Damato B, Dopierala JA, Coupland SE. Genotypic profiling of 452 choroidal melanomas with multiplex ligation-dependent probe amplification. Clin Cancer Res. 2010;16(24):6083–92.
19. Davis JL, Viciana AL, Ruiz P. Diagnosis of intraocular lymphoma by flow cytometry. Am J Ophthalmol. 1997;124:362–72.
20. Mehra S, de la Roza G, Tull J, Shrimpton A, Valente A, Zhang S. Detection of FOXO1 (FKHR) gene break-apart by fluorescence in situ hybridization in formalin-fixed, paraffin-embedded alveolar rhabdomyosarcomas and its clinicopathologic correlation. Diagn Mol Pathol. 2008;17(1):14–20.

21. Speicher MR, Prescher G, du Manoir S, Jauch A, Horsthemke B, Bornfeld N, Becher R, Cremer T. Chromosomal gains and losses in uveal melanomas detected by comparative genomic hybridization. Cancer Res. 1994;54(14):3817–23.

22. Onken MD, Worley LA, Person E, Char DH, Bowcock AM, Harbour JW. Loss of heterozygosity of chromosome 3 detected with single nucleotide polymorphisms is superior to monosomy 3 for predicting metastasis in uveal melanoma. Clin Cancer Res. 2007;13(10):2923–7.

23. https://documents.cap.org/protocols/cp-retinoblastoma-17protocol-4000.pdf

24. https://www.google.co.uk/search?q=RCPath+retinoblastoma+dataset&gws_rd=cr,ssl&dcr=0&ei=qITDWYzSOKWTgAbd1YOIAg

25. http://www.cap.org/ShowProperty?nodePath=/UCMCon/ContributionFolders/WebContent/pdf/cp-uveal-melanoma-17protocol-4000.pdf

26. https://www.rcpath.org/resourceLibrary/dataset-for-the-histopathological-reporting-of-uveal-melanoma%2D%2D3rd-edition-.html

27. https://www.google.co.uk/search?q=rcpath+basal+cell+carcinoma+dataset&gws_rd=cr,ssl&dcr=0&ei=lIHDWbX9FeTOgAbYspjwBw

28. Barr FG. Molecular genetics and pathogenesis of rhabdomyosarcoma. J Pediatr Hematol Oncol. 1997;19:483–91.

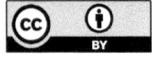

Appendices

Appendix A: American Joint Committee on Cancer (AJCC) 8th Edition Cancer Staging

From Amin MB, Edge SB, Greene FL, et al., eds. *AJCC Cancer Staging Manual.* 8th ed. New York: Springer; 2017. *Used with permission of the American College of Surgeons, Chicago, Illinois. The original and primary source for this information is the AJCC Cancer Staging Manual, Eighth Edition (2017) published by Springer International Publishing.*

Eyelid Tumors

Primary tumor (T)	
TX	Primary tumor cannot be assessed
T0	No evidence of primary tumor
Tis	Carcinoma in situ
T1	Tumor <10 mm in greatest dimension
T1a	Tumor does not invade the tarsal plate or eyelid margin
T1b	Tumor invades the tarsal plate or eyelid margin
T1c	Tumor involves full thickness of eyelid
T2	Tumor >10 mm but <20 mm in greatest dimension
T2a	Tumor does not invade the tarsal plate or eyelid margin
T2b	Tumor invades the tarsal plate or eyelid margin
T2c	Tumor involves full thickness of eyelid
T3	Tumor >20 mm but <30 mm in greatest dimensions
T3a	Tumor does not invade the tarsal plate or eyelid margin
T3b	Tumor invades the tarsal plate or eyelid margin
T3c	Tumor involves full thickness of eyelid
T4	Any eyelid tumor that invades adjacent ocular, orbital, or facial structures
T4a	Tumor invades ocular or intra-orbital structures
T4b	Tumor invades (or erodes through) the bony walls of the orbit or extends to the paranasal sinuses or invades the lacrimal sac/nasolacrimal duct or brain
Regional lymph node (N)	
NX	Regional lymph nodes cannot be assessed
N0	No evidence of lymph node involvement
N1	Metastasis in a single ipsilateral lymph node, <3 cm in greatest dimension
N1a	Metastasis in a single ipsilateral lymph node based on clinical evaluation or imaging findings
N1b	Metastasis in a single ipsilateral lymph node based on lymph node biopsy
N2	Metastasis in a single ipsilateral lymph node, >3 cm in greatest dimension, or in bilateral or contralateral lymph nodes
N2a	Metastasis documented based on clinical evaluation or imaging findings
N2b	Metastasis documented based on microscopic findings on lymph node biopsy
Distant metastasis (M)	
M0	No distant metastasis
M1	Distant metastasis

Conjunctival Carcinoma

Primary tumor (T)	
TX	Primary tumor cannot be assessed
T0	No evidence of primary tumor
Tis	Carcinoma in situ

© The Author(s) 2019
S. S. Chaugule et al. (eds.), *Surgical Ophthalmic Oncology*,
https://doi.org/10.1007/978-3-030-18757-6

T1	Tumor (<5 mm in greatest dimension) invades through the conjunctival basement membrane without invasion of adjacent structures
T2	Tumor (>5 mm in greatest dimension) invades through the conjunctival basement membrane without invasion of adjacent structures
T3	Tumor invades the adjacent structures (excluding the orbit)
T4	Tumor invades the orbit with or without further extension
T4a	Tumor invades orbital soft tissue without bone invasion
T4b	Tumor invades bone
T4c	Tumor invades adjacent paranasal sinuses
T4d	Tumor invades brain
Regional lymph node (N)	
NX	Regional lymph nodes cannot be assessed
N0	No evidence of lymph node involvement
N1	Regional lymph node metastasis
Distant metastasis (M)	
M0	No distant metastasis
M1	Distant metastasis

Conjunctival Melanoma

Primary tumor (T)	
Clinical tumor (cT)	
TX	Primary tumor cannot be assessed
T0	No evidence of primary tumor
T1	Tumor of the bulbar conjunctiva
T1a	<1 quadrant
T1b	>1 to <2 quadrant
T1c	>2 to <3 quadrant
T1d	>3 quadrants
T2	Tumor of nonbulbar (forniceal, palpebral, tarsal) conjunctiva, the tumor involving the caruncle
T2a	Noncaruncular, and <1 quadrant of nonbulbar conjunctiva involved
T2b	Noncaruncular, and >1 quadrant of nonbulbar conjunctiva involved
T2c	Caruncular, and <1 quadrant of the nonbulbar conjunctiva involved
T2d	Caruncular, and >1 quadrant of the nonbulbar conjunctiva involved
T3	Tumor of any size with local invasion
T3a	Globe
T3b	Eyelid
T3c	Orbit

T3d	Nasolacrimal duct and/or lacrimal sac and/or paranasal sinuses
T4	Tumor of any size with invasion of central nervous system
Pathological tumor (pT)	
TX	Primary tumor cannot be assessed
T0	No evidence of primary tumor
Tis	Melanoma confined to the conjunctival epithelium
T1	Tumor of the bulbar conjunctiva
T1a	Tumor of the bulbar conjunctiva with invasion of the substantia propria, not more than 2.0 mm in thickness
T1b	Tumor of the bulbar conjunctiva with invasion of the substantia propria, more than 2.0 mm in thickness
T2	Tumor of the nonbulbar (forniceal, palpebral, tarsal) conjunctiva, and tumor involving the caruncle
T2a	Tumor of the nonbulbar conjunctiva with invasion of the substantia propria, not more than 2.0 mm in thickness
T2b	Tumor of the nonbulbar conjunctiva with invasion of the substantia propria, more than 2.0 mm in thickness
T3	Tumor of any size with local invasion
T3a	Globe
T3b	Eyelid
T3c	Orbit
T3d	Nasolacrimal duct and/or lacrimal sac and/or paranasal sinuses
T4	Tumor of any size with invasion of paranasal sinuses and/or central nervous system
Regional lymph node (N)	
NX	Regional lymph nodes cannot be assessed
N0	No evidence of lymph node involvement
N1	Regional lymph node metastasis
Distant metastasis (M)	
M0	No distant metastasis
M1	Distant metastasis

Retinoblastoma

Clinical classification (cTNM)	
Primary tumor	
cTX	Unknown evidence of intraocular tumor
cT0	No evidence of intraocular tumor
cT1	Intraretinal tumor(s) with subretinal fluid <5 mm from base of any tumor
cT1a	Tumors ≤3 mm in size and > 1.5 mm away from the optic disc and fovea

cT1b	Tumors >3 mm in size and < 1.5 mm away from the optic disc and fovea
cT2	Intraretinal tumor(s) with retinal detachment, subretinal seeding/vitreous seeding
cT2a	Subretinal fluid >5 mm from the base of any tumor
cT2b	Tumors with vitreous seeding and/or subretinal seeding
cT3	Advanced intraocular tumor(s)
cT3a	Phthisis or pre-phthisis bulbi
cT3b	Tumor invasion of choroid, pars plana, ciliary body, lens, zonules, iris, or anterior chamber
cT3c	Raised intraocular pressure with neovascularization and/or buphthalmos
cT3d	Hyphema and/or massive vitreous hemorrhage
cT3e	Aseptic orbital cellulitis
cT4	Extraocular tumor(s) involving orbit, including optic nerve
cT4a	Radiological evidence of retrobulbar optic nerve involvement or thickening of optic nerve or involvement of orbital tissues
cT4b	Extraocular tumor clinically evident with proptosis and /or an orbital mass

Regional lymph node (cN)

cNX	Regional lymph nodes cannot be assessed
cN0	No regional lymph node involvement
cN1	Evidence of preauricular, submandibular, and cervical lymph node involvement

Distant metastasis (M)

cM0	No signs or symptoms of intracranial or distant metastasis
cM1	Distant metastasis without microscopic confirmation
cM1a	Tumor(s) involving any distant site (e.g., bone marrow, liver) on clinical or radiological tests
cM1b	Tumor involving the CNS on radiological imaging (not including trilateral retinoblastoma)
pM1	Distant metastasis with microscopic confirmation
pM1a	Pathological evidence of tumor at any distant site (e.g., bone marrow, liver, or other)
pM1b	Pathological evidence of tumor in the cerebrospinal fluid or CNS parenchyma

Heritable trait (H)

HX	Unknown or insufficient evidence of *RB1* gene constitutional mutation
H0	Normal *RB1* alleles in blood tested with demonstrated high-sensitivity assays
H1	Bilateral retinoblastoma, retinoblastoma with an intracranial primitive neuroectodermal tumor (i.e., trilateral retinoblastoma), family history of retinoblastoma, or molecular definition of constitutional *RB1* gene mutation

Pathological classification

Primary tumor (pT)

pTX	Unknown evidence of intraocular tumor
pT0	No evidence of intraocular tumor
pT1	Intraocular tumor(s) without any local invasion, focal choroidal invasion, or pre- or intralaminar involvement of the optic nerve head
pT2	Intraocular tumor(s) with local invasion
pT2a	Concomitant focal choroidal invasion and pre- or intralaminar involvement of the optic nerve head
pT2b	Tumor invasion of stroma of iris and/or trabecular meshwork and/or Schlemm's canal
pT3	Intraocular tumor(s) with significant local invasion
pT3a	Massive choroidal invasion (>3 mm in largest diameter, or multiple foci of focal choroidal involvement totaling >3 mm, or any full-thickness choroidal involvement)
pT3b	Retrolaminar invasion of the optic nerve head, not involving the transected end of the optic nerve
pT3c	Any partial-thickness involvement of the sclera within the inner two-thirds
pT3d	Full-thickness invasion into the outer third of the sclera and/or invasion into or around emissary channels
pT4	Evidence of extraocular tumor: tumor at the transected end of the optic nerve, tumor in the meningeal spaces around the optic nerve, full-thickness invasion of the sclera with invasion of the episclera, adjacent adipose tissue, extraocular muscle, bone, conjunctiva, or eyelids

Regional lymph node (pN)

pNX	Regional lymph node involvement cannot be assessed
pN0	No lymph node involvement
pN1	Regional lymph node involvement

Distant metastasis (M)

cM0	No signs or symptoms of intracranial or distant metastasis
cM1	Distant metastasis without microscopic confirmation
cM1a	Tumor(s) involving any distant site (e.g., bone marrow, liver) on clinical or radiological test

cM1b	Tumor involving the CNS on radiological imaging (not including trilateral retinoblastoma)
pM1	Distant metastasis with histopathologic confirmation
pM1a	Histopathologic confirmation of tumor at any distant site (e.g., bone marrow, liver, or others)
pM1b	Histopathologic confirmation of tumor in the cerebrospinal fluid or CNS parenchyma

Uveal Melanoma

Primary tumor (T)	
Iris melanomas	
T1	Tumor limited to the iris
T1a	Tumor limited to the iris, not more than 3 clock hours in size
T1b	Tumor limited to the iris, more than 3 clock hours in size
T1c	Tumor limited to the iris with secondary glaucoma
T2	Tumor confluent with or extending into ciliary body, choroid, or both
T2a	Tumor confluent with or extending into ciliary body, without secondary glaucoma
T2b	Tumor confluent with or extending into ciliary body and choroid, without secondary glaucoma
T2c	Tumor confluent with or extending into ciliary body, choroid, or both with secondary glaucoma
T3	Tumor confluent with or extending into the ciliary Body, choroid, or both, with scleral extension
T4	Tumor with extrascleral extension
T4a	Tumor with extrascleral extension <5 mm in largest diameter
T4b	Tumor with extrascleral extension >5 mm in largest diameter
Choroidal and ciliary body melanomas	
T1	Tumor size category 1
T1a	Tumor size category 1 without ciliary body involvement and extraocular extension
T1b	Tumor size category 1 with ciliary body involvement
T1c	Tumor size category 1 without ciliary body involvement but with extraocular extension <5 mm in largest diameter
T1d	Tumor size category 1 with ciliary body involvement but with extraocular extension <5 mm in largest diameter

T2	Tumor size category 2
T2a	Tumor size category 2 without ciliary body involvement and extraocular extension
T2b	Tumor size category 2 with ciliary body involvement
T2c	Tumor size category 2 without ciliary body involvement but with extraocular extension <5 mm in largest diameter
T2d	Tumor size category 2 with ciliary body involvement but with extraocular extension <5 mm in largest diameter
T3	Tumor size category 3
T3a	Tumor size category 3 without ciliary body involvement and extraocular extension
T3b	Tumor size category 3 with ciliary body involvement
T3c	Tumor size category 3 without ciliary body involvement but with extraocular extension <5 mm in largest diameter
T3d	Tumor size category 3 with ciliary body involvement but with extraocular extension <5 mm in largest diameter
T4	Tumor size category 4
T4a	Tumor size category 4 without ciliary body involvement and extraocular extension
T4b	Tumor size category 4 with ciliary body involvement
T4c	Tumor size category 4 without ciliary body involvement but with extraocular extension <5 mm in largest diameter
T4d	Tumor size category 4 with ciliary body involvement but with extraocular extension <5 mm in largest diameter
T4e	Any tumor size category with extraocular extension >5 mm in largest diameter
Regional lymph node (N)	
N1	Regional lymph node metastases or discrete tumor deposits in the orbit
N1a	Metastases in one or more regional lymph node (s)
N1b	No regional lymph nodes are positive, but there are discrete tumor deposits in the orbit that are not contiguous to the eye
Distant metastasis (M)	
M0	No distant metastasis by clinical classification
M1	Distant metastasis
M1a	Largest diameter of the largest metastasis <3.0 cm
M1b	Largest diameter of the largest metastasis 3.1–8.0 cm
M1c	Largest diameter of the largest metastasis >8.1 cm

Fig. A.1 Tumor size category

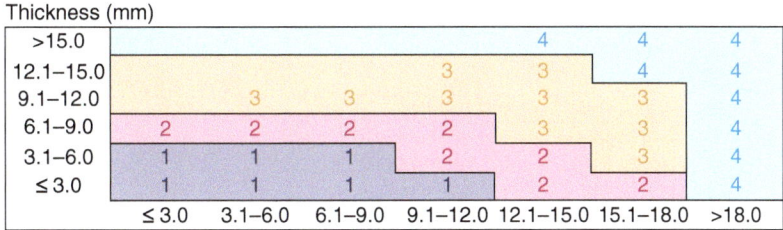

Thickness (mm)

>15.0					4	4	4
12.1–15.0				3	3	4	4
9.1–12.0		3	3	3	3	3	4
6.1–9.0	2	2	2	2	3	3	4
3.1–6.0	1	1	1	2	2	3	4
≤3.0	1	1	1	1	2	2	4
	≤3.0	3.1–6.0	6.1–9.0	9.1–12.0	12.1–15.0	15.1–18.0	>18.0

Largest basal diameter (mm)

Orbital Sarcoma

Primary tumor (T)

TX	Primary tumor cannot be assessed
T0	No evidence of primary tumor
T1	Tumor <2 cm in greatest dimension
T2	Tumor >2 cm in greatest diameter without invasion of bony walls or globe
T3	Tumor of any size with invasion of bony walls
T4	Tumor of any size with invasion of globe or periorbital structures, including eyelid, conjunctiva, temporal fossa, nasal cavity, paranasal sinuses, and/or central nervous system

Regional lymph node (N)

NX	Regional lymph nodes cannot be assessed
N0	No regional lymph node metastasis
N1	Regional lymph node metastasis

Distant metastasis (M)

M0	No distant metastasis
M1	Distant metastasis

Ocular Adnexal Lymphoma

Primary tumor (T)

TX	Lymphoma extent not specified
T0	No evidence of lymphoma
T1	Lymphoma involving the conjunctiva alone without eyelid or orbital involvement
T2	Lymphoma with orbital involvement with or without conjunctival involvement
T3	Lymphoma with pre-septal eyelid involvement with or without orbital involvement and with or without conjunctival involvement
T4	Orbital adnexal lymphoma and extraorbital lymphoma extending beyond the orbit to adjacent structures, such as bone, maxillofacial sinuses, and brain

Regional lymph node (N)

NX	Involvement of lymph nodes not assessed

N0	No evidence of regional lymph node involvement
N1	Involvement of lymph node region or regions draining the ocular adnexal structures and superior to the mediastinum (preauricular, parotid, submandibular, and cervical nodes)
N1a	Involvement of a single lymph node region superior to mediastinum
N1b	Involvement of two or more lymph node regions superior to mediastinum
N2	Involvement of lymph node regions of the mediastinum
N3	Diffuse or disseminated involvement of peripheral and central lymph node regions

Distant metastasis (M)

M0	No evidence of involvement of other extranodal sites
M1a	Noncontiguous involvement of tissues or organs external to the ocular adnexa (e.g., parotid glands, submandibular gland, lung, liver, spleen, kidney, breast)
M1b	Lymphomatous involvement of the bone marrow
M1c	Both M1a and M1b involvement

Lacrimal Gland Carcinoma

Primary tumor (T)

TX	Primary tumor cannot be assessed
T0	No evidence of primary tumor
T1	Tumor <2 cm in greatest dimension with or without extraglandular extension into the orbital soft tissue
T1a	No periosteal or bone involvement
T1b	Periosteal involvement only
T1c	Periosteal and bone involvement
T2	Tumor >2 cm and <4 cm in greatest diameter
T2a	No periosteal or bone involvement
T2b	Periosteal involvement only
T2c	Periosteal and bone involvement

T3	Tumor >4 cm in greatest dimension
T3a	No periosteal or bone involvement
T3b	Periosteal involvement only
T3c	Periosteal and bone involvement
T4	Involvement of adjacent structures, including sinuses, temporal fossa, pterygoid fossa, superior orbital fissure, cavernous sinus, or brain
T4a	Tumor <2 cm in greatest dimension
T4b	Tumor >2 cm and <4 cm in greatest dimension
T4c	Tumor >4 cm in greatest dimension
Regional lymph node (N)	
NX	Regional lymph nodes cannot be assessed
N0	No regional lymph node metastasis
N1	Regional lymph node metastasis
Distant metastasis (M)	
M0	No distant metastasis
M1	Distant metastasis

Appendix B: College of American Pathologists Protocol for the Examination of Specimens from Patients with Retinoblastoma

Version: Retinoblastoma 4.0.0.0	**Protocol Posting Date:** June 2017
Includes pTNM requirements from the 8th Edition, AJCC Staging Manual	

Reproduced by permission of the *College of American Pathologists (CAP)* © 2019. *The CAP* periodically revises the CAP Cancer Protocols, and the current versions may be retrieved from www.cap.org/cancerprotocols. The CAP does not permit reproduction of any substantial portion of these protocols without its written authorization. The CAP hereby authorizes use of these protocols by physicians and other healthcare providers in reporting on surgical specimens, in teaching, and in carrying out medical research for nonprofit purposes. This authorization does not extend to reproduction or other use of any substantial portion of these protocols for commercial purposes without the written consent of the CAP.

For accreditation purposes, this protocol should be used for the following procedures and tumor types:

Procedure	Description
Resection	Includes enucleation and partial or complete exenteration
Tumor type	**Description**
Retinoblastoma	

Authors

Hans E. Grossniklaus, MD, MBA[1]; Paul T. Finger, MD; J. William Harbour, MD; Tero Kivelä, MD

With guidance from the CAP Cancer and CAP Pathology Electronic Reporting Committees.

Accreditation Requirements

This protocol can be utilized for a variety of procedures and tumor types for clinical care purposes. For accreditation purposes, only the definitive primary cancer resection specimen is required to have the core and conditional data elements reported in a synoptic format.

- *Core data elements* are required in reports to adequately describe appropriate malignancies. For accreditation purposes, essential data elements must be reported in all instances, even if the response is "not applicable" or "cannot be determined."
- *Conditional data elements* are only required to be reported if applicable as delineated in the protocol. For instance, the total number of lymph nodes examined must be reported, but only if nodes are present in the specimen.
- *Optional data elements* are identified with "+" and although not required for CAP accreditation purposes, may be considered for reporting as determined by local practice standards.

The use of this protocol is not required for recurrent tumors or for metastatic tumors that are

---

[1]Denotes primary author. All other contributing authors are listed alphabetically.

resected at a different time than the primary tumor. Use of this protocol is also not required for pathology reviews performed at the second institution (i.e., secondary consultation, second opinion, or review of outside case at the second institution).

Synoptic Reporting

All core and conditionally required data elements outlined in the surgical case summary from this cancer protocol must be displayed in synoptic report format. Synoptic format is defined as:

- Data element: followed by its answer (response), outline format without the paired "Data element: Response" format is not considered synoptic.
- The data element must be represented in the report as it is listed in the case summary. The response for any data element may be modified from those listed in the case summary, including "Cannot be determined" if appropriate.
- Each diagnostic parameter pair (Data element: Response) is listed on a separate line or in a tabular format to achieve visual separation. The following exceptions are allowed to be listed on one line:
  - Anatomic site or specimen, laterality, and procedure
  - Pathologic Stage Classification (pTNM) elements
  - Negative margins, as long as all negative margins are specifically enumerated where applicable
- The synoptic portion of the report can appear in the diagnosis section of the pathology report, at the end of the report or in a separate section, but all data element: Responses must be listed together in one location.

Organizations and pathologists may choose to list the required elements in any order, use additional methods in order to enhance or achieve visual separation, or add optional items within the synoptic report. The report may have required elements in a summary format elsewhere in the report in addition to but not as replacement for the synoptic report, i.e., all required elements must be in the synoptic portion of the report in the format defined above.

CAP Laboratory Accreditation Program Protocol Required Use Date: March 2018[a]

[a]*Beginning January 1, 2018, the 8th edition AJCC Staging Manual should be used for reporting pTNM.*

CAP Retinoblastoma Protocol Summary of Changes

The following data elements were modified:

- Pathologic Stage Classification (pTNM, AJCC 8th Edition)
- Tumor Site
- Tumor Size
- Tumor Involvement of Other Ocular Structures
- Histologic Grade
- Additional Pathologic Findings

The following data element was added:

- Cytologic Features Suggesting *MYCN* Amplification

Surgical Pathology Cancer Case Summary

Protocol posting date: June 2017

Retinoblastoma
Select a single response unless otherwise indicated.

Procedure (Notes A, B, and C)
___ Enucleation
   Length of optic nerve (millimeters): ___ mm
___ Partial exenteration
___ Complete exenteration
___   Other   (specify):
_____
___ Not specified

Specimen Laterality
___ Right
___ Left
___ Not specified

Tumor Site (Macroscopic Examination/ Transillumination) (Select All that Apply) (Notes D and E)

___ Cannot be determined
___ Superotemporal quadrant of globe
___ Superonasal quadrant of globe
___ Inferotemporal quadrant of globe
___ Inferonasal quadrant of globe
___ Anterior chamber
___ Between ____ and ____ o'clock
___ Other (specify): _____

Tumor Size After Sectioning (Note F)

___ Cannot be determined
Greatest basal diameter (millimeters): ____ mm
+ Base at cut edge (millimeters): ____ mm
Greatest thickness (millimeters): ____ mm
+ Thickness at cut edge (millimeters): ____ mm

Tumor Site After Sectioning (Notes G and H)

___ Cannot be determined
___ Superonasal
___ Inferonasal
___ Superotemporal
___ Inferotemporal
+ Distance from anterior edge of tumor to limbus at cut edge (millimeters): ____ mm
+ Distance of posterior margin of tumor base from edge of optic disc (millimeters): ____ mm

Tumor Involvement of Other Ocular Structures (Select all that Apply) (Note I)

___ Cannot be determined
___ Cornea
___ Anterior chamber
___ Iris
___ Angle
___ Lens
___ Ciliary body
___ Vitreous
___ Retina
___ Subretinal space
___ Subretinal pigment epithelial space
___ Optic nerve head
___ Choroid, minimal (solid tumor nest less than 3 mm in maximum diameter [width or thickness])
___ Choroid, massive (solid tumor nest 3 mm or more in maximum diameter [width or thickness])
___ Sclera
___ Vortex vein
___ Orbit
___ Other (specify): _____
_____

Growth Pattern (Note J)

___ Cannot be determined
___ Endophytic
___ Exophytic
___ Combined endophytic/exophytic
___ Diffuse
___ Anterior diffuse

Extent of Optic Nerve Invasion

___ Cannot be determined
___ None
___ Anterior to lamina cribrosa
___ At lamina cribrosa
___ Posterior to lamina cribrosa but not to end of nerve
___ To cut end of optic nerve

Histologic Grade

___ G1: Tumor with areas of retinocytoma (fleurettes or neuronal differentiation)
___ G2: Tumor with many rosettes (Flexner-Wintersteiner or Homer Wright)
___ G3: Tumor with occasional rosettes (Flexner-Wintersteiner or Homer Wright)
___ G4: Tumor with poorly differentiated cells without rosettes and/or with extensive areas (more than half of tumor) of anaplasia
___ GX: Grade cannot be assessed

+ Anaplasia Grade (Note K)

Note: Grade based on the highest level of anaplasia in the tumor, with at least 30% of the tumor being able to be graded.

+ ___ Mild
+ ___ Moderate
+ ___ Severe
+ ___ Cannot be determined

+ Cytologic Features Suggesting MYCN Amplification (Note K)

Note: Unilateral retinoblastoma with a loose cellular pattern, round nuclei, and prominent multiple nucleoli

+ ___ Absent
+ ___ Present

Margins (Select All that Apply)

___ Cannot be assessed
___ No tumor at margins
___ Tumor present at surgical margin of optic nerve
___ Extrascleral extension (for enucleation specimens)
___ Other margin(s) involved (specify):
_____

Regional Lymph Nodes

___ No lymph nodes submitted or found

Lymph Node Examination (Required Only if Lymph Nodes Are Present in the Specimen)

Number of Lymph Nodes Involved: _____
___ Number cannot be determined (explain):
_____

Number of Lymph Nodes Examined: _____
___ Number cannot be determined (explain):
_____

Pathologic Stage Classification (pTNM, AJCC 8th Edition) (Note M)

Note: Reporting of pT, pN, and (when applicable) pM categories is based on information available to the pathologist at the time the report is issued. Only the applicable T, N, or M category is required for reporting; their definitions need not be included in the report. The categories (with modifiers when applicable) can be listed on one line or more than one line.

TNM Descriptors (Required Only if Applicable) (Select All That Apply)
___ m (multiple primary tumors)
___ r (recurrent)
___ y (posttreatment)

Primary Tumor (pT)
___ pTX: Unknown evidence of intraocular tumor
___ pT0: No evidence of intraocular tumor
___ pT1: Intraocular tumor(s) without any local invasion, focal choroidal invasion, or pre- or intralaminar involvement of the optic nerve head
___ pT2: Intraocular tumor(s) with local invasion
___ pT2a: Concomitant focal choroidal invasion and pre- or intralaminar involvement of the optic nerve head
___ pT2b: Tumor invasion of stroma of iris and/or trabecular meshwork and/or Schlemm's canal
___ pT3: Intraocular tumor(s) with significant local invasion
___ pT3a: Massive choroidal invasion (>3 mm in largest diameter, or multiple foci of focal choroidal involvement totaling >3 mm, or any full-thickness choroidal involvement)
___ pT3b: Retrolaminar invasion of the optic nerve head, not involving the transected end of the optic nerve
___ pT3c: Any partial-thickness involvement of the sclera within the inner two-thirds
___ pT3d: Full-thickness invasion into the outer third of the sclera and/or invasion into or around emissary channels
___ pT4: Evidence of extraocular tumor: tumor at the transected end of the optic nerve, tumor in the meningeal spaces around the optic nerve, full-thickness invasion of the sclera with invasion of the episclera, adjacent adipose tissue, extraocular muscle, bone, conjunctiva, or eyelids

Regional Lymph Nodes (pN)

___ pNX: Regional lymph nodes cannot be assessed

___ pN0: No regional lymph node involvement

___ pN1: Regional lymph node involvement

Distant Metastasis (pM) (Required Only if Confirmed Pathologically in This Case)

___ pM1: Distant metastasis with histopathologic confirmation

___ pM1a: Histopathologic confirmation of tumor at any distant site (e.g., bone marrow, liver, or others)

___ pM1b: Histopathologic confirmation of tumor in the cerebrospinal fluid or CNS parenchyma

Specify site(s), if known: _____

_____

+ Additional Pathologic Findings (Select All that Apply)

+ ___ None identified

+ ___ Calcifications

+ ___ Mitotic rate: Number of mitoses per 40 fields determined by using a 40x objective with a field area of 0.152 mm^2 (specify): ____

+ ___ Apoptosis

+ ___ Necrosis

+ ___ Basophilic vascular deposits

+ ___ Inflammatory cells

+ ___ Hemorrhage (specify site): _____

_____

+ ___ Retinal detachment

+ ___ Neovascularization (specify site): _____

_____

+ ___ Other (specify): _____

_____

Explanatory Notes

A. Cytology/Biopsy

Cytologic and biopsy specimens are rarely obtained from eyes with suspected retinoblastoma owing to the potential risk of tumor seeding. An anterior chamber paracentesis may be performed, if indicated by clinical findings, and is not associated with risk of tumor seeding [1, 2].

B. Fixation

The minimum recommended fixation time for whole globes with intraocular tumors is 48 hours. The globe should be fixed in an adequate volume of fixative with a 10:1 ratio of fixative volume to specimen volume recommended. Incisions or windows in the globe are not necessary for adequate penetration of fixative and are not recommended. Injection of fixative into the globe is also not recommended.

C. Additional Studies

Genetic studies may be requested on neoplastic tissue and should be harvested prior to fixation [3]. Identification of *RB1* mutations and other genetic studies in tumor tissue are difficult with formalin-fixed tissue.

The surgical margin of the optic nerve should be obtained prior to opening the globe (Note E). Once tissue is harvested for genetic studies, the globe can be fixed prior to completing macroscopic examination. The appropriate materials/medium required by the laboratory performing genetic testing should be obtained prior to the procedure.

D. Processing With Tumor Sampling

To collect the tumor specimen, the optic nerve should be removed before opening the globe to prevent the optic nerve from accidentally becoming contaminated with artifactual clumps of tumor cells (so-called "floaters"). The surgeon should first ink the surgical margin of the optic nerve, then cut the optic nerve stump off from the sclera with a sharp razor about 2 mm behind the globe. The optic nerve stump, which should be kept separate from the globe, should be placed into a jar of 10% buffered formaldehyde. Then, a sample of tumor should be obtained by opening a small sclero-choroidal window adjacent to the tumor near the equator with a 6- to 8-mm corneal trephine. Once the opening into the vitreous chamber is established, tumor tissue should be gently removed with forceps and scissors. It is best to leave a hinge on one side of the scleral flap so that it can be closed with one or two suture(s) following the removal of tumor sample. This is done in an attempt to maintain the overall spherical architecture of the specimen during fixation. The globe should be placed in the second jar of for-

malin (separate from the optic nerve stump) and be allowed to fix for at least 24 to 48 hours.

E. **Orientation of Globe**

The orientation of a globe may be determined by identifying extraocular muscle insertions, optic nerve, and other landmarks as illustrated in Fig. B.1. The terms *temporal* and *nasal* are

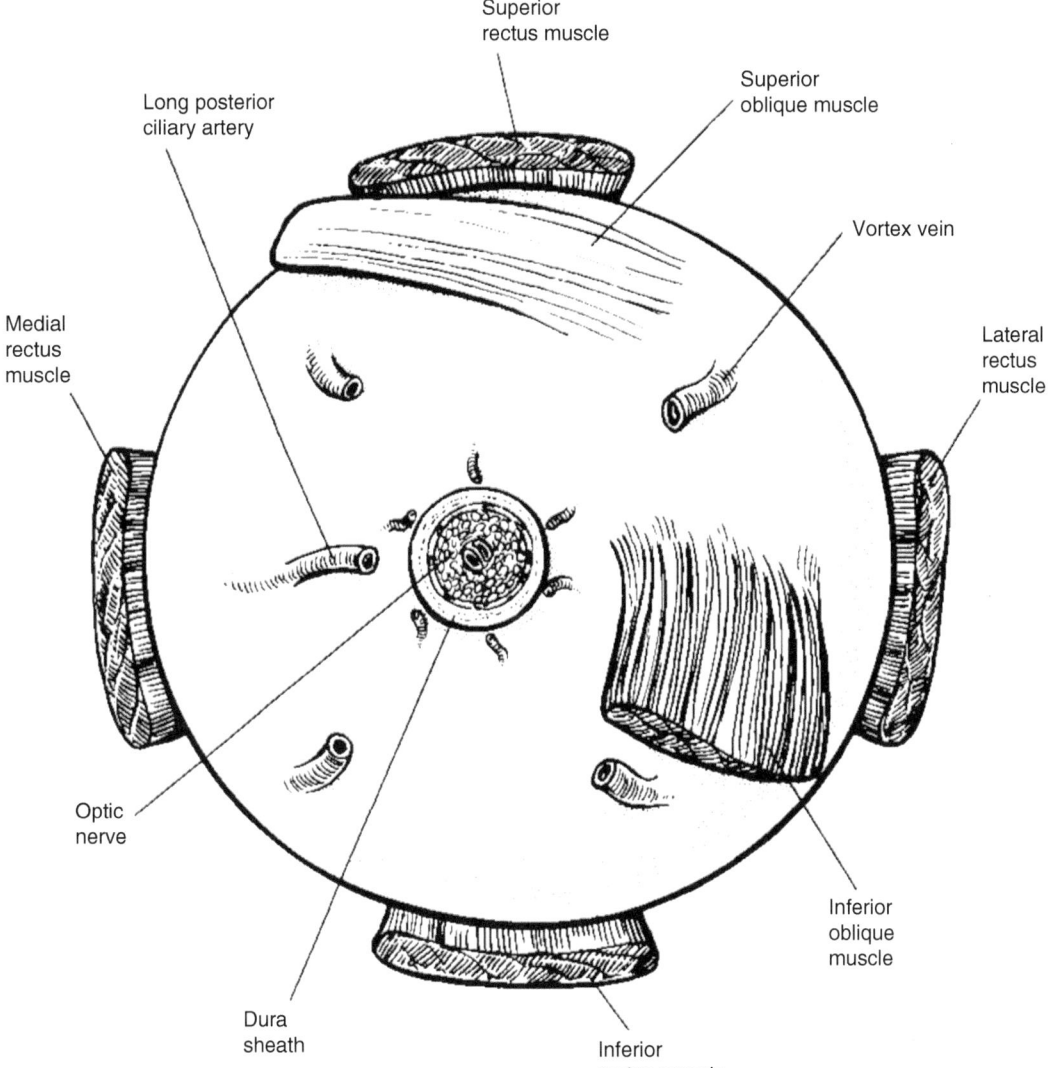

Fig. B.1 Anatomic landmarks of the posterior aspect of the globe (right eye). The position of the inferior oblique muscle relative to the optic nerve is most helpful in orienting the globe. The inferior oblique muscle insertion is located temporal (lateral) to the optic nerve on the sclera, and its fibers travel inferonasally from its insertion. The long posterior ciliary artery is often seen as a blue-gray line in the sclera on either side of the optic nerve and marks the horizontal meridian of the globe. (From [4] with permission)

generally used in place of *lateral* and *medial* with reference to ocular anatomy.

F. Processing Without Tumor Sampling

If there is no need for fresh tissue sampling, the enucleated globe should simply be fixed in 10% buffered formaldehyde for at least 24 and preferably 48 hours. When the fixed globe is examined by the pathologist, if the optic nerve was not previously amputated in the operative room, that should be performed first as described above. The surgical margin of the nerve stump should be embedded face down in paraffin for sectioning (i.e., thereby obtaining cross sections of the nerve, starting at the surgical margin). Then, the eye itself is sectioned. First, a section should be made that extends from pupil through the optic nerve (the "P-O" section), which contains the center of the optic nerve with all the optic nerve structures (optic nerve head, lamina cribrosa, and postlaminar optic nerve). Preferably this plane should bisect the largest dimension of the tumor, previously identified by transillumination and during clinical examination. When possible, the plane should avoid the scleral opening if one was made for fresh tumor sampling. This section is critical for evaluation of the optic nerve for tumor invasion. The P-O section and minor calottes are then embedded in paraffin. The embedded P-O calotte is then sectioned every 100–150 microns (each section being about 5 microns thick), for a total of about 10–20 sections. Additional sections should also be made anterior-posteriorly in a bread-loaf fashion through the minor callotes. These segments should be submitted in one cassette per calotte on edge to evaluate the choroid for invasion. Three levels of this block are usually sufficient for examination. In total, four cassettes are submitted: the optic nerve stump, the P-O section, and the two minor calottes (unless one or both of these have no visible tumor).

G. Sectioning the Globe

The globe is generally sectioned in the horizontal or vertical plane, with care to include the pupil and optic nerve in the cassette to be submitted for microscopic examination. If the mass cannot be included with horizontal or vertical sectioning, the globe is sectioned obliquely to include tumor, pupil, and optic nerve (Fig. B.2). The surgical margin of the optic nerve should be sectioned and submitted prior to sectioning the globe to ensure that intraocular malignant cells do not contaminate this important surgical margin [3]. Retinoblastoma is an extremely friable tumor.

Each calotte should also be sampled. The calottes should be bread-loafed and submitted in a cassette on edge for processing as shown in Fig. B.3.

H. Sections Submitted for Microscopic Examination

Multiple sections should be examined, with special attention to sections containing optic nerve and tumor. The nerve should be sectioned along the various levels to determine tumor extension.

I. Rules for Classification

Choroidal invasion: The presence and the extent (focal versus massive) of choroidal invasion by tumor should be stated. Differentiation should be made between true choroidal invasion and artifactual invasion due to seeding of fresh tumor cells during post-enucleation retrieval of tumor tissue and/or gross sectioning.

Artifactual invasion is identified when there are groups of tumor cells present in the open spaces among intraocular structures, extraocular tissues, and/or subarachnoid space.

True invasion is defined as one or more solid nests of tumor cells that fills or replaces the choroid and has pushing borders. Note: Invasion of the subretinal pigment epithelium (RPE) space, where tumor cells are present under the RPE (but not beyond Bruch's membrane into the choroid), is not choroidal invasion.

Focal choroidal invasion is defined as a solid nest of tumor that measures less than 3 mm in maximum diameter (width or thickness).

Fig. B.2 The most common methods of sectioning a globe. After transillumination, the tumor base is marked, if possible, and included in the pupil-optic (p-o) nerve section and submitted for processing. If tumor is found in either of the calottes, these may also be submitted for sectioning. The meridian in which the globe was sectioned should be included in the gross description of the pathology report. It is not uncommon to induce an artifactitious retinal detachment while sectioning the globe. This can be minimized by gentle handling and by avoiding a sawing motion with the blade. (From [4] with permission)

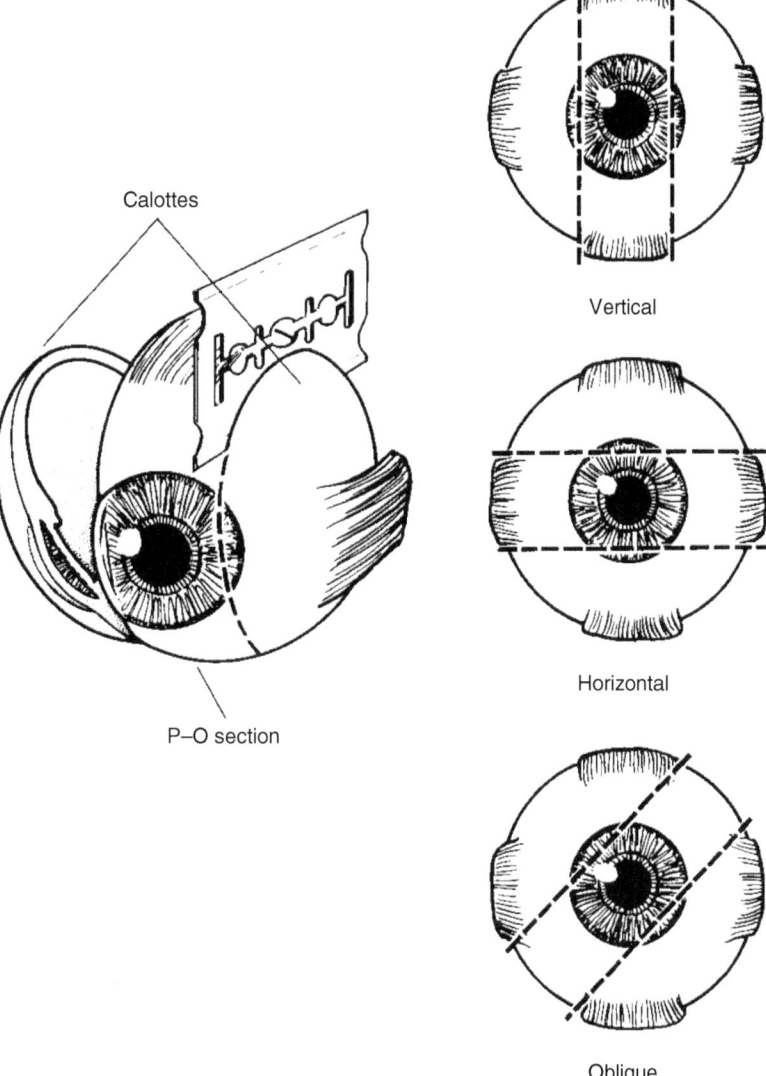

Massive choroidal invasion is defined as a solid tumor nest 3 mm or more in maximum diameter (width or thickness) in contact with the underlying sclera.

J. Growth Pattern

Endophytic growth pattern indicates growth from the inner retinal surface into the vitreous cavity. Exophytic tumors grow primarily from the outer surface of the retina into the subretinal space toward the choroid. Mixed growth pattern exhibits features of both endophytic and exo-phytic growths. Diffuse infiltrating tumors grow laterally within the retina without significant thickening.

K. Histologic Features

Histopathologic features of retinoblastoma include small round cells staining blue on hematoxylin-eosin. Flexner-Wintersteiner rosettes (typical for retinoblastoma) and Homer Wright rosettes (characteristic of neuroectodermal tumors) both occur. Tumors with many Flexner-Wintersteiner rosettes are graded as moderately

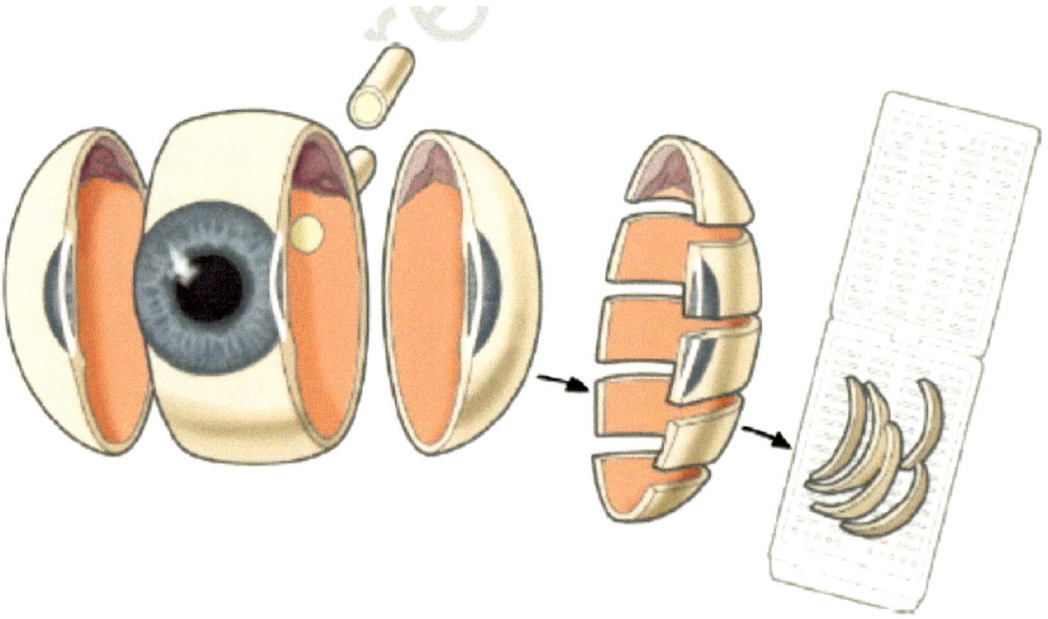

Fig. B.3 Calotte sampling. (From Grossniklaus HE [5] with kind permission of Springer Science+Business Media)

differentiated. Some tumors show photoreceptor-like differentiation (fleurettes) or neuronal differentiation without mitoses or apoptosis, which is evidence of an underlying premalignant lesion: retinocytoma [6, 7]. It is not uncommon to find a retinocytomatous area at the base of the tumor [8]. Retinocytomatous areas are more resistant to chemotherapy and, occasionally, only the retinocytomatous part may remain viable, surrounded by calcifications and debris from the regressed retinoblastoma that it spawned. Tumors that show no fleurettes or rosettes are graded as poorly differentiated. The nuclei of poorly differentiated tumors may show anaplasia [9]. Rarely, unilateral retinoblastoma tumors show a loose cellular pattern with round nuclei and prominent multiple nucleoli indicative of *MYCN* amplification and normal *RB1* alleles [10]. Retinoblastoma undergoes pathognomonic dystrophic calcification. Small tumors initially are limited by the retinal boundaries (Bruch's membrane and the inner limiting membrane). As the tumor grows, it spreads into the adjacent vitreous, subretinal space, underlying choroid, optic nerve, or anterior segment (iris, trabecular meshwork, or Schlemm's canal).

L. Histologic Features of Additional Prognostic Significance

Histologic features with prognostic significance for survival include the following: invasion of optic nerve, particularly if tumor is present at the surgical margin (most important feature); invasion of sclera; invasion of choroid; tumor size; basophilic staining of tumor vessels; seeding of vitreous; degree of differentiation; involvement of anterior segment; and growth pattern [11–17]. This list should not be confused with the Reese-Ellsworth classification, which is intended as a predictor for visual outcome, not survival [18].

M. Pathologic Stage Classification

The American Joint Committee on Cancer (AJCC) and the International Union Against Cancer (UICC) TNM staging system for retinoblastoma is shown below [19].

By AJCC/UICC convention, the designation "T" refers to a primary tumor that has not been previously treated. The symbol "p" refers to the pathologic classification of the TNM, as opposed to the clinical classification, and is based on gross and microscopic examination. pT entails a resection of the primary tumor or biopsy adequate to evaluate the highest pT category, pN entails removal of nodes adequate to validate lymph node metastasis, and pM implies microscopic examination of distant lesions. It is not uncommon to receive an eye of histopathologic examination that has been enucleated after failed conservative treatment such as chemoreduction or intra-arterial chemosurgery combined with focal treatments and radiotherapy. In such cases, the symbol "y" referring to a treated tumor and/or the symbol "r" referring to a recurrent tumor may be added. Clinical classification (cTNM) is usually carried out by the referring physician before treatment during initial evaluation of the patient or when pathologic classification is not possible.

Pathologic staging is usually performed after surgical resection of the primary tumor. Pathologic staging depends on pathologic documentation of the anatomic extent of disease, whether or not the primary tumor has been completely removed. If a biopsied tumor is not resected for any reason (e.g., when technically unfeasible) and if the highest T and N categories or the M1 category of the tumor can be confirmed microscopically, the criteria for pathologic classification and staging have been satisfied without total removal of the primary cancer.

TNM Descriptors

For identification of special cases of TNM or pTNM classifications, the "m" suffix and "y," "r," and "a" prefixes are used. Although they do not affect the stage grouping, they indicate cases needing separate analysis.

The "m" suffix indicates the presence of multiple primary tumors in a single site and is recorded in parentheses: pT(m)NM.

The "y" prefix indicates those cases in which classification is performed during or following initial multimodality therapy (i.e., neoadjuvant chemotherapy, radiation therapy, or both chemotherapy and radiation therapy). The cTNM

or pTNM category is identified by a "y" prefix. The ycTNM or ypTNM categorizes the extent of tumor actually present at the time of that examination. The "y" categorization is not an estimate of tumor prior to multimodality therapy (i.e., before initiation of neoadjuvant therapy).

The "r" prefix indicates a recurrent tumor when staged after a documented disease-free interval, and is identified by the "r" prefix: rTNM.

The "a" prefix designates the stage determined at autopsy: aTNM.

Additional Descriptors
Residual Tumor (R)

Tumor remaining in a patient after therapy with curative intent (e.g., surgical resection for cure) is categorized by a system known as R classification, as shown below.

RX	Presence of residual tumor cannot be assessed
R0	No residual tumor
R1	Microscopic residual tumor
R2	Macroscopic residual tumor

For the surgeon, the R classification may be useful to indicate the known or assumed status of the completeness of a surgical excision. For the pathologist, the R classification is relevant to the status of the margins of a surgical resection specimen. That is, tumor involving the resection margin on pathologic examination may be assumed to correspond to residual tumor in the patient and may be classified as macroscopic or microscopic according to the findings at the specimen margin(s).

T Category Considerations
Lymph-Vascular Invasion (LVI)

LVI indicates whether microscopic lymph-vascular invasion is identified in the pathology report. LVI includes lymphatic invasion, vascular invasion, or lymph-vascular invasion. By AJCC/UICC convention, LVI does not affect the T category indicating local extent of tumor unless specifically included in the definition of a T category.

Clinical TNM Classifications

Primary tumor (T)

TX	Primary tumor cannot be assessed
T0	No evidence of primary tumor
cT1	Intraretinal tumor(s) with subretinal fluid ≤5 mm from the base of any tumor
cT1a	Tumors ≤3 mm and further than 1.5 mm from disc and fovea
cT1b	Tumors >3 mm or closer than 1.5 mm from disc or fovea
cT2	Intraocular tumor(s) with retinal detachment, vitreous seeding, or subretinal seeding
cT2a	Subretinal fluid >5 mm from the base of any tumor
cT2b	Vitreous seeding and/or subretinal seeding
cT3	Advanced intraocular tumor(s)
cT3a	Phthisis or pre-phthisis bulbi
cT3b	Tumor invasion of choroid, pars plana, ciliary body, lens, zonules, iris, or anterior chamber
cT3c	Raised intraocular pressure with neovascularization and/or buphthalmos
cT3d	Hyphema and/or massive vitreous hemorrhage
cT3e	Aseptic orbital cellulitis
cT4	Extraocular tumor(s) involving orbit, including optic nerve
cT4a	Radiologic evidence of retrobulbar optic nerve involvement or thickening of optic nerve or involvement of orbital tissues
cT4b	Extraocular tumor clinically evident with proptosis and/or an orbital mass

Regional lymph nodes (N)

cNX	Regional lymph nodes cannot be assessed
cN0	No regional lymph node involvement
cN1	Regional lymph node involvement (preauricular, cervical, submandibular)

Metastasis (M)

cM0	No metastasis
cM1	Distant metastasis without microscopic confirmation
cM1a	Tumor(s) involving any distant site (e.g., bone marrow, liver) on clinical or radiologic tests
cM1b	Tumor involving the CNS on radiologic imaging (not including trilateral retinoblastoma)

Definition of heritable trait (H)

HX	Unknown or insufficient evidence of a constitutional RB1 gene mutation
H0	Normal *RB1* alleles in blood tested with demonstrated high-sensitivity assays
H1	Bilateral retinoblastoma, any retinoblastoma with an intracranial primitive neuroectodermal tumor (i.e., trilateral retinoblastoma), patient with family history of retinoblastoma, or molecular definition of a constitutional *RB1* gene mutation

TNM Prognostic Stage Groupings
Clinical Stage (cTNM)

When cT is…	And N is…	And M is…	And H is…	Then the clinical stage group is…
cT1, cT2, cT3	cN0	cM0	Any	I
cT4a	cN0	cM0	Any	II
cT4b	cN0	cM0	Any	III
Any	cN1	cM0	Any	III
Any	Any	cM1 or pM1	Any	IV

Pathologic Stage (pTNM)

When pT is…	And N is…	And M is…	And H is…	Then the pathologic stage group is…
pT1, pT2, pT3	pN0	cM0	Any	I
pT4	pN0	cM0	Any	II
Any	pN1	cM0	Any	III
Any	Any	cM1 or pM1	Any	IV

WHO Classification of Tumors

International Agency for Research on Cancer, World Health Organization. International Classification of Diseases for Oncology. ICD-O-3-Online. http://codes.iarc.fr/home. Accessed May 15, 2016.

Code	Description
9510	Retinoblastoma, NOS
9511	Retinoblastoma, differentiated

Code	Description
9512	Retinoblastoma, undifferentiated
9513	Retinoblastoma, diffuse

Appendix C: College of American Pathologists Protocol for the Examination of Specimens from Patients with Uveal Melanoma

Version: UvealMelanoma 4.0.0.0	Protocol Posting Date: June 2017
Includes pTNM requirements from the 8th Edition, AJCC Staging Manual	

Reproduced by permission of the *College of American Pathologists (CAP)* © 2019. *The CAP* periodically revises the CAP Cancer Protocols and the current versions may be retrieved from www.cap.org/cancerprotocols. The CAP does not permit reproduction of any substantial portion of these protocols without its written authorization. The CAP hereby authorizes use of these protocols by physicians and other healthcare providers in reporting on surgical specimens, in teaching, and in carrying out medical research for nonprofit purposes. This authorization does not extend to reproduction or other use of any substantial portion of these protocols for commercial purposes without the written consent of the CAP.

For accreditation purposes, this protocol should be used for the following procedures and tumor types:

Procedure	Description
Resection	Includes local resection, enucleation, and partial or complete exenteration
Tumor type	**Description**
Uveal melanoma	

The following tumor types should not be reported using this protocol:

Tumor type
Cutaneous melanoma (consider skin melanoma protocol)

Authors

Hans E. Grossniklaus, MD, MBA[2]; Paul T. Finger, MD; J. William Harbour, MD; Tero Kivelä, MD
    With guidance from the CAP Cancer and CAP Pathology Electronic Reporting Committees.

Accreditation Requirements

This protocol can be utilized for a variety of procedures and tumor types for clinical care purposes. For accreditation purposes, only the definitive primary cancer resection specimen is required to have the core and conditional data elements reported in a synoptic format.

- *Core data elements* are required in reports to adequately describe appropriate malignancies. For accreditation purposes, essential data elements must be reported in all instances, even if the response is "not applicable" or "cannot be determined."
- *Conditional data elements* are only required to be reported if applicable as delineated in the protocol. For instance, the total number of lymph nodes examined must be reported, but only if nodes are present in the specimen.
- *Optional data elements* are identified with "+" and although not required for CAP accreditation purposes, may be considered for reporting as determined by local practice standards.

---

[2]Denotes primary author. All other contributing authors are listed alphabetically.

The use of this protocol is not required for recurrent tumors or for metastatic tumors that are resected at a different time than the primary tumor. Use of this protocol is also not required for pathology reviews performed at the second institution (i.e., secondary consultation, second opinion, or review of outside case at the second institution).

Synoptic Reporting

All core and conditionally required data elements outlined in the surgical case summary from this cancer protocol must be displayed in synoptic report format. Synoptic format is defined as:

- Data element: followed by its answer (response), outline format without the paired "Data element: Response" format is not considered synoptic.
- The data element must be represented in the report as it is listed in the case summary. The response for any data element may be modified from those listed in the case summary, including "Cannot be determined" if appropriate.
- Each diagnostic parameter pair (Data element: Response) is listed on a separate line or in a tabular format to achieve visual separation. The following exceptions are allowed to be listed on one line:
  - Anatomic site or specimen, laterality, and procedure
  - Pathologic Stage Classification (pTNM) elements
  - Negative margins, as long as all negative margins are specifically enumerated where applicable
- The synoptic portion of the report can appear in the diagnosis section of the pathology report, at the end of the report or in a separate section, but all data element: Responses must be listed together in one location.

Organizations and pathologists may choose to list the required elements in any order, use additional methods in order to enhance or achieve visual separation, or add optional items within the synoptic report. The report may have required elements in a summary format elsewhere in the report in addition to but not as replacement for the synoptic report, i.e., all required elements must be in the synoptic portion of the report in the format defined above.

**CAP Laboratory Accreditation Program Protocol
Required Use Date: March 2018[a]**

[a]*Beginning January 1, 2018, the 8th edition AJCC Staging Manual should be used for reporting pTNM.*

CAP Uveal Melanoma Protocol Summary of Changes

The following data elements were modified:

- Pathologic Stage Classification (pTNM, AJCC 8th Edition)
- Tumor Site
- Tumor Size
- Tumor Involvement of Other Ocular Structures
- Microscopic Tumor Extension
- Additional Pathologic Findings

Surgical Pathology Cancer Case Summary

Protocol posting date: June 2017

**Uveal Melanoma
Select a single response unless otherwise indicated.**

Procedure (Note A)
___ Local resection
___ Enucleation
___ Limited exenteration
___ Complete exenteration
___   Other   (specify):
_____
___ Not specified

Specimen Laterality
___ Right
___ Left
___ Not specified

Tumor Site (Macroscopic Examination/Transillumination) (Select All that Apply) (Note B)

___ Cannot be determined
___ Superotemporal quadrant of globe
___ Superonasal quadrant of globe
___ Inferotemporal quadrant of globe
___ Inferonasal quadrant of globe
___ Anterior chamber
___ Between ____ and ____ o'clock
___ Other (specify): _____
  _____

Tumor Size After Sectioning (Note C)

___ Cannot be determined
Greatest basal diameter (millimeters): ____ mm
+ Base at cut edge (millimeters): ____ mm
Greatest thickness (millimeters): ____ mm
+ Thickness at cut edge (millimeters): ____ mm

Tumor Site After Sectioning (Note D)

___ Cannot be determined
___ Superonasal
___ Inferonasal
___ Superotemporal
___ Inferotemporal
+ Distance from anterior edge of tumor to limbus at cut edge (millimeters): ___ mm
+ Distance of posterior margin of tumor base from edge of optic disc (millimeters): ___ mm

Tumor Involvement of Other Ocular Structures (Select All that Apply)

___ Sclera
___ Vortex vein(s)
___ Optic nerve head
___ Vitreous
___ Choroid
___ Ciliary body
___ Iris
___ Lens
___ Anterior chamber
___ Extrascleral extension (anterior)
___ Extrascleral extension (posterior)
___ Angle/Schlemm's canal
___ Optic nerve

___ Retina
+ ___ Cornea
___ Other (specify): _____
  _____
___ Cannot be assessed

Growth Pattern

___ Cannot be determined
___ Solid mass
___ Dome shape
___ Mushroom shape
___ Diffuse (ciliary body ring)
___ Diffuse (flat)

Histologic Type (Note E)

___ Spindle cell melanoma (>90% spindle cells)
___ Mixed cell melanoma (>10% epithelioid cells and < 90% spindle cells)
___ Epithelioid cell melanoma (>90% epithelioid cells)

Tumor Extension

+ Tumor Location
+ ___ Anterior margin between ciliary body and iris
+ ___ Anterior margin between equator and ciliary body
+ ___ Anterior margin between disc and equator
+ ___ Posterior margin between ciliary body and iris
+ ___ Posterior margin between equator and ciliary body
+ ___ Posterior margin between disc and equator
+ ___ Cannot be determined
+ ___ Other (specify): _____

Scleral Involvement

___ None
___ Intrascleral
___ Extrascleral (≤5 mm largest diameter)
___ Extrascleral (>5 mm largest diameter)
___ Cannot be determined

Margins
___ Cannot be assessed

___ No melanoma at margins

___ Extrascleral extension (for enucleation specimens)

___ Other margin(s) involved (specify):

_____

Regional Lymph Nodes
___ No lymph nodes submitted or found

Lymph Node Examination (Required Only if Lymph Nodes Are Present in the Specimen)

Number of Lymph Nodes Involved: _____
___ Number cannot be determined (explain):

_____

Number of Lymph Nodes Examined: _____
___ Number cannot be determined (explain):

_____

Pathologic Stage Classification (pTNM, AJCC 8th Edition) (Note F)
Note: Reporting of pT, pN, and (when applicable) pM categories is based on information available to the pathologist at the time the report is issued. Only the applicable T, N, or M category is required for reporting; their definitions need not be included in the report. The categories (with modifiers when applicable) can be listed on one line or more than one line.

TNM Descriptors (Required Only if Applicable) (Select All That Apply)
___ m (multiple primary tumors)

___ r (recurrent)

___ y (posttreatment)

Primary Tumor (pT)
Iris

___ pTX: Primary tumor cannot be assessed

___ pT0: No evidence of primary tumor

___ pT1: Tumor limited to the iris

___ pT1a: Tumor limited to the iris not more than 3 clock hours in size

___ pT1b: Tumor limited to the iris more than 3 clock hours in size

___ pT1c: Tumor limited to the iris with secondary glaucoma

___ pT2: Tumor confluent with or extending into the ciliary body, choroid, or both

___ pT2a: Tumor confluent with or extending into the ciliary body, without secondary glaucoma

___ pT2b: Tumor confluent with or extending into the ciliary body and choroid, without secondary glaucoma

___ pT2c: Tumor confluent with or extending into the ciliary body, choroid, or both, with secondary glaucoma

___ pT3: Tumor confluent with or extending into the ciliary body, choroid, or both, with scleral extension

___ pT4: Tumor with extrascleral extension

___ pT4a: Tumor with extrascleral extension ≤5 mm in largest diameter

___ pT4b: Tumor with extrascleral extension >5 mm in largest diameter

Note: Iris melanomas originate from, and are predominantly located in, this region of the uvea. If less than half the tumor volume is located within the iris, the tumor may have originated in the ciliary body, and consideration should be given to classifying it accordingly.

Ciliary Body and Choroid

___ pTX: Primary tumor cannot be assessed

___ pT0: No evidence of primary tumor

___ pT1: Tumor size category 1

___ pT1a: Tumor size category 1 without ciliary body involvement and extraocular extension

___ pT1b: Tumor size category 1 with ciliary body involvement

___ pT1c: Tumor size category 1 without ciliary body involvement but with extraocular extension ≤5 mm in largest diameter

___ pT1d: Tumor size category 1 with ciliary body involvement and extraocular extension ≤5 mm in largest diameter

___ pT2: Tumor size category 2

___ pT2a: Tumor size category 2 without ciliary body involvement and extraocular extension

___ pT2b: Tumor size category 2 with ciliary body involvement

___ pT2c: Tumor size category 2 without ciliary body involvement but with extraocular extension ≤5 mm in largest diameter

___ pT2d: Tumor size category 2 with ciliary body involvement and extraocular extension ≤5 mm in largest diameter

___ pT3: Tumor size category 3

___ pT3a: Tumor size category 3 without ciliary body involvement and extraocular extension

___ pT3b: Tumor size category 3 with ciliary body involvement

___ pT3c: Tumor size category 3 without ciliary body involvement but with extraocular extension ≤5 mm in largest diameter

___ pT3d: Tumor size category 3 with ciliary body involvement and extraocular extension ≤5 mm in largest diameter

___ pT4: Tumor size category 4

___ pT4a: Tumor size category 4 without ciliary body involvement and extraocular extension

___ pT4b: Tumor size category 4 with ciliary body involvement

___ pT4c: Tumor size category 4 without ciliary body involvement but with extraocular extension ≤5 mm in largest diameter

___ pT4d: Tumor size category 4 with ciliary body involvement and extraocular extension ≤5 mm in largest diameter

___ pT4e: Any tumor size category with extraocular extension >5 mm in largest diameter

Notes:

1. *Primary ciliary body and choroidal melanomas are classified according to the four tumor size categories defined in* Fig. C.1.

2. *In clinical practice, the largest tumor basal diameter may be estimated in optic disc diameters (DD; average: 1 DD = 1.5 mm), and tumor thickness may be estimated in diopters (average: 2.5 diopters = 1 mm). Ultrasonography and fundus photography are used to provide more accurate measurements.*

3. *When histopathologic measurements are recorded after fixation, tumor diameter and thickness may be underestimated because of tissue shrinkage.*

Regional Lymph Nodes (pN)

___ pNX: Regional lymph nodes cannot be assessed

___ pN0: No regional lymph node metastasis

___ pN1: Regional lymph node metastasis or discrete tumor deposits in the orbit

___ pN1a: Metastasis in one or more regional lymph node(s)

___ pN1b: No regional lymph nodes are positive, but there are discrete tumor deposits in the orbit that are not contiguous to the eye (choroidal and ciliary body).

Distant Metastasis (pM) (Required Only if Confirmed Pathologically in This Case)

___ pM1: Distant metastasis

___ pM1a: Largest diameter of the largest metastasis ≤3 cm

___ pM1b: Largest diameter of the largest metastasis 3.1–8.0 cm

___ pM1c: Largest diameter of the largest metastasis ≥8.1 cm

Fig. C.1 Tumor size categories. (From [19] with permission)

Thickness (mm)	≤3.0	3.1–6.0	6.1–9.0	9.1–12.0	12.1–15.0	15.1–18.0	>18.0
>15.0					4	4	4
12.1–15.0				3	3	4	4
9.1–12.0		3	3	3	3	3	4
6.1–9.0	2	2	2	2	3	3	4
3.1–6.0	1	1	1	2	2	3	4
≤3.0	1	1	1	1	2	2	4

Largest basal diameter (mm)

Specify sites(s), if known: _____

_____

+ Additional Pathologic Findings (Select All that Apply) (Note G)

+ ___ None identified

+ ___ Mitotic rate (number of mitoses per 40 fields determined by using a 40X objective with a field area of 0.152 mm^2) (specify): _____

+ ___ Extravascular matrix pattern (extracellular closed loops and networks, the latter defined as at least three back-to-back closed loops, are associated with death from metastatic disease)

+ ___ Vascular invasion (tumor vessels or other vessels)

+ ___ Degree of pigmentation

+ ___ Inflammatory cells/tumor infiltrating lymphocytes and macrophages

+ ___ Drusen

+ ___ Retinal detachment

+ ___ Invasion of Bruch's membrane

+ ___ Nevus

+ ___ Hemorrhage (specify site): _____

+ ___ Neovascularization

+ ___ Other (specify): _____

+ Comment(s)

Note: Chromosome 3 and 8 loss or gain, immunohistochemical staining for the presence or absence of BAP1 protein immunoreactivity, and/ or gene expression profile may be included in the report.

Explanatory Notes

A. Fixative

The minimum recommended fixation time for whole globes with intraocular tumors is 48 hours. The globe should be fixed in an adequate volume of fixative, with a 10:1 ratio of fixative volume to specimen volume recommended. Incisions or windows in the globe are not necessary for adequate penetration of fixative and are not recommended. Injection of fixative into the globe is also not recommended.

B. Orientation

The orientation of a globe may be determined by identification of extraocular muscle insertions, the optic nerve, and other landmarks, as illustrated in Fig. C.2. The terms *temporal* and *nasal* are generally used in place of *lateral* and *medial* with reference to ocular anatomy.

C. Tumor Size

Tumor size has prognostic significance. Many studies of choroidal and ciliary body melanoma have defined small tumors as being less than 10 mm in greatest diameter [4]. More recently, an ongoing study started in 1986, the Collaborative Ocular Melanoma Study [20, 21], defined the following size classification based on clinical measurements.

Small tumors[a]	Smaller than medium or large tumors defined below
Medium tumors	Greater than or equal to 2.5 mm, less than or equal to 10 mm in height, and less than or equal to 16 mm in basal diameter
Large tumors	Greater than 10 mm in height *or*
	Greater than 2 mm in height and greater than 16 mm in basal diameter *or*
	Greater than 8 mm in height with optic nerve involvement

[a]Small tumors have a more favorable prognosis [22, 23]

Since then, the AJCC TNM system defined empirically four tumor sizes (Fig. C.1)—small (T1), medium (T2), large (T3), and very large (T4)—that differ significantly in survival prognosis [24, 25]. This size classification was externally validated and is now recommended.

D. Sectioning the Globe

The globe is generally sectioned in the horizontal or vertical plane, with care to include the

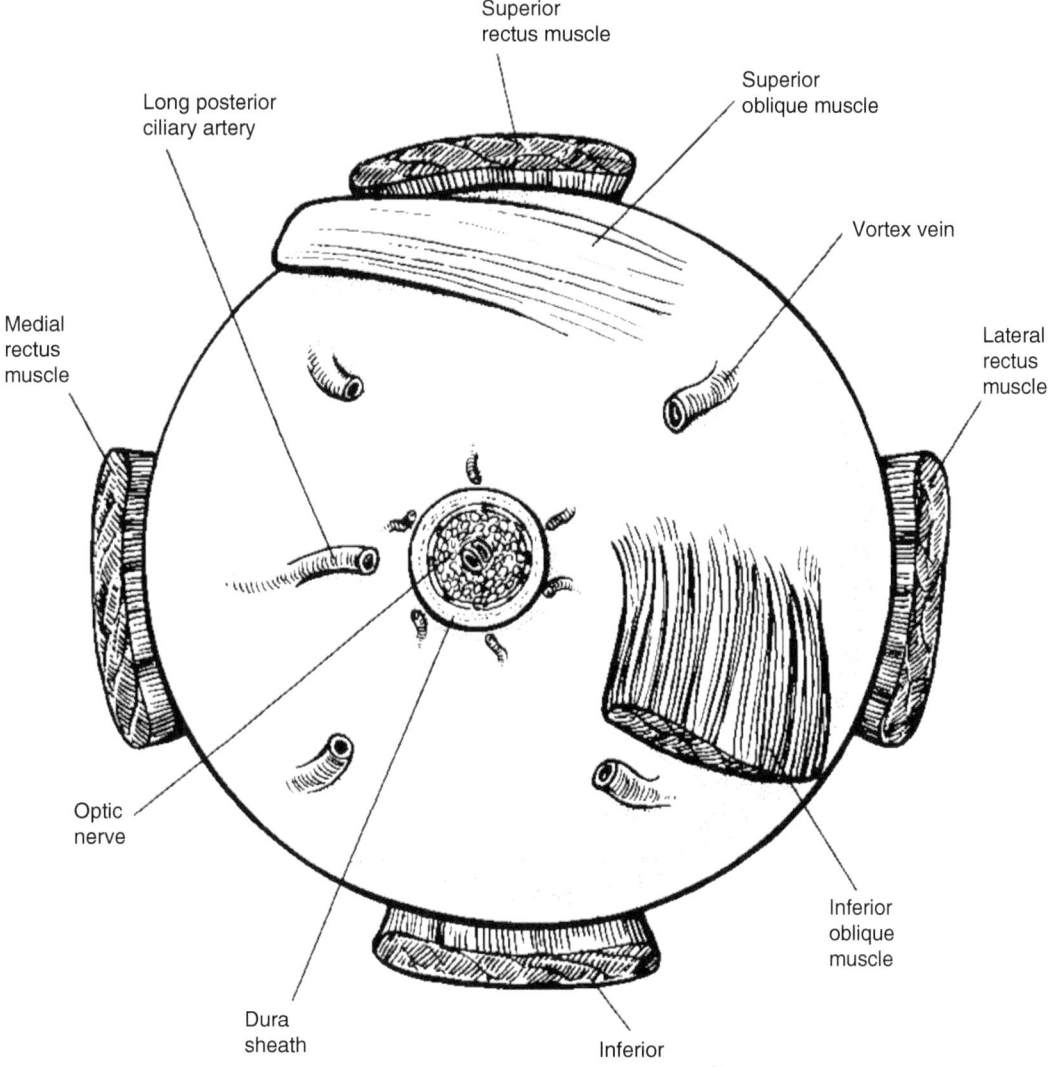

Superior
rectus muscle

Long posterior
ciliary artery

Superior
oblique muscle

Vortex vein

Medial
rectus
muscle

Lateral
rectus
muscle

Optic
nerve

Inferior
oblique
muscle

Dura
sheath

Inferior
rectus muscle

Fig. C.2 Anatomic landmarks of the posterior aspect of the globe (right eye). The position of the inferior oblique muscle relative to the optic nerve is most helpful in orienting the globe. The inferior oblique muscle insertion is located temporal (lateral) to the optic nerve on the sclera, and its fibers travel inferonasally from its insertion. The long posterior ciliary artery is often seen as a blue-gray line in the sclera on either side of the optic nerve and marks the horizontal meridian of the globe. (From [4] with permission)

pupil and optic nerve in the section to be submitted for microscopic examination. If the mass cannot be included with horizontal or vertical sectioning, the globe is sectioned obliquely to include the tumor, pupil, and optic nerve, as illustrated in Fig. C.3. Alternative methods of sectioning have been described [24].

E. **Histologic Type**

The modified Callender classification shown below is used for determining cell type but has prognostic significance only for tumors of the choroid and ciliary body, not those of the iris, which generally have a benign course unless they

Fig. C.3 The most
common methods of
sectioning a globe. After
transillumination, the
tumor base is marked, if
possible, and included in
the pupil-optic (p-o) nerve
section and submitted for
processing. If tumor is
found in either of the
calottes, these may also be
submitted for sectioning.
The meridian in which the
globe was sectioned should
be included in the gross
description of the
pathology report. It is not
uncommon to induce an
artifactitious retinal
detachment while
sectioning the globe. This
can be minimized by
gentle handling and by
avoiding a sawing motion
with the blade. (From [4]
with permission)

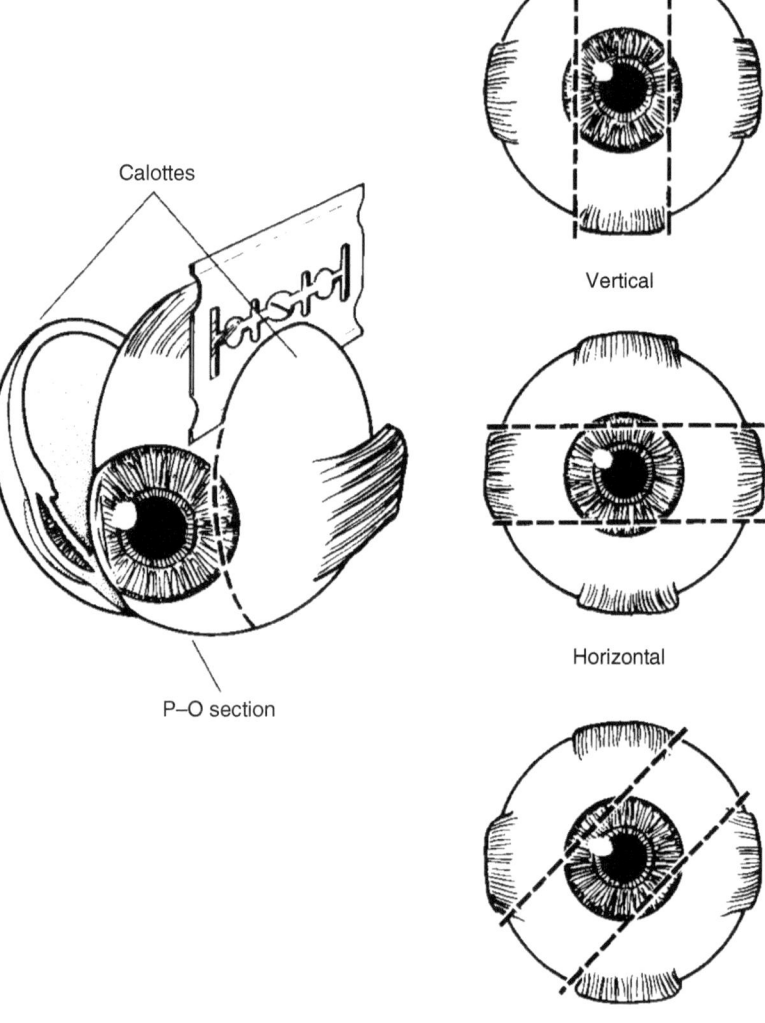

invade the chamber angle [4, 26–29]. The
American Joint Committee on Cancer (AJCC)
defined the histopathologic types[3] as follows [28]:

- Spindle cell melanoma (>90% spindle cells)
- Mixed cell melanoma (>10% epithelioid cells
  and <90% spindle cells)
- Epithelioid cell melanoma (>90% epithelioid
  cells)

---

[3]Spindle cell melanomas have the most favorable prognosis, and epithelioid cell melanomas the least favorable in
terms of survival.

Histologic Grade (G)

G	G definition
GX	Grade cannot be assessed
G1	Spindle cell melanoma (>90% spindle cells)
G2	Mixed cell melanoma (>10% epithelioid cells and < 90% spindle cells)
G3	Epithelioid cell melanoma (>90% epithelioid cells)

*Note: Because of the lack of universal agreement regarding
which proportion of epithelioid cells classifies a tumor as
mixed or epithelioid, some ophthalmic pathologists currently combine grades 2 and 3 (nonspindle, i.e., epithelioid
cells detected) and contrast them with grade 1 (spindle, i.e.,
no epithelioid cells detected) or even tumors that have no
epithelioid cells with those that have any epithelioid cells*

F. **Pathologic Stage Classification**

The American Joint Committee on Cancer (AJCC) and the International Union Against Cancer (UICC) TNM staging systems for uveal melanoma of the iris, ciliary body, and choroid are shown below [19].

By AJCC/UICC convention, the designation "T" refers to a primary tumor that has not been previously treated. The symbol "p" refers to the pathologic classification of the TNM, as opposed to the clinical classification, and is based on gross and microscopic examination. pT entails a resection of the primary tumor or biopsy adequate to evaluate the highest pT category, pN entails removal of nodes adequate to validate lymph node metastasis, and pM implies microscopic examination of distant lesions. Clinical classification (cTNM) is usually carried out by the referring physician before treatment during initial evaluation of the patient or when pathologic classification is not possible.

Pathologic staging is usually performed after surgical resection of the primary tumor. Pathologic staging depends on pathologic documentation of the anatomic extent of disease, whether or not the primary tumor has been completely removed. If a biopsied tumor is not resected for any reason (e.g., when technically unfeasible) and if the highest T and N categories or the M1 category of the tumor can be confirmed microscopically, the criteria for pathologic classification and staging have been satisfied without total removal of the primary cancer.

TNM Descriptors

For identification of special cases of TNM or pTNM classifications, the "m" suffix and "y," "r," and "a" prefixes are used. Although they do not affect the stage grouping, they indicate cases needing separate analysis.

The "m" suffix indicates the presence of multiple primary tumors in a single site and is recorded in parentheses: pT(m)NM.

The "y" prefix indicates those cases in which classification is performed during or following initial multimodality therapy (i.e., neoadjuvant chemotherapy, radiation therapy, or both chemotherapy and radiation therapy). The cTNM or pTNM category is identified by a "y" prefix. The ycTNM or ypTNM categorizes the extent of tumor actually present at the time of that examination. The "y" categorization is not an estimate of tumor prior to multimodality therapy (i.e., before initiation of neoadjuvant therapy).

The "r" prefix indicates a recurrent tumor when staged after a documented disease-free interval, and is identified by the "r" prefix: rTNM.

The "a" prefix designates the stage determined at autopsy: aTNM.

Additional Descriptors
Residual Tumor (R)

Tumor remaining in a patient after therapy with curative intent (e.g., surgical resection for cure) is categorized by a system known as R classification, as shown below.

RX	Presence of residual tumor cannot be assessed
R0	No residual tumor
R1	Microscopic residual tumor
R2	Macroscopic residual tumor

For the surgeon, the R classification may be useful to indicate the known or assumed status of the completeness of a surgical excision. For the pathologist, the R classification is relevant to the status of the margins of a surgical resection specimen. That is, tumor involving the resection margin on pathologic examination may be assumed to correspond to residual tumor in the patient and may be classified as macroscopic or microscopic according to the findings at the specimen margin(s).

T Category Considerations

Iris melanomas originate from, and are predominantly located in, this region of the uvea. If less than half of the tumor volume is located within the iris, the tumor may have originated in the ciliary body, and consideration should be given to classifying it accordingly.

Ciliary Body and Choroid

Primary ciliary body and choroidal melanomas are classified according to the four tumor size categories in Fig. C.1 [19]:

In clinical practice, the largest tumor basal diameter may be estimated in optic disc diameters (dd, average: 1 dd = 1.5 mm). Tumor thickness may be estimated in diopters (average: 2.5 diopters = 1 mm). However, techniques such as ultrasonography and fundus photography are used to provide more accurate measurements. Ciliary body involvement can be evaluated by the slit lamp, ophthalmoscopy, gonioscopy, and transillumination. However, high-frequency ultrasonography (ultrasound biomicroscopy) is used for more accurate assessment. Extension through the sclera is evaluated visually before and during surgery, and with ultrasonography, computed tomography, or magnetic resonance imaging.

When histopathologic measurements are recorded after fixation, tumor diameter and thickness may be underestimated because of tissue shrinkage.

Lymph-Vascular Invasion (LVI)

LVI indicates whether microscopic lymph-vascular invasion is identified in the pathology report. LVI includes lymphatic invasion, vascular invasion, or lymph-vascular invasion. By AJCC/UICC convention, LVI does not affect the T category indicating local extent of tumor unless specifically included in the definition of a T category. It should be noted that regional lymph node involvement is rare in uveal melanoma, but metastasis to the liver and direct extension into the orbit are more common [19].

Stage Grouping

Stage I	T1a	N0	M0
Stage IIA	T1b-d	N0	M0
	T2a	N0	M0
Stage IIB	T2b	N0	M0
	T3a	N0	M0
Stage IIIA	T2c-d	N0	M0
	T3b-c	N0	M0

	T4a	N0	M0
Stage IIIB	T3d	N0	M0
	T4b-c	N0	M0
Stage IIIC	T4d-e	N0	M0
Stage IV	Any T	N1	M0
	Any T	Any N	M1a-c

G. Other Pathologic Features of Prognostic Significance

Other histologic features with prognostic significance in choroidal and ciliary body melanoma include the number of mitoses in 40 high-powered fields, pigmentation, degree of inflammation, number of tumor-infiltrating macrophages, growth pattern (diffuse choroidal melanomas and ring melanomas of the ciliary body have a much less favorable prognosis), location of anterior margin of tumor, degree and patterns of vascularity, blood vessel invasion (both tumor vessels and normal vessels), tumor necrosis, extraocular extension, optic nerve involvement, and lack of nuclear BAP1 immunostaining [4, 30–44].

References

1. Karcioglu ZA, Gordon RA, Karcioglu GL. Tumor seeding in ocular fine needle aspiration biopsy. Ophthalmology. 1985;92:1763–7.
2. Stevenson KE, Hungerford J, Garner A. Local extraocular extension of retinoblastoma following intraocular surgery. Br J Ophthalmol. 1989;73:739–42.
3. Shields JA, Shields CL, De Potter P. Enucleation technique for children with retinoblastoma. J Pediatr Ophthalmol Strabismus. 1992;29:213–5.
4. Zimmerman LE. Malignant melanoma of the uveal tract. In: Spencer WH, editor. Ophthalmic pathology: an atlas and textbook. 3rd ed. Philadelphia: WB Saunders Co; 1986. p. 2072–139.
5. Brown HH, Wells JR, Grossniklaus HE. Chapter 11. Tissue preparation for pathologic examination. In: Grossniklaus HE, editor. Pocket guide to ocular oncology and pathology. Heidelberg: Springer; 2013.
6. Gallie BL, Ellsworth RM, Abramson DH, Phillips RA. Retinoma: spontaneous regression of retinoblastoma or benign manifestation of the mutation? Br J Cancer. 1982;45(4):513–21.
7. Dimaras H, Khetan V, Halliday W, et al. Loss of RB1 induces non-proliferative retinoma: increasing genomic instability correlates with progression to retinoblastoma. Hum Mol Genet. 2008;17(10):1363–72.

8. Eagle RC Jr. High-risk features and tumor differentiation in retinoblastoma: a retrospective histopathologic study. Arch Pathol Lab Med. 2009;133(8):1203–9.

9. Mendoza PR, Specht CS, Hubbard GB, et al. Histopathologic grading of anaplasia in retinoblastoma. Am J Ophthalmol. 2015;159(4):764–76.

10. Rushlow DE, Mol BM, Kennett JY, et al. Characterisation of retinoblastomas without RB1 mutations: genomic, gene expression, and clinical studies. Lancet Oncol. 2013;14(4):327–34.

11. Redler LD, Ellsworth RM. Prognostic importance of choroidal invasion in retinoblastoma. Arch Ophthalmol. 1973;90:294–6.

12. Kopelman JE, McLean IW. Multivariate analysis of clinical and histological risk factors for metastasis in retinoblastoma [abstract]. Invest Ophthalmol Vis Sci. 1983;24(ARVO suppl):50.

13. Kopelman JE, McLean IW. Multivariate analysis of risk factors for metastasis in retinoblastoma treated by enucleation. Ophthalmology. 1987;94:371–7.

14. Haik BG, Dunleavy SA, Cooke C, et al. Retinoblastoma with anterior chamber extension. Ophthalmology. 1987;94:367–70.

15. Magramm I, Abramson DH, Ellsworth RM. Optic nerve involvement in retinoblastoma. Ophthalmology. 1989;96:217–22.

16. Shields CL, Shields JA, Baez KA, Cater J, De Potter PV. Choroidal invasion of retinoblastoma: metastatic potential and clinical risk factors. Br J Ophthalmol. 1993;77:544–8.

17. Shields CL, Shields JA, Baez K, Cater JR, De Potter P. Optic nerve invasion of retinoblastoma: metastatic potential and clinical risk factors. Cancer. 1994;73:692–8.

18. Reese AB, Ellsworth RM. The evaluation and current concept of retinoblastoma therapy. Trans Am Acad Ophthalmol Otolaryngol. 1963;67:164–72.

19. Amin MB, Edge SB, Greene FL, et al., editors. *AJCC cancer staging manual*. 8th ed. New York: Springer; 2017.

20. The Collaborative Ocular Melanoma Study Group. Design and methods of a clinical trial for a rare condition: COMS report no. 3. The Collaborative Ocular Melanoma Study Group. Control Clin Trials. 1993;14:362–91.

21. Collaborative Ocular Melanoma Study Group. COMS manual of procedures. Springfield: National Technical Information Service; 1989. NTIS Accession No. PB90-115536.

22. McLean IW, Foster WD, Zimmerman LE. Prognostic factors in small malignant melanomas of choroid and ciliary body. Arch Ophthalmol. 1977;95:48–58.

23. Affeldt JC, Minckler DS, Azen SP, Yeh L. Prognosis in uveal melanoma with extraocular extension. Arch Ophthalmol. 1980;98:1975–9.

24. Kujala E, Damato B, Coupland SE, et al. Staging of ciliary body and choroidal melanomas based on anatomic extent. J Clin Oncol. 2013;31:2825–31.

25. AJCC Ophthalmic Oncology Task Force. International validation of the American Joint Committee on cancer's 7th edition classification of uveal melanoma. JAMA Ophthalmol. 2015;133:376–83.

26. Folberg R, Verdick R, Weingeist TA, Montague PR. The gross examination of eyes removed for choroidal and ciliary body melanomas. Ophthalmology. 1986;93:1643–7.

27. Callender GR. Malignant melanotic tumors of the eye: a study of histologic types in 111 cases. Trans Am Acad Ophthalmol Otolaryngol. 1931;36:131–42.

28. McLean IW, Zimmerman LE, Evans RM. Reappraisal of Callender's spindle A type of malignant melanoma of choroid and ciliary body. Am J Ophthalmol. 1978;86:557–64.

29. McLean IW, Foster WD, Zimmerman LE. Modifications of Callender's classification of uveal melanoma at the Armed Forces Institute of Pathology. Am J Ophthalmol. 1983;96:502–9.

30. Font RL, Spaulding AG, Zimmerman LE. Diffuse malignant melanoma of the uveal tract: a clinicopathologic report of 54 cases. Trans Am Acad Ophthalmol Otolaryngol. 1968;72:877–94.

31. McLean IW, Foster WD, Zimmerman LE. Uveal melanoma: location, size, cell type, and enucleation as risk factors in metastasis. Hum Pathol. 1982;13:123–32.

32. Weinhaus RS, Seddon JM, Albert DM, Gragoudas ES, Robinson N. Prognostic factor study of survival after enucleation for juxtapapillary melanomas. Arch Ophthalmol. 1985;103:1673–7.

33. Gamel JW, McCurdy JB, McLean IW. A comparison of prognostic covariates for uveal melanoma. Invest Ophthalmol Vis Sci. 1992;33:1919–22.

34. Folberg R, Peer J, Gruman LM, et al. The morphologic characteristics of tumor blood vessels as a marker of tumor progression in primary human uveal melanoma: a matched case-control study. Hum Pathol. 1992;23:1298–305.

35. Coleman K, Baak JP, Van Diest P, Mullaney J, Farrell M, Fenton M. Prognostic factors following enucleation of 111 uveal melanomas. Br J Ophthalmol. 1993;77:688–92.

36. Folberg R, Rummelt V, Parys-Van Ginderdeuren R, et al. The prognostic value of tumor blood vessel morphology in primary uveal melanoma. Ophthalmology. 1993;100:1389–98.

37. Folberg R, Rummelt V, Gruman LM, et al. Microcirculation architecture of melanocytic nevi and malignant melanomas of the ciliary body and choroid: a comparative histopathologic and ultrastructural study. Ophthalmology. 1994;101:718–27.

38. Rummelt V, Folberg R, Woolson RF, Hwang T, Peíer J. Relation between the microcirculation architecture and the aggressive behavior of ciliary body melanomas. Ophthalmology. 1995;102:844–51.

39. Finger PT. Intraocular melanoma. In: DeVita Jr VT, Lawrence TS, Rosenberg SA, editors. DeVita, Hellman, and Rosenberg's cancer: principles & practice of oncology. 10th ed. Riverwoods: Wolters Kluwer Health; 2015.

40. Mäkitie T, Summanen P, Tarkkanen A, Kivelä T. Tumor-infiltrating macrophages (CD68(+) cells)

and prognosis in malignant uveal melanoma. Invest Ophthalmol Vis Sci. 2001;42:1414–141.

41. Bronkhorst IH, Ly LV, Jordanova ES, Vrolijk J, Versluis M, Luyten GP, Jager MJ. Detection of M2-macrophages in uveal melanoma and relation with survival. Invest Ophthalmol Vis Sci. 2011;52:643–50.

42. Koopmans AE, Verdijk RM, Brouwer RW, et al. Clinical significance of immunohistochemistry for detection of BAP1 mutations in uveal melanoma. Mod Pathol. 2014;27:1321–30.

43. Kalirai H, Dodson A, Faqir S, Damato BE, Coupland SE. Lack of BAP1 protein expression in uveal melanoma is associated with increased metastatic risk and has utility in routine prognostic testing. Br J Cancer. 2014;111:1373–80.

44. van de Nes JA, Nelles J, Kreis S, et al. Comparing the prognostic value of *BAP1* mutation pattern, chromosome 3 status, and BAP1 immunohistochemistry in uveal melanoma. Am J Surg Pathol. 2016;40:796–805.

Index